Vascular Medicine: Research and Practice

Vascular Medicine: Research and Practice

Edited by Connor Smith

hayle
medical

New York

Hayle Medical,
750 Third Avenue, 9th Floor,
New York, NY 10017, USA

Visit us on the World Wide Web at:
www.haylemedical.com

ISBN: 978-1-63241-558-5

Cataloging-in-Publication Data

Vascular medicine : research and practice / edited by Connor Smith.
    p. cm.
Includes bibliographical references and index.
ISBN 978-1-63241-558-5
1. Blood-vessels--Diseases. 2. Peripheral vascular diseases. 3. Cardiology.
I. Smith, Connor.
RC691 .V38 2019
616.13--dc23

Table of Contents

Preface XI

Chapter 1   Postoperative "Chimney" for Unintentional Renal Artery Occlusion after EVAR 1
            Marco Franchin, Federico Fontana, Filippo Piacentino, Matteo Tozzi and
            Gabriele Piffaretti

Chapter 2   Successful Endovascular Treatment of Iatrogenic Thyrocervical Trunk
            Pseudoaneurysm with Concomitant Arteriovenous Fistula using 0.010-Inch
            Detachable Microcoils 5
            Kohei Hamamoto, Mitsunori Nakano, Kiyoka Omoto, Masahiko Tsubuku,
            Emiko Chiba, Tomohisa Okochi, Katsuhiko Matsuura and Osamu Tanaka

Chapter 3   Successful Treatment of Iatrogenic Vertebral Pseudoaneurysm using
            Pipeline Embolization Device 11
            Sudheer Ambekar, Mayur Sharma, Donald Smith and Hugo Cuellar

Chapter 4   Surgical Treatment for Profunda Femoris Artery Aneurysms 15
            Kimihiro Igari, Toshifumi Kudo, Takahiro Toyofuku and Yoshinori Inoue

Chapter 5   Successful Obliteration of a Pseudoaneurysm from Post-CEA Repair
            Secondary to a Pruitt-Inahara Shunt using a Stent Graft 20
            Vishal Dahya and Prasad Chalasani

Chapter 6   Exercise Induced Left Bundle Branch Block Treated with Cardiac Rehabilitation 23
            Nathan S. Anderson, Alexies Ramirez, Ahmad Slim and Jamil Malik

Chapter 7   Anomalous Left Main Coronary Artery: Case Series of Different Courses 27
            Adam T. Marler, Jamil A. Malik and Ahmad M. Slim

Chapter 8   Modification of the No-Touch Technique during Renal Artery Stenting 32
            John A. Stathopoulos

Chapter 9   Successful use of the MYNXGRIP Closure Device during Repeated
            Transbrachial Percutaneous Peripheral Intervention 35
            Klaus Hertting and Werner Raut

Chapter 10   Concomitant Deep Venous Thrombosis, Femoral Artery Thrombosis and
            Pulmonary Embolism after Air Travel 39
            Salim Abunnaja, Marshall Clyde, Andrea Cuviello, Robert A. Brenes
            and Giuseppe Tripodi

Chapter 11   Chimney-Graft as a Bail-Out Procedure for Endovascular Treatment of
            an Inflammatory Juxtarenal Abdominal Aortic Aneurysm 43
            Francesca Fratesi, Ashok Handa, Raman Uberoi and Ediri Sideso

Chapter 12   Adverse Outcome of Early Recurrent Ischemic Stroke Secondary to Atrial Fibrillation after Repeated Systemic Thrombolysis.. 47
Luciano A. Sposato, Valeria Salutto, Diego E. Beratti, Paula Monti,
Patricia M. Riccio and Claudio Mazia

Chapter 13   Cerebral Hyperperfusion Syndrome following Protected Carotid Artery Stenting...51
Rainer Knur

Chapter 14   Giant Pseudoaneurysm Associated with Arteriovenous Fistula of the Brachial and Femoral Arteries following Gunshot Wounds: Report of Two Cases 55
Handy Eone Daniel, Ankouane Firmin, Pondy O. Angele,
Minka Ngom Esthelle, Bombah Freddy and Ngo Nonga Bernadette

Chapter 15   Right Upper Lobe Partial Anomalous Pulmonary Venous Connection........................ 59
Christos Tourmousoglou, Christina Kalogeropoulou, Efstratios Koletsis,
Nikolaos Charoulis, Christos Prokakis, Panagiotis Alexopoulos,
Emmanoil Margaritis and Dimitrios Dougenis

Chapter 16   Pulmonary-Esophageal Variceal Bleeding: A Unique Presentation of Partial Cor Triatriatum Sinistrum.. 62
Fortune O. Alabi, Manuel Hernandez, Francis G. Christian, Fred Umeh and
Maximo Lama

Chapter 17   Periodontal Disease and Late-Onset Aortic Prosthetic Vascular Graft Infection.................................... 65
Stephanie Thomas, Jonathan Ghosh, Johnathan Porter, Adele Cockcroft and
Riina Rautemaa-Richardson

Chapter 18   Multiple Aneurysms of the Inferior Pancreaticoduodenal Artery: A Rare Complication of Acute Pancreatitis 68
Chris Klonaris, Emmanouil Psathas, Athanasios Katsargyris,
Stella Lioudaki, Achilleas Chatziioannou and Theodore Karatzas

Chapter 19   Endovascular Repair of a Large Profunda Femoris Artery Pseudoaneurysm 73
Ahsan Syed Khalid, Omar M. Ghanem and Seyed Mojtaba Gashti

Chapter 20   Successful Implantation of a Coronary Stent Graft in a Peripheral Vessel.................................... 77
Alexander Hess, Britta Vogel, Benedikt Kohler, Oliver J. Müller,
Hugo A. Katus and Grigorios Korosoglou

Chapter 21   Onyx Embolization of Ruptured Intracranial Aneurysm Associated with Behçet's Disease.. 81
Maher Kurdi, Saleh Baeesa, Mohammed Bin-Mahfoodh and Khalil Kurdi

Chapter 22   Medial Clavicular Osteophyte: A Novel Cause of Paget-Schroetter Syndrome...................................... 88
Keagan Werner-Gibbings and Steven Dubenec

Chapter 23   A Giant Pseudoaneurysm of the Forearm as Unusual Complication of Bacterial Endocarditis.. 91
Michele Arcopinto, Teresa Russo, Antonio Ruvolo, Antonio Cittadini,
Luigi Saccà and Raffaele Napoli

Chapter 24   **Upper Limb Ischemic Gangrene as a Complication of Hemodialysis Access** 94
Shamir O. Cawich, Emil Mohammed, Marlon Mencia and Vijay Naraynsingh

Chapter 25   **Unique Nutcracker Phenomenon Involving the Right Renal Artery and
Portal Venous System** 99
Maximilian Stephens, Sarah Kate Ryan and Roger Livsey

Chapter 26   **Treatment with Aortic Stent Graft Placement for Stanford B-Type Aortic
Dissection in a Patient with an Aberrant Right Subclavian Artery** 103
Yohei Kawatani, Yujiro Hayashi, Yujiro Ito, Hirotsugu Kurobe,
Yoshitsugu Nakamura, Yuji Suda and Takaki Hori

Chapter 27   **Critical Limb Ischemia in a Young Man: Saddle Embolism or Unusual
Presentation of Thromboangiitis Obliterans?** 108
Federico Bucci, Adriano Redler and Leslie Fiengo

Chapter 28   **Surgical Treatment of Cystic Adventitial Disease of the Popliteal Artery** 112
Kimihiro Igari, Toshifumi Kudo, Takahiro Toyofuku and Yoshinori Inoue

Chapter 29   **The Infrapopliteal Arterial Occlusions Similar to Buerger Disease** 118
Kimihiro Igari, Toshifumi Kudo, Takahiro Toyofuku,
Yoshinori Inoue and Takehisa Iwai

Chapter 30   **Mediastinal B-Cell Lymphoma Presenting with Jugular-Subclavian
Deep Vein Thrombosis as the First Presentation** 122
Sherif Ali Eltawansy, Mana Rao, Sidney Ceniza and David Sharon

Chapter 31   **Occult Bacteraemia and Aortic Graft Infection: A Wolf in Sheep's Clothing** 126
E. Trautt, S. Thomas, J. Ghosh, P. Newton and A. Cockcroft

Chapter 32   **A Novel Technique of Stenting of the Renal Artery In-Stent Restenosis with
GuideLiner through Radial Approach** 129
Maheedhar Gedela, Shenjing Li, Tomasz Stys and Adam Stys

Chapter 33   **Typical Asthmatic Presentation of Congenital Vascular Ring can
Masquerade a General Physician** 132
Naveen Swami, Georgey Koshy, Maan Jamal, Thair S. Abdulla and
Abdulaziz Alkhulaifi

Chapter 34   **Iatrogenic IVC Perforation after Successful Catheter-Directed Thrombolysis** 135
Ata Firoozi, Jamal Moosavi, Omid Shafe and Parham Sadeghipour

Chapter 35   **Endovascular Treatment of Infrarenal Abdominal Aortic Aneurysm with
Short and Angulated Neck in High-Risk Patient** 139
Stylianos Koutsias, Georgios Antoniou, Christos Karathanos, Vassileios Saleptsis,
Konstantinos Stamoulis and Athanasios D. Giannoukas

Chapter 36   **Right Aortic Arch and Kommerell's Diverticulum Repaired without
Reconstruction of Aberrant Left Subclavian Artery** 143
Hiroshi Osawa, Daisuke Shinohara, Kouan Orii, Shigeru Hosaka,
Shoji Fukuda, Okihiko Akashi and Hiroshi Furukawa

Chapter 37   **Sandwich EVAR occludes Celiac and Superior Mesenteric Artery for
Infected Suprarenal Abdominal Aortic Aneurysm Treatment** 146
Supatcha Prasertcharoensuk, Narongchai Wongkonkitsin, Parichat Tunmit,
Su-a-pa Theeragul and Anucha Ahooja

Chapter 38   **Pulmonary Endarterectomy in a Patient with Immune Thrombocytopenic
Purpura** 151
Bedrettin Yıldızeli, Mehmed Yanartaş, Sibel Keskin,
Işık Atagündüz and Ece Altınay

Chapter 39   **Novel Visceral-Anastomosis-First Approach in Open Repair of a Ruptured
Type 2 Thoracoabdominal Aortic Aneurysm: Causes behind a Mortal Outcome** 154
Einar Dregelid and Alireza Daryapeyma

Chapter 40   **Cystic Adventitial Disease of Popliteal Artery with Venous Aneurysm of
Popliteal Vein: Two-Year Follow-Up after Surgery** 158
Koki Takizawa, Hiroshi Osawa, Atsuo Kojima, Samuel J. K. Abraham and
Shigeru Hosaka

Chapter 41   **A Case of Successful Coil Embolization for a Late-Onset Type Ia
Endoleak after Endovascular Aneurysm Repair with the Chimney Technique**................... 162
Kimihiro Igari, Toshifumi Kudo, Takahiro Toyofuku and Yoshinori Inoue

Chapter 42   **Successful Endovascular Repair of an Iatrogenic Perforation of the Superficial
Femoral Artery using Self-Expanding Nitinol Supera Stents in a Patient with
Acute Thromboembolic Limb Ischemia** 166
Tom Eisele, Benedikt M. Muenz and Grigorios Korosoglou

Chapter 43   **High Output Cardiac Failure Resolving after Repair of AV Fistula in
a Six-Month-Old**.. 170
Uygar Teomete, Rubee Anne Gugol, Holly Neville, Ozgur Dandin and
Ming-Lon Young

Chapter 44   **Endovascular Management of Right Subclavian Artery Pseudoaneurysm
due to War Injury in Adolescent Patient** 174
Onur Saydam, Deniz Ferefli, Mehmet Atay and Cengiz Sert

Chapter 45   **A Case of Superficial Femoral Arteriovenous Fistula and Severe Venous
Stasis Ulceration, Managed with an Iliac Extender Prosthesis** 178
Nicole Ilonzo, Selena Goss, Chun Yang and Michael Dudkiewicz

Chapter 46   **Endovascular Management of Middle Aortic Syndrome Presenting with
Uncontrolled Hypertension**.. 181
Owen S. Glotzer, Kathryn Bowser, F. Todd Harad and Sandra Weiss

Chapter 47   **Anomalous Right Subclavian Artery-Esophageal Fistulae**.. 185
Courtney Brooke Shires and Michael J. Rohrer

Chapter 48   **Recurrent Upper Extremity Thrombosis Associated with
Overactivity: A Case of Delayed Diagnosis of Paget-Schroetter Syndrome** 190
Himani Sharma and Abhinav Tiwari

Chapter 49   **Left Brachiocephalic Vein Stenosis due to the Insertion of a Temporal Right Subclavian Hemodialysis Catheter** 194
Eleni I. Skandalou, Fani D. Apostolidou-Kiouti, Ilias D. Minasidis and Ioannis K. Skandalos

Chapter 50   **A Case of Unusual Vascularization of Upper Abdominal Cavity Organs** 197
Natalia Mazuruc, Serghei Covantev and Olga Belic

Chapter 51   **A Case of Atrioventricular Block Potentially Associated with Right Coronary Artery Lesion and Ticagrelor Therapy Mediated by the Increasing Adenosine Plasma Concentration** 203
Xiaoye Li, Ying Xue and Hongyi Wu

Chapter 52   **Haematochezia from a Splenic Artery Pseudoaneurysm Communicating with Transverse Colon** 206
James O'Brien, Francesca Muscara, Aser Farghal and Irshad Shaikh

Chapter 53   **Upper Extremity Deep Vein Thromboses: The Bowler and the Barista** 211
Seth Stake, Anne L. du Breuil and Jeremy Close

Chapter 54   **A Rare Case of Intermittent Claudication Associated with Impaired Arterial Vasodilation** 215
J. J. Posthuma, K. D. Reesink, M. Schütten, C. Ghossein, M. E. Spaanderman, H. ten Cate and G. Schep

Permissions

List of Contributors

Index

Preface

The world is advancing at a fast pace like never before. Therefore, the need is to keep up with the latest developments. This book was an idea that came to fruition when the specialists in the area realized the need to coordinate together and document essential themes in the subject. That's when I was requested to be the editor. Editing this book has been an honour as it brings together diverse authors researching on different streams of the field. The book collates essential materials contributed by veterans in the area which can be utilized by students and researchers alike.

Vascular medicine is a specialization in the field of medicine that is concerned with the management, treatment, prevention and diagnosis of diseases of the circulatory system and the lymphatic system. The lymphatic system is made up of the veins, arteries and lymphatic vessels. Disorders of the arteries or arterial diseases affect the aorta and arteries that supply blood to the hands, legs, brain, kidneys and intestines. Some arterials disorders are aneurysms, embolism, arterial thrombosis, vasospastic disorders and vasculitides. Venous diseases may include varicose veins, venous thrombosis and chronic venous insufficiency. Lymphatic diseases include varied forms of lymphedema as well as modification of cardiovascular disease risk factors such as high blood pressure and high cholesterol. This book covers in detail some existing theories and innovative concepts revolving around vascular medicine. It presents this complex subject in the most comprehensible language. A number of latest researches have been included to keep the readers up-to-date with the global concepts in this area of study.

Each chapter is a sole-standing publication that reflects each author's interpretation. Thus, the book displays a multi-facetted picture of our current understanding of application, resources and aspects of the field. I would like to thank the contributors of this book and my family for their endless support.

Editor

Postoperative "Chimney" for Unintentional Renal Artery Occlusion after EVAR

Marco Franchin,[1] Federico Fontana,[2] Filippo Piacentino,[2]
Matteo Tozzi,[1] and Gabriele Piffaretti[1]

[1] Vascular Surgery, Department of Surgery and Morphological Sciences, Circolo University Hospital,
University of Insubria School of Medicine, Via Guicciardini 9, 21100 Varese, Italy
[2] Interventional Radiology, Department of Surgery and Morphological Sciences, Circolo University Hospital,
University of Insubria School of Medicine, Via Guicciardini 9, 21100 Varese, Italy

Correspondence should be addressed to Gabriele Piffaretti; gabriele.piffaretti@uninsubria.it

Academic Editor: Atila Iyisoy

Renal artery obstruction during endovascular repair of abdominal aortic aneurysm using standard device is a rare but life-threatening complication and should be recognized and repaired rapidly in order to maintain renal function. Both conventional surgery and endovascular stenting have been reported. We report a case of late postoperative bilateral "chimney" to resolve a bilateral thrombosis of the renal artery following an uncomplicated endovascular aortic repair.

1. Introduction

Acute kidney injury (AKI) remains a known complication after endovascular abdominal aortic aneurysm repair (EVAR): multiple factors may be involved in postoperative AKI including contrast-induced nephropathy, atheroembolism, occlusion of accessory renal arteries, or unintentional overstenting of the renal arteries [1, 2].

Generally, renal artery occlusion due to endograft (EG) overstenting is recognized rapidly and could be treated immediately during the procedure; in contrast, unexpected renal artery occlusion may lead to prolonged ischemic damage and potential permanent injury requiring hemodialysis [3, 4].

In this report, we describe the occurrence of an unintentional and unexpected bilateral renal artery overstenting successfully managed with a bilateral renal artery "chimney" stenting in the late postoperative course.

2. Case Report

A 73-year-old man was admitted to our department with a diagnosis of an asymptomatic 57 mm fusiform abdominal aortic aneurysm (AAA). Medical history was notable for obesity, hypertension, chronic depressed (<30%) left heart dysfunction, and chronic obstructive pulmonary disease. Preoperative computed tomography angiography (CT-A) highlighted the presence of a hostile proximal aortic neck characterized by a reversed tapered shape (Figures 1(a) and 1(b)) plus an acute β-angle > 60° (Figure 1(c)). In the operating room, a 28 mm transrenal bifurcated EG (Endurant-Medtronic; Santa Rosa-CA; USA) was implanted through conventional bilateral groin cut-down. Final angiography confirmed the complete exclusion of the AAA with no evidence of proximal or distal endoleak, as well as the visualization of the renal arteries (Figures 2(a) and 2(b)). The immediate postoperative serum creatinine level was 1.48 mg/dL (range, 0.6–1.3 mg/dL; preoperative level: 1.36 mg/dL). Twelve hours later, a progressive reduction of urine output was noted; at that time, serum creatinine level increased to 3.26 mg/dL, configuring a grade 4 AKI according to the Aneurysm Renal Injury Score (ARISe) [5]. Angiography was performed immediately thereafter: it showed the occlusion of the renal artery, bilaterally. During the same procedure, we attempted an endovascular revascularization of the renal

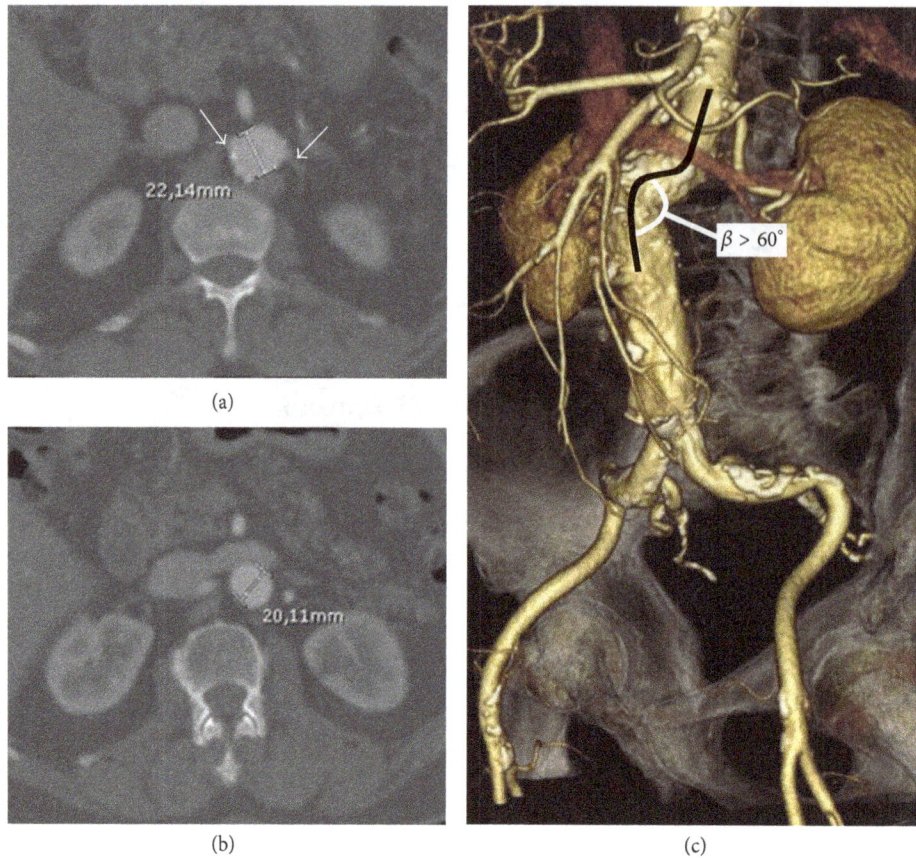

FIGURE 1: Preliminary CT-A showing (a, b) the reversed tapered shape of the proximal neck (arrows: renal arteries origin) and the severe β-angle (c).

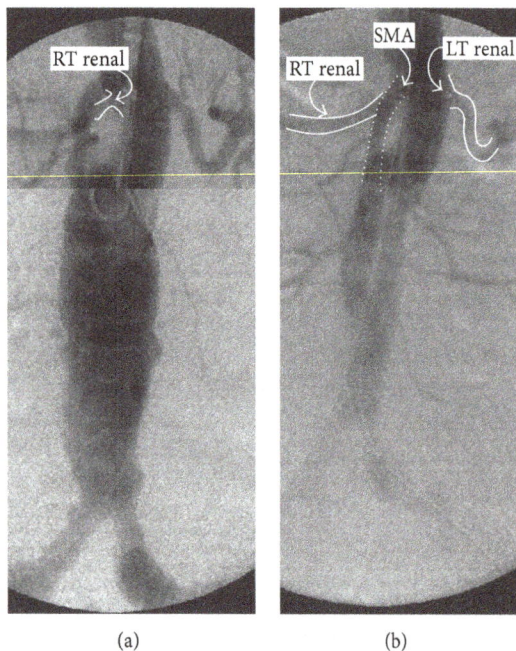

FIGURE 2: Predeployment preliminary angiography (a). Final control (b) showed the patency of both the renal arteries (arrows).

arteries, which failed because of the acute onset of a high-response atrial fibrillation causing hemodynamic instability and acute respiratory distress. The patient was transferred in the intensive care unit and started a temporary renal replacement therapy and amiodarone (Cordarone-Sanofi-Aventis; Milano-Italy) intravenously. Four days later, hemodynamic stability was recovered; at that time, a percutaneous left transbrachial approach was used to catheterize selectively the renal arteries (Figure 3(a)) with a 0.014″ guidewire (Stabilizer-Cordis, Miami Lakes, FL, USA) coupled with a 4F vertebral catheter (Cordis; Miami Lakes-FL; USA). A 5 × 15 mm bare metal stent (Genesis-Cordis; Miami Lakes-FL; USA) was used bilaterally with the complete restoration of renal flow into the parenchyma (Figure 3(b)). The subsequent postoperative course was uneventful: the urine output improved progressively. He was discharged on day 6 postoperatively on acetylsalicylic acid (Cardioaspirin-Bayer; Milano-Italy) 100 mg/die *ad infinitum*. He was last seen eighteen months later; the patient is still alive, asymptomatic, and the follow-up CT-A confirmed the complete exclusion of the aneurysm without endoleaks and the patency of the renal stents with preservation of visceral flow (Figures 3(c) and 3(d)). At that time serum creatinine level was 1.38 mg/dL.

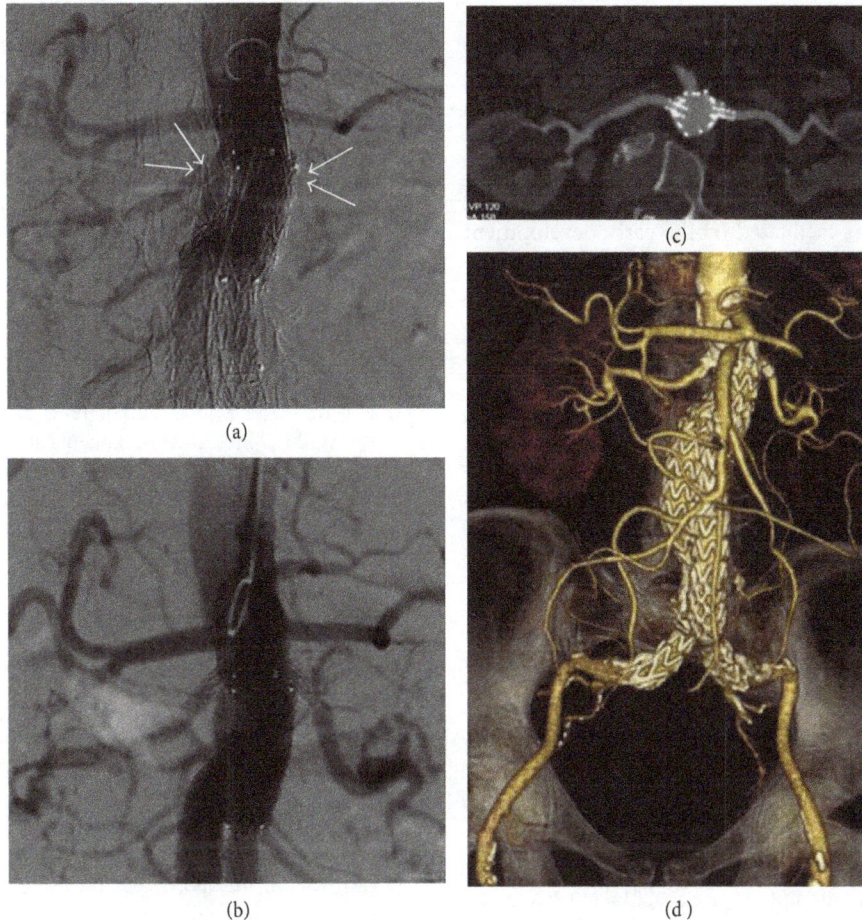

FIGURE 3: Selective angiography at the proximal extremity of the EG (a) showed the overstenting (arrows) of the origin of both the renal arteries. Complete revascularization after bilateral stenting (b). Follow-up CT-A: complete reperfusion of the parenchyma (c) as well as persistent exclusion of the aneurysm and absence of endoleak (d).

3. Discussion

The starting points for discussion of our case are either technical or clinical: they concern the underhanded pathogenesis of the renal artery occlusion, the feasibility of a postoperative "chimney" technique to overcome the renal artery ostia overstenting, and the recovery of the renal function 96 hours after the onset of the acute kidney injury.

As all the innovative techniques, even EVAR has brought new complications such as endoleaks and migration; some others are shared with conventional aortic repair such as renal artery occlusion [6]. Acute kidney injury is a serious complication and harbinger of poor prognosis after EVAR [7, 8]: despite renal artery occlusion during EVAR remaining an uncommon complication, as EVAR gains popularity, the incidence of EVAR-associated renal artery obstruction may increase.

EVAR-related renal artery occlusion is generally found intraoperatively following an EG maldeployment; however, it has been suggested that also those occlusions detected during the follow-up could be considered occluded since the initial operation [9–11]. Inan et al. [12] described a case of intraoperative bilateral renal artery occlusion: the cause was a proximal migration of a bifurcated EG, an event that is anecdotal and mainly due to an iatrogenic upward thrust of the device during contralateral cannulation. When suprarenal stents were first introduced, there was concern that they would induce hyperplasia and narrow the renal orifices; up to date, insufficient high-level evidence has decreed for or against proximal transrenal fixation on EVAR-related renal occlusion [13–15]. In our case, as probably occurs in most of the cases, the mechanism that caused the renal artery thrombosis was an underhanded partial obstruction that can be difficult to identify on intraoperative angiograms. We had an uncomplicated deployment with visualization of the renal arteries at completion angiography: the reason that may explain the delayed onset of the thrombosis of the renal arteries can be ascribed to the imperceptible filling defect in the renal artery profile even when the EG covers much of the orifice so that the renal artery lumen often fills with contrast-enhanced blood. Furthermore, the partial obstructions of renal arteries by the graft material or the struts of the suprarenal hooks were potentially masked by intraoperative anticoagulation.

Currently, there is no consensus about the treatment strategy of operative treatment and outcomes after prolonged renal artery occlusion. We believe that an attempt to revascularize the overstented renal arteries should have been mandatory in our case. Twine and Boyle [5] reported the occlusion of both renal arteries in the early postoperative period of an ordinary infrarenal EVAR resulting in dialysis-dependent kidney injury. Our case shows that urgent revascularization could be effective for this type of complication. Maybe the favorable outcome was facilitated by the early development of a rich collateral circulation that has been studied to come up most commonly from the periureteral, peripelvic, and adrenal vessels and that can maintain viability of nephrons at sub-filtration arterial pressures; furthermore, it provides the rationale for rescue intervention after total renal artery occlusion, even when the diagnosis has been delayed [16, 17].

Both open and endovascular techniques may be used as procedures to treat this uncommon, but important, especially if we consider the rapid and steady increase of EVARs either to treat conventional anatomies or complex aortic necks [18]. Open conversion still remains an option: when they covered the renal arteries for a number of weeks Adu et al. [18] proposed a flowchart with specific vascular bypasses depending on the patency status of the celiac trunk. In contrast, endovascular revascularization is primarily determined by accessibility of the renal orifices [4, 10, 12]. Similar to our case, Hedayati et al. [11] reported two cases of renal artery occlusion treated one week after a transrenal EVAR with renal artery stenting using a transfemoral approach which led to symptom resolution and recovery of renal function. In the present case the femoral approach has not been successful; in contrast, the second attempt using a brachial approach has led to an easier and more rapid catheterization of both renal arteries, perhaps more so for the presence of the transrenal bare fixation and despite the greater length of the shaft affecting its maneuverability.

4. Conclusion

Lessons learned from our case are never settled on the contrast effect into renal arteries at the time of completion angiography, and revascularization is still an option even when EVAR-related occlusion of the renal arteries has a delayed onset. Postoperative "chimney" might be considered a viable alternative if the renal artery overstenting is not completely occlusive also because it does not preclude a subsequent conventional bypass attempt.

References

[1] R. Wald, S. S. Waikar, O. Liangos, B. J. G. Pereira, G. M. Chertow, and B. L. Jaber, "Acute renal failure after endovascular vs open repair of abdominal aortic aneurysm," *Journal of Vascular Surgery*, vol. 43, no. 3, pp. 460–466, 2006.

[2] M. Antonello, M. Menegolo, M. Piazza, L. Bonfante, F. Grego, and P. Frigatti, "Outcomes of endovascular aneurysm repair on renal function compared with open repair," *Journal of Vascular Surgery*, vol. 58, no. 4, pp. 886–893, 2013.

[3] P. Cao, F. Verzini, S. Zannetti et al., "Device migration after endoluminal abdominal aortic aneurysm repair: analysis of 113 cases with a minimum follow-up period of 2 years," *Journal of Vascular Surgery*, vol. 35, no. 2, pp. 229–235, 2002.

[4] B. T. Katzen, A. A. MacLean, and H. E. Katzman, "Retrograde migration of an abdominal aortic aneurysm endograft leading to postoperative renal failure," *Journal of Vascular Surgery*, vol. 42, no. 4, pp. 784–787, 2005.

[5] C. P. Twine and J. R. Boyle, "Renal dysfunction after EVAR: time for a standard definition," *Journal of Endovascular Therapy*, vol. 20, no. 3, pp. 331–333, 2013.

[6] W. Grande and S. W. Stavropoulos, "Treatment of complications following endovascular repair of abdominal aortic aneurysms," *Seminars in Interventional Radiology*, vol. 23, no. 2, pp. 156–164, 2006.

[7] B. Wisniowski, M. Barnes, J. Jenkins, N. Boyne, A. Kruger, and P. J. Walker, "Predictors of outcome after elective endovascular abdominal aortic aneurysm repair and external validation of a risk prediction model," *Journal of Vascular Surgery*, vol. 54, no. 3, pp. 644–653, 2011.

[8] G. T. Pisimisis, C. F. Bechara, N. R. Barshes, P. H. Lin, W. S. Lai, and P. Kougias, "Risk factors and impact of proximal fixation on acute and chronic renal dysfunction after endovascular aortic aneurysm repair using glomerular filtration rate criteria," *Annals of Vascular Surgery*, vol. 27, no. 1, pp. 16–22, 2013.

[9] B. Thomas and L. Sanchez, "Proximal migration and endoleak: impact of endograft design and deployment techniques," *Seminars in Vascular Surgery*, vol. 22, no. 3, pp. 201–206, 2009.

[10] P. H. Lin, R. L. Bush, and A. B. Lumsden, "Endovascular rescue of a maldeployed aortic stent-graft causing renal artery occlusion: technical considerations," *Vascular and Endovascular Surgery*, vol. 38, no. 1, pp. 69–73, 2004.

[11] N. Hedayati, P. H. Lin, A. B. Lumsden, and W. Zhou, "Prolonged renal artery occlusion after endovascular aneurysm repair: endovascular rescue and renal function salvage," *Journal of Vascular Surgery*, vol. 47, no. 2, pp. 446–449, 2008.

[12] K. Inan, A. Ucak, B. Onan, V. Temizkan, M. Ugur, and A. T. Yilmaz, "Bilateral renal artery occlusion due to intraoperative retrograde migration of an abdominal aortic aneurysm endograft," *Journal of Vascular Surgery*, vol. 51, no. 3, pp. 720–724, 2010.

[13] S. K. Subedi, A. M. Lee, and G. S. Landis, "Suprarenal fixation barbs can induce renal artery occlusion in endovascular aortic aneurysm repair," *Annals of Vascular Surgery*, vol. 24, no. 1, pp. 113.e7–113.e10, 2010.

[14] A. Saratzis, P. Sarafidis, N. Melas et al., "Suprarenal graft fixation in endovascular abdominal aortic aneurysm repair is associated with a decrease in renal function," *Journal of Vascular Surgery*, vol. 56, no. 3, pp. 594–600, 2012.

[15] G. N. Kouvelos, I. Boletis, N. Papa, A. Kallinteri, M. Peroulis, and M. I. Matsagkas, "Analysis of effects of fixation type on renal function after endovascular aneurysm repair," *Journal of Endovascular Therapy*, vol. 20, no. 3, pp. 334–344, 2013.

[16] M. Hamish, G. Geroulakos, D. A. Hughes, S. Moser, A. Shepherd, and A. D. Salama, "Delayed hepato-spleno-renal bypass for renal salvage following malposition of an infrarenal aortic stent-graft," *Journal of Endovascular Therapy*, vol. 17, no. 3, pp. 326–331, 2010.

[17] B. Williams, J. Feehally, A. R. Attard, and P. R. F. Bell, "Recovery of renal function after delayed revascularisation of acute occlusion of the renal artery," *The British Medical Journal*, vol. 296, no. 6636, pp. 1591–1592, 1988.

Successful Endovascular Treatment of Iatrogenic Thyrocervical Trunk Pseudoaneurysm with Concomitant Arteriovenous Fistula Using 0.010-Inch Detachable Microcoils

Kohei Hamamoto,[1] Mitsunori Nakano,[2] Kiyoka Omoto,[3] Masahiko Tsubuku,[4] Emiko Chiba,[1] Tomohisa Okochi,[1] Katsuhiko Matsuura,[1] and Osamu Tanaka[1]

[1]*Department of Radiology, Saitama Medical Center, Jichi Medical University, 1-847 Amanuma-cho, Omiya-ku, Saitama 330-8503, Japan*
[2]*Department of Cardiovascular Surgery, Saitama Medical Center, Jichi Medical University, 1-847 Amanuma-cho, Omiya-ku, Saitama 330-8503, Japan*
[3]*Department of Laboratory Medicine, Diagnostic Ultrasound Division, Saitama Medical Center, Jichi Medical University, 1-847 Amanuma-cho, Omiya-ku, Saitama 330-8503, Japan*
[4]*Department of Radiology, Maruyama Memorial General Hospital, 2-10-5 Hon-cho, Iwatsuki-ku, Saitama 339-8521, Japan*

Correspondence should be addressed to Kohei Hamamoto; hkouhei917@gmail.com

Academic Editor: Konstantinos A. Filis

Pseudoaneurysms (PsA) and arteriovenous fistulae (AVF) of the thyrocervical trunk and its branches are rare complications of traumatic or iatrogenic arterial injuries. Most such injuries are iatrogenic and are associated with central venous catheterization. Historically, thyrocervical trunk PsA and AVF have been managed with open surgical repair; however, multiple treatment modalities are now available, including ultrasound-guided compression repair, ultrasound-guided thrombin injection, and endovascular repair with covered stent placement. We report a case of a 65-year-old woman with an iatrogenic thyrocervical trunk PsA with concomitant AVF that developed after attempted internal jugular vein cannulation for hemodialysis access. The PsA was successfully treated by transcatheter coil embolization using 0.010-inch detachable microcoils. Our case is the first published instance of a thyrocervical trunk PsA with concomitant AVF that was successfully treated by endovascular procedure.

1. Introduction

Pseudoaneurysms (PsA) and arteriovenous fistulae (AVF) of the thyrocervical trunk and its branches are rare complications of traumatic or iatrogenic arterial injuries. Most of these injuries are caused by iatrogenic needle puncture of the thyrocervical trunk at the time of attempted internal jugular vein catheterization. The typical clinical symptom of PsA is a pulsatile mass with bruit at the injured site, while the typical clinical symptoms of AVF are bruit and cardiac insufficiency [1–14]. A PsA usually requires intervention because of the risk of complications including pain, a mass effect involving adjacent structures, and rupture; in contrast, an AVF infrequently requires intervention because it often resolves spontaneously [15].

Historically, thyrocervical trunk PsA and AVF have been managed with open surgical repair. In recent years, however, endovascular interventional procedures have often served as the first-line therapy for PsA and AVF in other locations, such as the femoral artery [16]. Although several cases of successful treatment by percutaneous and endovascular procedures have also been reported in the thyrocervical trunk region [9, 11, 12, 14], most of these reports described branched lesions of the thyrocervical trunk or solitary lesions without AVF. Therefore, this approach to cases involving main trunk lesions or concomitant PsA and AVF remains challenging. We herein

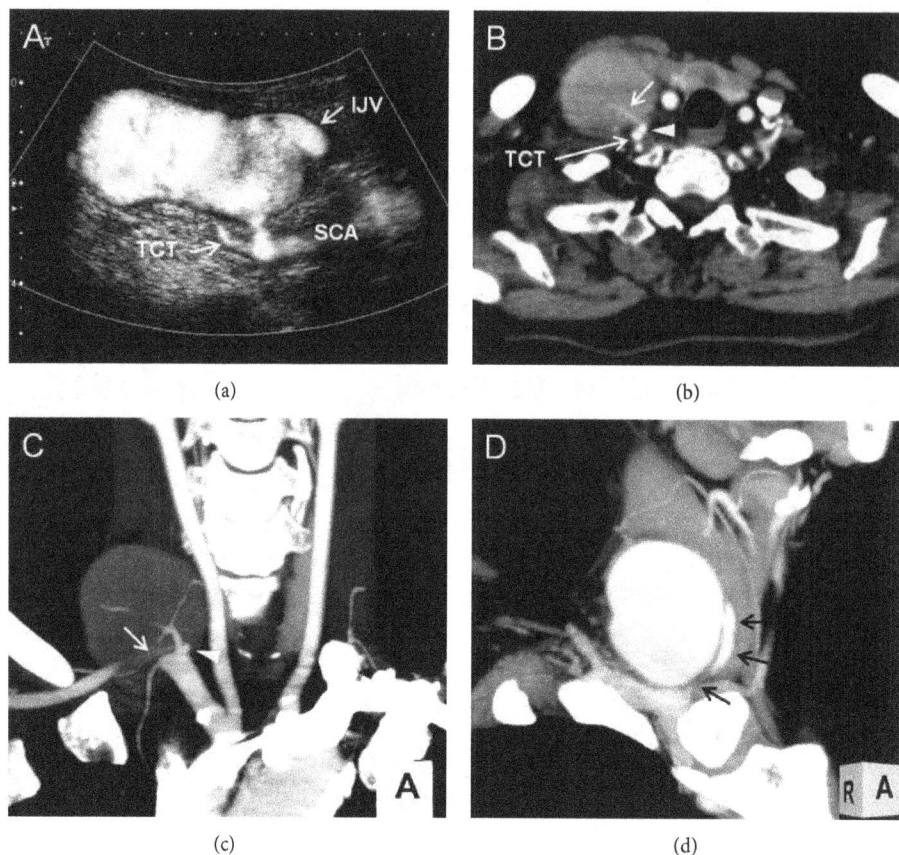

FIGURE 1: (a) Duplex ultrasound in the longitudinal plane at the level of the right supraclavicular fossa. The PsA communicated with the root of the thyrocervical trunk (TCT) with inner turbulent flow via the short, narrow neck. Continuity between the PsA and the internal jugular vein (IJV) was also noted. SCA: subclavian artery. (b) Contrast-enhanced computed tomography angiography showed a high-density-flow jet of contrast agent shunting from the TCT (arrow) into the aneurysmal sac via the short neck (arrowhead). (c) Maximum-intensity projection (MIP) image in the arterial phase clearly showed the anatomical relationship between the TCT and PsA neck (arrowhead). A flow jet within the PsA was also shown (arrow). (d) MIP image in the venous phase showed continuity between the aneurysmal sac and internal jugular vein (arrows).

describe a case of an iatrogenic thyrocervical trunk PsA with concomitant AVF involving the internal jugular vein after central venous catheter insertion for hemodialysis. Successful coil embolization of the PsA and AVF was achieved using 0.010-inch detachable microcoils.

2. Case Report

A 65-year-old woman was referred to our interventional radiology department for investigation of a palpable mass and irritating audible bruit on her right neck. Two months prior to this visit, she had developed an acute exacerbation of chronic renal failure secondary to viral gastroenteritis and underwent temporary hemodialysis using a central venous catheter placed in her right jugular vein. Upon arrival at our hospital, a 50×30 mm soft mass was palpable over the right side of her neck, and systolic bruit was heard during auscultation. Laboratory data showed elevated levels of serum creatinine and blood urea nitrogen at 155.6 μmol/L and 10.0 mmol/L, respectively. Duplex ultrasonography evaluation of the neck was performed, which showed a $48 \times 27 \times 46$ mm aneurysmal

sac that connected the craniomedial side of the thyrocervical trunk via a short narrow neck approximately 3 mm in length and 2.5 mm in diameter (Figure 1(a)). The aneurysmal sac also continued to the internal jugular vein, and the cranial aspect of the internal jugular vein was occluded by a thrombus. Computed tomography angiography of the neck showed a high-density-flow jet of contrast agent shunting from the thyrocervical trunk into the aneurysmal sac via the short neck in the arterial phase (Figures 1(b) and 1(c)). Continuity between the aneurysmal sac and internal jugular vein was also noted (Figure 1(d)). Based on these findings, the diagnosis of iatrogenic PsA of the thyrocervical trunk with an AVF involving the internal jugular vein was made. We discussed surgical versus endovascular intervention with the patient, and the latter was elected. A 4-Fr sheath (Terumo, Tokyo, Japan) was inserted through the right brachial artery, and the right subclavian artery was selectively catheterized by a 4.2-Fr Judkins Right 4.0 angiographic catheter (Goodman, Nagoya, Japan). Selective digital subtraction angiography of the right subclavian artery showed a PsA originating from the thyrocervical trunk root; the PsA had a short

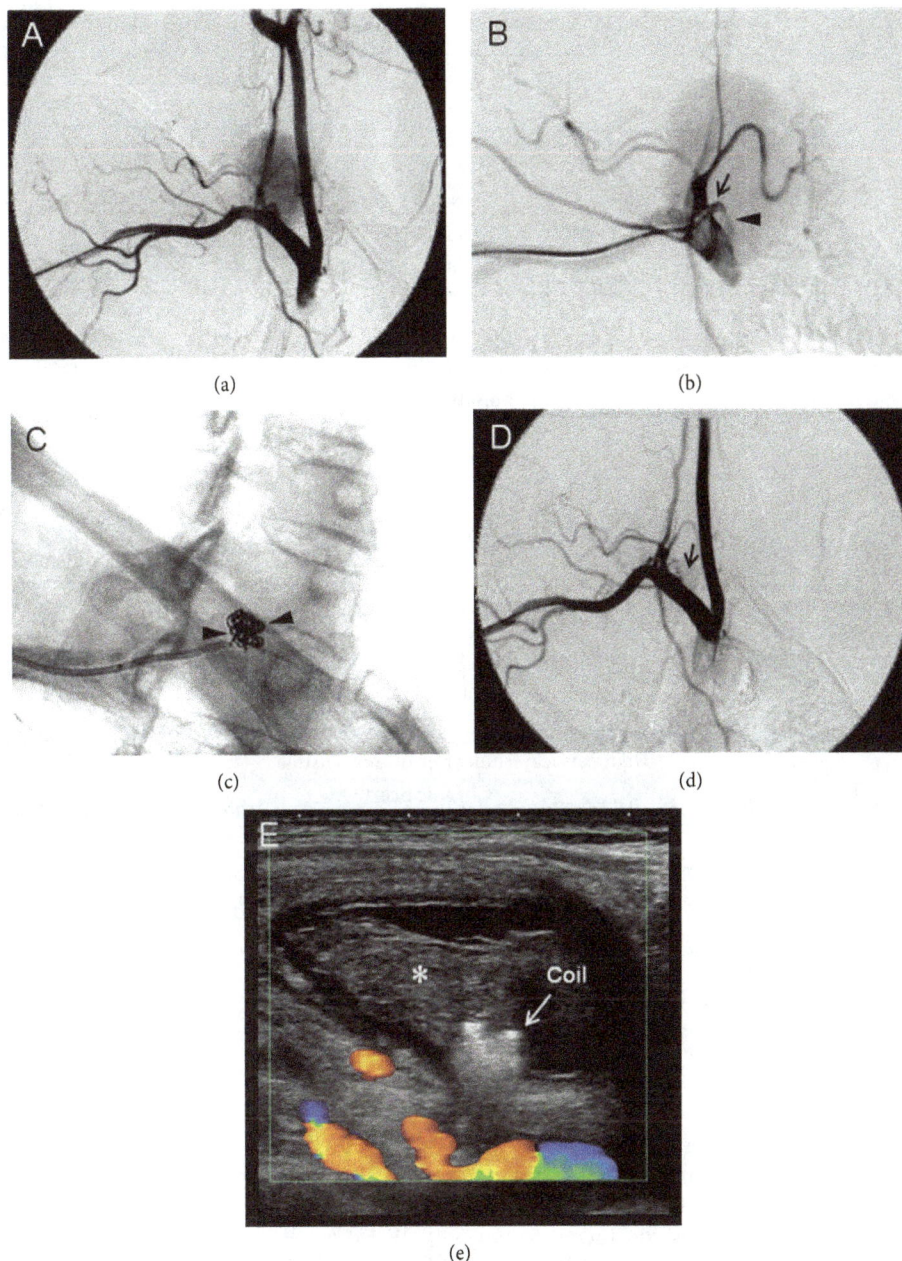

FIGURE 2: (a) Digital subtraction angiogram (DSA) in the right anterior oblique view showed a large PsA originating from the TCT. (b) Selective DSA of the PsA neck clearly showed the short narrow neck originating from the proximal side of the TCT root. (c) Coil embolization of the PsA. Arrowheads indicate the coils corresponding to the PsA neck. (d) DSA after coil embolization showed the near disappearance of the PsA, but faintly residual contrast dye was noted near the coil (arrowhead). (e) Duplex ultrasound following 15 min ultrasound-guided compression. Complete disappearance of blood flow within the PsA and thrombus formation (asterisk) was observed.

narrow neck that connected it to the internal jugular vein (Figures 2(a) and 2(b)). Based on the angiographic findings, we decided to perform coil embolization of the PsA neck because this method was likely to reduce the blood flow of the PsA while preserving the flow of the subclavian artery and other branches of the thyrocervical trunk. Using the abovementioned Judkins Right catheter and a 0.035-inch hydrophilic wire (Radifocus; Terumo, Tokyo, Japan), selective catheterization of the ostium of the PsA neck was achieved.

A 2.0-Fr microcatheter (Excelsior1080; Stryker Neurovascular, Fremont, CA, USA) was then introduced coaxially over a 0.016-inch-diameter guide wire (Meister; Asahi Intecc, Nagoya, Japan) and placed into the proximal site of the PsA via its neck. Four 0.010-inch detachable coils (Target Helical Ultra; Stryker Neurovascular) measuring 3.0 mm × 8.0 cm, 2.5 mm × 6.0 cm, 2.0 mm × 6.0 cm, and 2.0 mm × 4.0 cm were sequentially placed across the PsA neck (Figure 2(c)). Subclavian angiography after coil embolization revealed

TABLE 1: Chart review of pseudoaneurysm and arteriovenous fistula of thyrocervical trunk.

Reference	Side	Location	Age	Etiology	Symptoms	Time to onset of symptoms after injury	Treatment	Outcome
					Thyrocervical trunk pseudoaneurysms			
Shield III et al. [1]	R	Main trunk	54	Iatrogenic	Pulsatile mass	3 months	Surgical resection	Successful
	R	Main trunk	16	Iatrogenic	Nonpulsatile mass	6 weeks	Surgical resection	Successful
den Hollander and Slapak [3]	R	Main trunk	16	Iatrogenic	Pulsatile mass with bruit	5 weeks	Surgical resection	Successful
Abrokwah et al. [5]	R	Main trunk	78	Iatrogenic	Horner's syndrome	1 day	Surgical resection	Successful
Elariny et al. [6]	R	Main trunk	78	Iatrogenic	Pain, bruit	2 days	Surgical resection	Successful
Houshian and Poulsen [7]	R	Main trunk	26	Traumatic	Pulsatile mass with bruit	4 months	Surgical resection	Successful
Peces et al. [8]	R	Main trunk	57	Iatrogenic	Pulsatile mass with bruit	3 months	Surgical resection	Successful
Majeski [10]	R	Main trunk	36	Traumatic	Pain, pulsatile mass	2 months	Surgical resection	Successful
Cuhaci et al. [9]	R	Branch	46	Iatrogenic	Pain, pulsatile mass	2 weeks	Coil embolization	Successful
Ramsay and McAuliffe [11]	L	Branch	36	Traumatic	Pain, pulsatile mass	4 hours	Coil embolization	Successful
Dwivedi et al. [12]	R	Branch	67	Iatrogenic	Pain, pulsatile mass	2 days	Coil embolization	Successful
Mazzei et al. [13]	R	Branch	71	Iatrogenic	Pulsatile mass	3 months	Surgical resection	Successful
Mehta et al. [14]	R	Branch	56	Traumatic	Pain, pulsatile mass	4 months	UGTI	Successful
					Thyrocervical trunk arteriovenous fistula			
Glaser et al. [2]	R	Main trunk	53	Iatrogenic	Chronic heart failure	2 months	Surgical resection	Successful
	R	N.D.	N.D.	Iatrogenic	Bruit, cardiac insufficiency	N.D.	Occluded by DBC	Successful
Herbreteau et al. [4]	R	N.D.	N.D.	Iatrogenic	Bruit	N.D.	Occluded by DBC	Successful
	R	N.D.	N.D.	Iatrogenic	None	N.D.	Occluded by DBC	Successful
	R	N.D.	N.D.	Iatrogenic	Bruit, chronic heart failure	N.D.	Occluded by DBC	Successful

N.D.: not described precisely; R: right; DBC: detachable balloon catheter; UGTI: ultrasound-guided thrombin injection.

faintly residual flow of contrast medium in the sac, but the flow volume was obviously reduced (Figure 2(d)). The blood flow of the thyrocervical trunk and its branches had been preserved. Additional coil placement was considered to be likely to achieve complete occlusion but possible undesirable embolization of the thyrocervical trunk. Ultrasonographic reevaluation revealed thrombus formation and an obvious decrease in the shunting flow within the PsA. Additionally, the diameter of the PsA was reduced. We determined that the coil embolization was effective, and ultrasound-guided compression repair was performed for 15 min to achieve complete occlusion. Finally, the turbulent flow in the aneurismal sac completely disappeared (Figure 2(e)), and the procedure was thus finished. Ultrasonography performed the next day showed a reduction in the size of the PsA with thrombolization. The patient was discharged 3 days after embolotherapy without worsening of renal function. In the reevaluation of 6 months after embolization, no mass or bruit was detected on her neck. Duplex ultrasonography showed complete thrombolization of the aneurysmal sac with partial cystic change. The size of the aneurysmal sac had been further reduced to 10 × 11 × 8 mm.

3. Discussion

In the present report, we describe a case of iatrogenic thyrocervical trunk PsA with concomitant AVF involving the internal jugular vein that was successfully treated by transcatheter coil embolization. Although PsA and AVF are well-documented complications of traumatic and iatrogenic arterial injuries, the occurrence of this condition in the thyrocervical trunk region is rare, as this structure is well protected and is located deep in the neck. Following a literature search performed using PubMed, we noted that only thirteen cases of PsAs [1, 3, 5–11, 14] and five cases of AVFs [2, 4] that were successfully treated with surgical repair or endovascular procedures have been reported (Table 1). To our knowledge, there is no report in the literature of a case with the coexistence of these conditions or a main trunk PsA that was successfully treated with an endovascular procedure.

The PsAs and AVFs of the thyrocervical trunk and its branches are usually iatrogenic in origin and are presumably caused by needle puncture of the thyrocervical trunk at the time of attempted catheterization of the internal jugular vein. A reported risk factor for iatrogenic PsA of the thyrocervical trunk is the use of a lower or lateral approach to the internal jugular vein [1]. Overanticoagulation, age, atherosclerosis, hypertension, and anatomical variation of the internal jugular vein are additional risk factors of central venous catheterization-related PsA [17]. Several treatment options are available for PsA and AVF, including surgical resection, ultrasound-guided compression (USGC), ultrasound-guided thrombin injection (UGTI), and endovascular procedures such as stent placement and embolization by using a metallic coil or vascular plug. In recent years, endovascular interventional procedures have often served as the first-line therapy as these methods are less invasive.

The treatment of PsAs and AVFs of the thyrocervical trunk is dependent on their location, anatomical form of the PsA neck or AVF tract, and the presence or absence of these coexisting conditions. In cases with solitary and branch lesions, relatively simple percutaneous or endovascular procedures such as USGC, UGTI, and coil embolization of culprit arteries can be employed [9–12, 14]. However, the occurrence of PsAs located at the root of the thyrocervical trunk and AVF, as in the present case, is believed to be more complex, and there is no established treatment. Historically, PsAs developing in this region have been managed with open surgical repair [1, 3, 5–8, 10]. Although USGC and USTI are less invasive techniques, they may be difficult to apply in cases with main trunk lesions. USGC, by itself, cannot achieve hemostasis, because the root of the thyrocervical trunk is located deep within the soft tissue of the neck. Moreover, UGTI is associated with an increased risk for systemic thrombosis or embolization in cases where the PsA originates from the adjacent area of the thyrocervical trunk root or is accompanied by AVF [18].

The closure of peripherally located PsAs and AVFs using detachable coils is a well-established and effective procedure; this was believed to be the most suitable treatment in the present case, as specific embolic materials can be specifically chosen to control the embolization. In the present case, a short-segment embolization of the PsA neck was required to preserve the flow in the other branches of the thyrocervical trunk while avoiding coil migration to the venous circulation; hence, we used 0.010-inch detachable microcoils. These coils are thin and highly flexible, and coil movement can be easily controlled by slowly pushing the delivery wire back and forth. This enabled the placement of tightly overlapping coils during coil embolization, thus facilitating the treatment of the short segments of small target vessels even in the critically limited area of the embolization. Although USGC was also needed, we achieved complete blood flow occlusion of the PsA and AVF without any unintended embolization of nontargeted vessels or coil migration into the venous circulation.

Other materials can also be used for PsA and AVF occlusion, such as the Amplatzer vascular plug or N-butyl cyanoacrylate glue. However, both approaches were believed to be unsuitable in the present case because of anatomical complexity of the PsA neck and coexistence of AVF. Covered or uncovered stent placement in the thyrocervical trunk is another alternative endovascular procedure; however, it is not an ideal procedure because of the risk of restenosis.

Additionally, patients should undergo long-term treatment with antiplatelet drugs to prevent restenosis.

4. Conclusion

Thyrocervical trunk PsA and AVF following central venous catheterization are a rare complication and can manifest days to months after the initial injury. Transcatheter coil embolization is a safe and effective treatment for PsA, even in cases accompanied by AVF or main trunk lesions. This is the first report of transcatheter coil embolization of a thyrocervical trunk PsA with concomitant AVF involving the internal jugular vein.

References

[1] C. F. Shield III, J. D. Richardson, C. J. Buckley, and C. O. Hagood Jr., "Pseudoaneurysm of the brachiocephalic arteries: a complication of percutaneous internal jugular vein catheterization," *Surgery*, vol. 78, no. 2, pp. 190–194, 1975.

[2] R. L. Glaser, D. McKellar, and K. S. Scher, "Arteriovenous fistulas after cardiac catheterization," *Archives of Surgery*, vol. 124, no. 11, pp. 1313–1315, 1989.

[3] D. den Hollander and M. Slapak, "False aneurysm of the thyrocervical trunk," *Nephrology, Dialysis, Transplantation*, vol. 6, no. 10, pp. 747–748, 1991.

[4] D. Herbreteau, A. Aymard, M. H. Khayata et al., "Endovascular treatment of arteriovenous fistulas arising from branches of the subclavian artery," *Journal of Vascular and Interventional Radiology*, vol. 4, no. 2, pp. 237–240, 1993.

[5] J. Abrokwah, K. N. Shenoy, and R. H. Armour, "False aneurysm of the thyrocervical trunk: an unconventional surgical approach," *European Journal of Vascular and Endovascular Surgery*, vol. 11, no. 3, pp. 373–374, 1996.

[6] H. A. Elariny, D. Crockett, and J. L. Hussey, "False aneurysm of the thyrocervical trunk," *Southern Medical Journal*, vol. 89, no. 5, pp. 519–521, 1996.

[7] S. Houshian and T. D. Poulsen, "Aneurysm of the thyrocervical trunk after blunt cervical injury," *Injury*, vol. 29, no. 1, pp. 77–78, 1998.

[8] R. Peces, R. A. Navascués, J. Baltar, A. S. Laurés, and J. Alvarez-Grande, "Pseudoaneurysm of the thyrocervical trunk complicating percutaneous internal jugular-vein catheterization for haemodialysis," *Nephrology Dialysis Transplantation*, vol. 13, no. 4, pp. 1009–1011, 1998.

[9] B. Cuhaci, P. Khoury, and R. Chvala, "Transverse cervical artery pseudoaneurysm: a rare complication of internal jugular vein cannulation," *American Journal of Nephrology*, vol. 20, no. 6, pp. 476–482, 2000.

[10] J. Majeski, "Traumatic pseudoaneurysm of the thyrocervical trunk," *Southern Medical Journal*, vol. 94, no. 4, pp. 380–382, 2001.

[11] D. W. Ramsay and W. McAuliffe, "Traumatic pseudoaneurysm and high flow arteriovenous fistula involving internal jugular vein and common carotid artery. Treatment with covered stent

and embolization," *Australasian Radiology*, vol. 47, no. 2, pp. 177–180, 2003.

[12] A. J. Dwivedi, C. Cherukupalli, R. Dayal, and K. V. Krishansastry, "Endovascular treatment of false aneurysm of the thyrocervical trunk," *Vascular and Endovascular Surgery*, vol. 41, no. 1, pp. 77–79, 2007.

[13] V. Mazzei, D. Benvenuto, M. Gagliardi, S. Guarracini, and M. Di Mauro, "Thyrocervical trunk pseudoaneurysm following central venous catheterization," *Journal of Cardiac Surgery*, vol. 26, no. 6, pp. 617–618, 2011.

[14] K. Mehta, E. England, J. Apgar, J. Moulton, A. Javadi, and R. Wissman, "Post-traumatic pseudoaneurysm of the thyrocervical trunk," *Skeletal Radiology*, vol. 42, no. 8, pp. 1169–1172, 2013.

[15] C. Thalhammer, A. S. Kirchherr, F. Uhlich, J. Waigand, and C. M. Gross, "Postcatheterization pseudoaneurysms and arteriovenous fistulas: repair with percutaneous implantation of endovascular covered stents," *Radiology*, vol. 214, no. 1, pp. 127–131, 2000.

[16] M. Dzijan-Horn, N. Langwieser, P. Groha et al., "Safety and efficacy of a potential treatment algorithm by using manual compression repair and ultrasound-guided thrombin injection for the management of iatrogenic femoral artery pseudoaneurysm in a large patient cohort," *Circulation: Cardiovascular Interventions*, vol. 7, no. 2, pp. 207–215, 2014.

[17] A. Najafi, R. S. Moharari, M. R. Khajavi, J. Salimi, and P. Khashayar, "A giant subclavian pseudoaneurysm following central venous catheterization," *Journal of Anesthesia*, vol. 23, no. 4, pp. 628–629, 2009.

[18] W. D. Middleton, A. Dasyam, and S. A. Teefey, "Diagnosis and treatment of iatrogenic femoral artery pseudoaneurysms," *Ultrasound Quarterly*, vol. 21, no. 1, pp. 3–17, 2005.

3

Successful Treatment of Iatrogenic Vertebral Pseudoaneurysm Using Pipeline Embolization Device

Sudheer Ambekar,[1] Mayur Sharma,[2] Donald Smith,[1] and Hugo Cuellar[1]

[1] *Department of Neurosurgery, Louisiana State University Health Sciences Center, 1501 Kings Highway, Shreveport, LA 71103, USA*
[2] *Center of Neuromodulation, Wexner Medical Center, The Ohio State University, Columbus, OH 43210, USA*

Correspondence should be addressed to Hugo Cuellar; hcuell@lsuhsc.edu

Academic Editor: Andreas Zirlik

Traumatic pseudoaneurysms are uncommon and one of the most difficult lesions to treat. Traditional treatment methods have focused on parent vessel sacrifice with or without revascularization. We report the case of a patient who underwent successful treatment of an iatrogenic extracranial vertebral artery pseudoaneurysm using the Pipeline Embolization Device. A 47-year-old man sustained an inadvertent injury to the left vertebral artery during C1-C2 fixation. Subsequent imaging revealed an iatrogenic vertebral artery pseudoaneurysm. Immediate angiogram was normal. A repeat angiogram done after 3 days of the surgery revealed a vertebral artery pseudoaneurysm. He underwent aneurysm exclusion and vascular reconstruction using the Pipeline Embolization Device. Although flow-diverting stents are currently not being used for treating traumatic pseudoaneurysms, their use may be considered in such cases if active bleeding has ceased. In our case, the patient did well and the aneurysm was excluded from circulation while reconstructing the vessel wall.

1. Introduction

Vertebral artery pseudoaneurysms may arise due to penetrating or blunt trauma, arterial dissection, associated collagen vascular disease, or following surgery. The extracranial segment (V3) of the vertebral artery is the most vulnerable to iatrogenic injury due to its course outside the transverse foramen and close proximity to C1. The incidence of vertebral artery (VA) injury during craniocervical fusion surgery has been reported between 0% and 5.8% [1, 2]. VA injury during these procedures may lead to massive hemorrhage, arterial infarction, and, sometimes, death. In a few cases, delayed formation of pseudoaneurysm may be observed. Although spontaneous resolution of these pseudoaneurysms has been reported, rupture is observed in about 31% to 54% of patients [3]. Therefore, prompt identification and management of these lesions are paramount to successful outcome.

Various treatment strategies for treatment of iatrogenic pseudoaneurysms have focused on open or endovascular parent artery sacrifice with or without revascularization [3, 4]. Coil or onyx embolization and use of stent grafts or covered stents have also been described in literature [5–8]. Recently, the use of flow-diverting stents in the management of traumatic pseudoaneurysms has been described [9]. We report a case of iatrogenic vertebral artery pseudoaneurysm that was successfully treated using the Pipeline Embolization Device (PED) (Ev3 Neurovascular, Irvine, CA), thus obtaining vascular reconstruction and excluding the aneurysm from circulation without compromising blood flow through the parent artery.

2. Case Report

A 47-year-old man presented with pseudofusion following an old odontoid fracture. The patient was planned for posterior C1-C2 fixation using screws and rods. During dissection around the C1 lateral mass, on the right side, sudden brisk arterial bleeding was encountered. Immediate packing was done and hemostasis achieved. Vertebral angiography revealed patent VAs without any evidence of lumen compromise or active extravasation of contrast. A small irregularity on the wall was identified as the possible area of injury

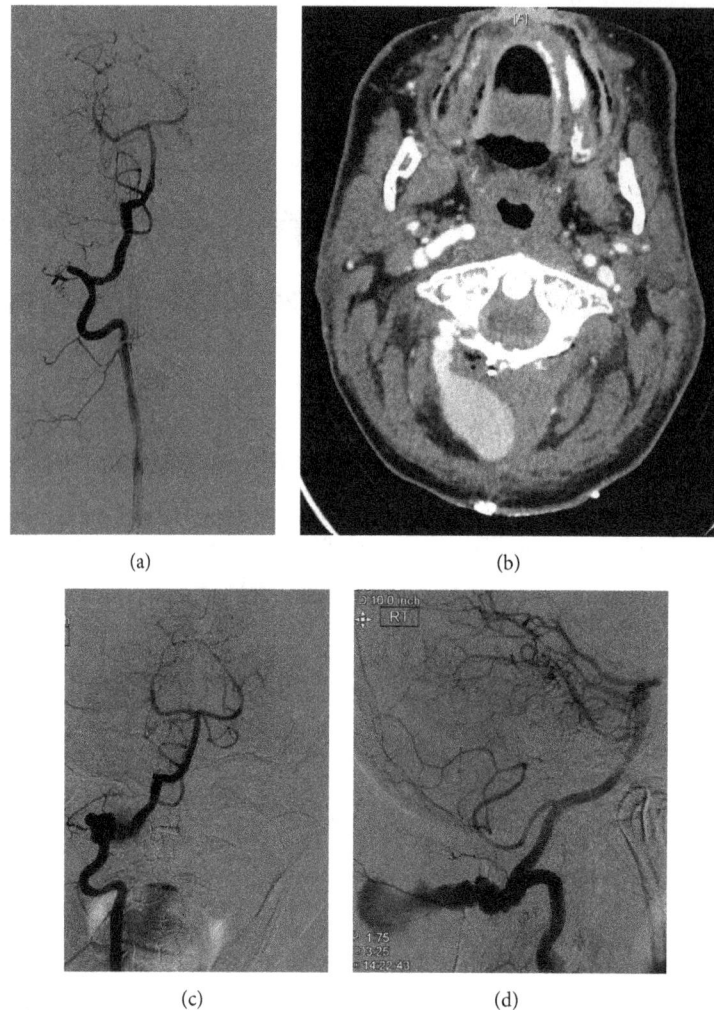

FIGURE 1: (a) shows normal filling of the right vertebral artery immediately following intraoperative injury: a small irregularity in the wall can be seen. (b) (CT angiogram) and (c) and (d) (digital subtraction angiogram) show a large saccular pseudoaneurysm arising from the V3 segment of the vertebral artery. The imaging was performed on the third postoperative day.

although no intimal flaps or flow limiting lesion was observed (Figure 1(a)). The patient underwent sublaminar wiring of C1 and C2 and was taken to the intensive care unit in a stable condition. Two days after the surgery, he developed a pulsatile swelling at the operative site. CT angiogram revealed a 5.5 × 2.0 cm pseudoaneurysm arising from the right vertebral artery (V3 segment), just superior to the posterior arch of C1 (Figure 1(b)). The patient was counseled regarding open and endovascular treatment options including parent artery sacrifice and vessel lumen reconstruction. Parent artery sacrifice was strongly considered; however, after discussion with the patient an attempt to preserve blood flow through the vertebral artery while excluding the aneurysm was decided upon.

3. Endovascular Treatment

The patient received a dose of 600 mg Plavix PO 1 day and 3 hrs prior to the procedure. The procedure was performed using 1% lidocaine as local anesthetic and standard Seldinger technique to access the left femoral artery and to place 5-French sheath. A 5F Envoy catheter was advanced over a 0.035 guidewire and placed at the distal cervical segment of the right vertebral artery. A DSA run showed the pseudoaneurysm arising from the V3 segment and measuring approximately 30 mm long × 10 mm high with a 6 mm neck (Figures 1(c) and 1(d)). A Marksman microcatheter (Ev3 Neurovascular, Irvine, CA) was then advanced over a 0.012 microguidewire and selectively placed distal to the neck of the pseudoaneurysm. A 5 × 18 mm Pipeline Embolization Device was deployed over the neck of the pseudoaneurysm obtaining immediate complete occlusion of the pseudoaneurysm (Figure 2(a)). The sheath was removed and a 6-French Angio-Seal is used as a closure device. The patient remained on Plavix 75 mg PO daily for 6 months and was then switched to aspirin 81 mg indefinitely. The patient did well and is asymptomatic at the last follow-up 10 months after the procedure (Figure 2(b)).

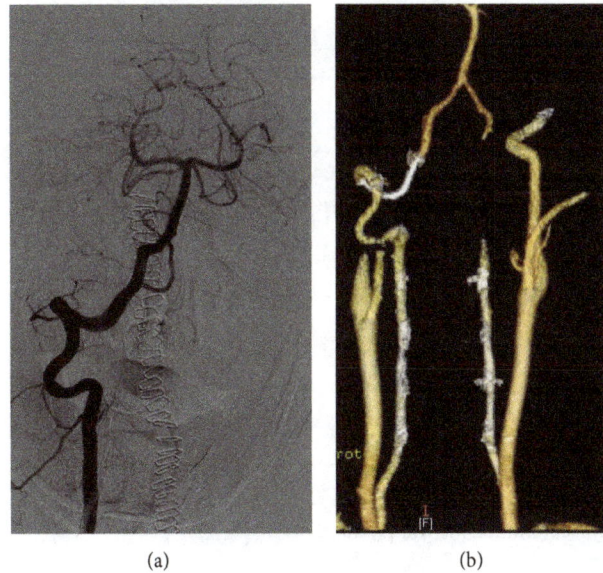

(a) (b)

FIGURE 2: (a) shows right vertebral injection image immediately after deployment of the Pipeline Embolization Device. There is nonfilling of the pseudoaneurysm while the vertebral artery fills normally. (b) shows stable complete pseudoaneurysm occlusion and patent right vertebral artery in the CT angiogram performed at 10-month follow-up.

4. Discussion

Pseudoaneurysms typically lack a true wall and are covered by a friable layer of connective tissue. Two types of iatrogenic pseudoaneurysms are reported, saccular and fusiform. Saccular pseudoaneurysms result from a focal, transmural injury to the vessel wall whereas fusiform pseudoaneurysms occur following dissection of the vessel resulting in thinning of adventitia and dilatation of the vessel [10]. Because of the lack of true neck, surgical or endovascular treatments have traditionally focused on parent vessel sacrifice with or without revascularization. Recently, management of these lesions has shifted from vessel destructive to vessel reconstructive strategies and various endovascular techniques are being employed to exclude the aneurysm from circulation while maintaining vessel patency [5, 6, 8].

The micropore flow-diverting stents are the most recent development in endovascular therapy of intracranial aneurysms. They were designed to obtain a greater change in aneurysm hemodynamics resulting in a diversion of flow within the stent. The SILK (SFD, Balt Extrusion, Montmorency, France) and Pipeline Embolization Device (PED, Covidien Vascular Therapies, Mansfield, MA, USA) promote flow diversion while preserving patency of branch vessels and perforating arteries. These flow-diverting devices have a larger metallic surface, thus having a greater potential to induce thrombosis within the aneurysm and endothelization of the neck of the aneurysm. In a recent systematic review, PED achieved 82.9% aneurysm obliteration at 6 months. The incidences of periprocedural complications and mortality were 6.3% and 1.5%, respectively [11].

Flow diversion has also been used in the management of dissecting carotid and vertebral artery aneurysms with occlusion rates up to 87.5% [12]. Amenta et al. reported a case of traumatic carotid pseudoaneurysm successfully treated using the PED [9]. Although flow-diversion stents have not been used earlier for treatment of traumatic vertebral pseudoaneurysms, we believe that they can be used to exclude the pseudoaneurysm while maintaining vessel patency. A caveat to the statement is that there is a higher possibility of successful outcome if the acute bleeding from the pseudoaneurysm has ceased at the time of treatment since the success of flow diversion is dependent on lack of significant pressure gradient across the wall of the pseudoaneurysm. Hence, use of a PED in actively bleeding traumatic pseudoaneurysms is likely not useful and potentially contraindicated. Since the flow-diversion technique causes thrombosis within the aneurysm over a period of time, there remains a risk of rupture of the pseudoaneurysm in the immediate postprocedure period. Further investigation into the blood flow hemodynamics of pseudoaneurysms following PED treatment is warranted to be able to treat these lesions more effectively and safely.

5. Conclusion

Iatrogenic pseudoaneurysms are rare, challenging lesions. The Pipeline Embolization Device, which has been effectively used in the management of complex aneurysms, may effectively be used in the management of these lesions while maintaining vessel lumen patency.

References

[1] M. Neo, S. Fujibayashi, M. Miyata, M. Takemoto, and T. Naka-mura, "Vertebral artery injury during cervical spine surgery: a survey of more than 5600 operations," *Spine*, vol. 33, no. 7, pp. 779–785, 2008.

[2] J. S. Yeom, J. M. Buchowski, K. W. Park, B. S. Chang, C. K. Lee, and K. D. Riew, "Undetected vertebral artery groove and foramen violations during C1 lateral mass and C2 pedicle screw placement," *Spine*, vol. 33, no. 25, pp. E942–E949, 2008.

[3] P. S. Larson, A. Reisner, D. J. Morassutti, B. Abdulhadi, and J. E. Harpring, "Traumatic intracranial aneurysms," *Neurosurgical Focus*, vol. 8, no. 1, article e4, 2000.

[4] B. Holmes and R. E. Harbaugh, "Traumatic intracranial aneurysms: a contemporary review," *The Journal of Trauma*, vol. 35, no. 6, pp. 855–860, 1993.

[5] T. E. Lempert, V. V. Halbach, R. T. Higashida et al., "Endovascular treatment of pseudoaneurysms with electrolytically detachable coils," *The American Journal of Neuroradiology*, vol. 19, no. 5, pp. 907–911, 1998.

[6] D. Maras, C. Lioupis, G. Magoufis, N. Tsamopoulos, K. Moulakakis, and V. Andrikopoulos, "Covered stent-graft treatment of traumatic internal carotid artery pseudoaneurysms: a review," *CardioVascular and Interventional Radiology*, vol. 29, no. 6, pp. 958–968, 2006.

[7] R. Medel, R. W. Crowley, D. K. Hamilton, and A. S. Dumont, "Endovascular obliteration of an intracranial pseudoaneurysm: the utility of Onyx," *Journal of Neurosurgery: Pediatrics*, vol. 4, no. 5, pp. 445–448, 2009.

[8] J. C. Méndez and F. González-Llanos, "Endovascular treatment of a vertebral artery pseudoaneurysm following posterior C1-C2 transarticular screw fixation," *CardioVascular and Interventional Radiology*, vol. 28, no. 1, pp. 107–109, 2005.

[9] P. S. Amenta, R. M. Starke, P. M. Jabbour et al., "Successful treatment of a traumatic carotid pseudoaneurysm with the Pipeline stent: case report and review of the literature," *Surgical Neurology International*, vol. 3, article 160, 2012.

[10] L. N. Sutton, "Vascular complications of surgery for craniopharyngioma and hypothalamic glioma," *Pediatric Neurosurgery*, vol. 21, no. 1, pp. 124–128, 1994.

[11] G. K. Leung, A. C. Tsang, and W. M. Lui, "Pipeline embolization device for intracranial aneurysm: a systematic review," *Clinical Neuroradiology*, vol. 22, no. 4, pp. 295–303, 2012.

[12] M. B. De Barros Faria, R. N. Castro, J. Lundquist et al., "The role of the pipeline embolization device for the treatment of dissecting intracranial aneurysms," *The American Journal of Neuroradiology*, vol. 32, no. 11, pp. 2192–2195, 2011.

4

Surgical Treatment for Profunda Femoris Artery Aneurysms

Kimihiro Igari, Toshifumi Kudo, Takahiro Toyofuku, and Yoshinori Inoue

Division of Vascular and Endovascular Surgery, Department of Surgery, Tokyo Medical and Dental University,
1-5-45 Yushima, Bunkyo-ku, Tokyo 113-8519, Japan

Correspondence should be addressed to Kimihiro Igari; igari.srg1@tmd.ac.jp

Academic Editor: Konstantinos A. Filis

Profunda femoris artery aneurysm (PFAA) is an extremely rare entity, with most cases being asymptomatic, which makes obtaining an early diagnosis difficult. We herein report a case series of PFAA, in which more than half of the PFAAs, which presented with no clinical symptoms, were discovered incidentally. All PFAAs were treated surgically with aneurysmectomy with or without vascular reconstruction. In cases involving a patent superficial femoral artery (SFA), graft replacement of the profunda femoris artery (PFA) is not mandatory; however, preserving the blood flow of the PFA is necessary to maintain lower extremity perfusion in patients with occlusion of the SFA. Therefore, the treatment of PFAAs should include appropriate management of both the aneurysmectomy and graft replacement, if possible.

1. Introduction

Profunda femoris artery aneurysm (PFAA) is an uncommon condition, accounting for only 0.5% of peripheral aneurysms and only 1–2.6% of all femoral artery aneurysms [1]. Most PFAAs are pseudoaneurysms resulting from iatrogenic injury or trauma [2], while true aneurysms of the profunda femoris artery (PFA) are much less frequent. Aneurysmal changes in PFA have been reported to be rare because several muscles cover the PFA in this anatomical location [3]. Based on the anatomical location, diagnosing small and asymptomatic PFAAs is difficult. PFAAs may cause symptoms of local venous and nerve compression, which may lead to distal venous congestion and local pain. Furthermore, these aneurysms are occasionally complicated with distal embolism, limb-threatening ischemia, and rupture [4]. We herein report the results of our experience with surgical treatment for true PFAAs.

2. Case Presentation

2.1. Patients and Methods. A retrospective review was performed on all patients with a diagnosis of PFAA who underwent surgical treatment at Tokyo Medical and Dental University Hospital between January 2005 and December 2014. All subjects provided their informed consent, and approval was obtained from our Institutional Review Board for a retrospective review of the patients' medical records and images. The inclusion criterion was aneurysmal dilatation of a PFA of more than 20 mm, based on preoperative imaging findings. Cases of pseudoaneurysms of PFAA due to trauma were excluded, and only true aneurysms were included. The medical records were abstracted to include basic demographic information, preoperative symptoms, aneurysm size measurements, intraoperative findings, perioperative complications, and long-term imaging findings. The characteristic features of the patients are given in Table 1.

2.2. Case 1. A 76-year-old asymptomatic male presented for follow-up magnetic resonance imaging (MRI) after open surgical repair of an abdominal aortic aneurysm (AAA). MRI showed a PFAA measuring 45 × 40 mm on the right side of the thigh. The aneurysm was successfully resected under general anesthesia without vascular reconstruction, as the superficial femoral artery (SFA) was patent, and the distal portion of the PFA was very small, making it unsuitable for revascularization. The patient's postoperative course was uneventful,

TABLE 1: Patients characteristics.

Pt	Gender	Age	PFAA Laterality	PFAA Size (mm)	Clinical symptoms	Diagnostic modality	Other aneurysms	Comorbidity
1	M	76	Rt	45 × 40	None	MRI, angiography	AAA	HT, Af, CHF, smoker
2	F	69	Bil	(Rt) 25 × 22 (Lt) 34 × 24	(Rt) None (Lt) Swelling, pain	CT	Bil CFAA	Smoker
3	M	73	Rt	25 × 22	None	CT	TAA, AAA, Bil CIAA	HT, smoker
4	F	65	Rt	26 × 25	None	US, CT	None	Smoker
5	M	70	Lt	86 × 78	Pulsatile mass, pain	CT	None	HT, smoker

*Pt: patient; M: male; F: female; Rt: right; Lt: left; Bil: bilateral; MRI: magnetic resonance imaging; CT: computed tomography; US: ultrasonography; PFAA: profunda femoris artery aneurysm; CFAA: common femoral artery aneurysm; TAA: thoracic aortic aneurysm; AAA: abdominal aortic aneurysm; CIAA: common iliac artery aneurysm; HT: hypertension; Af: atrial fibrillation; CHF: chronic heart failure.

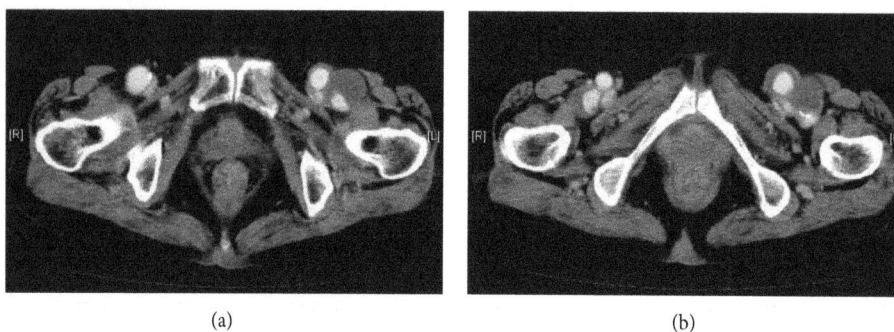

(a)   (b)

FIGURE 1: Computed tomography showed bilateral common femoral artery aneurysms (a) and bilateral profunda femoris artery aneurysms (b).

and the postoperative ankle brachial pressure was within the normal limits without any lower limb ischemia.

2.3. Case 2. A 69-year-old female presented with pain and swelling of the left thigh. Computed tomography (CT) showed a left PFAA measuring 34 × 24 mm. Furthermore, CT detected a right PFAA measuring 25 × 22 mm, without clinical symptoms, and the bilateral common femoral arteries (CFAs) showed aneurysmal changes (Figure 1). The bilateral CFA aneurysms (CFAAs) and PFAAs were resected under general anesthesia, and resected bilateral CFAAs were interposed using the prosthesis measuring 8 mm in size. Bilaterally, bypass grafting was performed from the interposed prosthesis which measured 8 mm in size to the distal part of PFA by a vascular prosthesis measuring 6 mm in size. The patient's postoperative course was uneventful, without any evidence of lower limb ischemia.

2.4. Case 3. A 73-year-old asymptomatic male presented for follow-up CT after open surgical repair of AAA and bilateral common iliac artery aneurysms and an assessment of an untreated thoracic artery aneurysm measuring 40 mm in size. CT exhibited a PFAA measuring 25 × 22 mm on the right side of the thigh (Figure 2(a)). The aneurysm was successfully resected under general anesthesia with revascularization from the proximal to the distal part of the PFA using an 8 mm prosthesis (Figure 2(b)). The patient developed a wound infection after the operation; however, it healed with conservative treatment.

2.5. Case 4. A 65-year-old asymptomatic female presented for the ultrasonography to evaluate the varicose vein. US showed the 25 mm sized mass on her right groin. Further contrast enhanced CT scanning showed the right PFAA measuring 26 × 25 mm. Under general anesthesia, the SFA and the proximal and distal part of PFAA were well controlled; the aneurysmectomy was successfully performed with the interposed 8 mm prosthetic graft placed between the proximal and distal PFA (Figure 3). Postoperative course was uneventful, without lower limb ischemia.

2.6. Case 5. A 70-year-old male presented with a palpable mass and pain in the left thigh. Contrast enhanced CT revealed a left PFAA measuring 86 × 76 mm (Figure 4). The aneurysm was successfully resected under general anesthesia without revascularization, as the distal portion of the PFA was very small, meaning that it was too difficult to revascularize, and the SFA was patent. The patient's postoperative course was uneventful, without any evidence of lower limb ischemia.

2.7. Surgical Procedures and Postoperative Results (Tables 2 and 3). A total of six PFAAs were resected in five patients. The mean operative time was 130 minutes (range: 81–210 minutes) and the mean amount of intraoperative blood loss was 122 mL (range: 15–594 mL); therefore, none of the patients required a blood transfusion. Four of the six PFAAs were interposed with a prosthetic graft, and, in case 2, the bilateral PFAAs and CFAAs were resected simultaneously with revascularization. Two of the six PFAAs were treated with ligation without

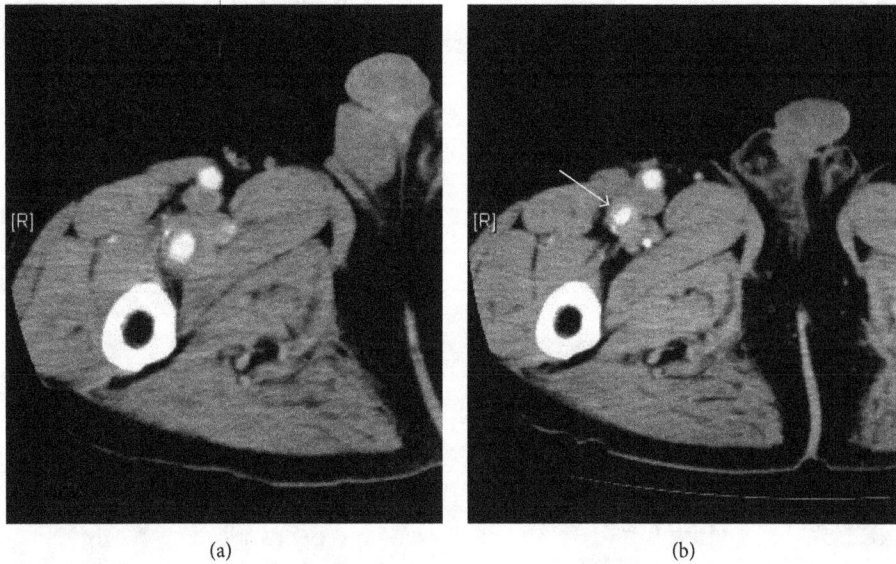

(a)   (b)

FIGURE 2: (a) Preoperative computed tomography exhibited a 22 mm right profunda femoris artery aneurysm with an intraluminal thrombus. (b) Postoperative computed tomography revealed a patent replaced prosthetic graft (white arrow).

TABLE 2: Surgical procedures and intra- and postoperative findings.

Pt	Surgical procedure	Conduit	Operative time (min)	Intraoperative blood loss (mL)	Pathology
1	Aneurysmectomy	None	149	122	Degenerative
2	(Rt) Aneurysmectomy + revascularization (Lt) Aneurysmectomy + revascularization	(Rt) 8 mm ePTFE + 6 mm ePTFE (Lt) 8 mm ePTFE + 6 mm ePTFE	210	502	(Rt) Degenerative (Lt) Degenerative
3	Aneurysmectomy + revascularization	8 mm Dacron	87	15	Degenerative
4	Aneurysmectomy + revascularization	8 mm ePTFE	130	86	Degenerative
5	Aneurysmectomy	None	81	594	Degenerative

*Pt: patient; ePTFE: expanded polytetrafluoroethylene.

TABLE 3: Postoperative and long-term follow-up results.

Pt	Postoperative morbidity	Postoperative (<30 days) mortality	Follow-up (month)	Limb ischemia	Graft patency
1	None	Alive	8	None	—
2	None	Alive	76	None	Patent
3	Wound infection, relief	Alive	18	None	Patent
4	None	Alive	12	None	Patent
5	None	Alive	35	None	—

*Pt: patient.

revascularization because the distal part of each PFAA was located too far to achieve revascularization. The pathological findings of the resected aneurysms showed degenerative and atherosclerotic changes in all six PFAAs.

None of the patients exhibited lower limb ischemia after the surgical procedures and all were discharged successfully. During the long-term follow-up period (median: 18 months, range: 8–76 months), no patients presented with signs of lower limb ischemia, and all of the interposed grafts remained patent.

3. Discussion

Previous reviews of published cases have indicated that patients with PFAA often have synchronous aneurysms, occurring in 65–75% of cases, including AAA and popliteal

(a)

(b)

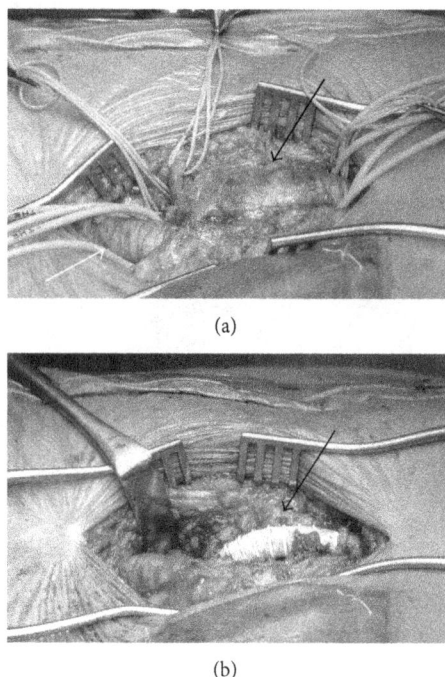

FIGURE 3: (a) The intraoperative findings showed the controlled profunda femoris artery (black arrow) and superficial femoral artery (white arrow), and (b) the aneurysmectomy was performed with graft interposition (black arrow). The patient's head was to the right.

(a)

(b)

FIGURE 4: Computed tomography showed a 78 × 86 mm left profunda femoris artery (PFA) (a), which extended to the distal part of the left PFA (white arrow) (b).

artery aneurysms [5]. Bilateral PFAAs occur in only 5% of patients with PFAAs, in contrast to femoral artery aneurysms, which occur bilaterally in the majority of cases [2]. In our case series, three of five patients with PFAAs had other synchronous aneurysms (60%), and bilateral PFAAs were noted in one case (20%); these findings are compatible with those of previous reviews. Cutler and Darling classified femoral artery aneurysms according to the relationship between the CFA and CFA bifurcation. Type I involves aneurysmal changes localized in the CFA, whereas, in type II, the aneurysmal changes extend to the proximal part of the superficial femoral artery (SFA) and PFA [6]. According to this classification, the current case 2 can be classified as type II.

It has been reported that PFAAs are much more common in males (92–100%) than in females, and most PFAAs are discovered in the sixth to seventh decades of life [3]. Furthermore, it has been reported that most patients with PFAAs have a decades-long history of smoking and hypertension [7]. In the current study, the details of our cases are comparable to those of previous reports concerning epidemiological findings, in particular, that all of the patients had a smoking habit, which may exhibit a significant correlation with the onset of PFAA.

Although patients with PFAAs usually remain asymptomatic and the lesions are discovered incidentally, such patients may present with symptoms related to local compression, thrombosis, or embolism, with consequent rupture. Compression-related symptoms include groin swelling, pain, and pulsatile masses [2]. In our cases, four of the six PFAAs were asymptomatic and found incidentally, and the other

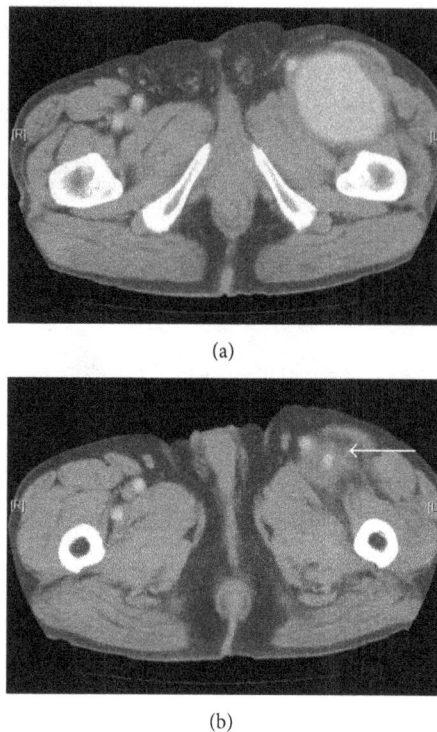

two presented with local compressive symptoms. However, PFAAs may present with acute ischemic symptoms due to thrombosis and/or embolism of distal vessels [8]. Furthermore, rupture is believed to be a more common presentation for PFAAs than other peripheral aneurysms [1] and may carry a high risk of limb loss and even mortality. Therefore, early diagnosis and treatment are essential in such cases.

Following the diagnosis of PFAA, elective surgical repair is recommended whenever the patient's general condition allows for surgical intervention [3]. A reasonable recommendation is to repair PFAAs measuring over 20 mm in diameter [1]. However, a recent study reported that acute complications are rare in cases of femoral artery aneurysms < 35 mm in diameter and that the repair criteria for asymptomatic femoral artery aneurysms should be >35 mm [9]. Furthermore, the presence of an intraluminal thrombus in cases of femoral artery aneurysms is an additional indication for elective repair and may cause ischemic complications [9]. Therefore, surgical decisions must be individualized according to the size of the aneurysm, symptoms, cause of complications, and the patient's general condition. Our surgical indication for elective repair of PFAA is a diameter over 20 mm or symptomatic PFAAs. All patients with PFAAs in this series were treated surgically, and we did not experience any cases of PFAAs that were managed conservatively.

The aim of surgical treatment for PFAAs is to eliminate the risk of complications, including distal ischemia and rupture, and maintain perfusion to the lower extremities. Therefore, surgical repair consists of aneurysmectomy with or without graft replacement [1, 10]. When the superficial femoral artery (SFA) is patent, reconstruction of the PFA is not mandatory; however, in cases with occlusion of the SFA and distal vessels, the PFA serves as an important collateral vessel to the lower extremities and reconstruction is necessary in order to maintain an optimal blood supply. Furthermore, preserving the PFA blood flow may have a positive effect for future limb salvage, as the PFA is less frequently damaged by atherosclerotic changes [3]. Therefore, cases of PFAAs should be treated with both aneurysmectomy and vascular reconstruction, if possible. If the PFAA is located in the distal part of the PFA and/or reconstruction is difficult due to the anatomical location, it may be adequate to excise the aneurysm. Endovascular treatment with stent graft placement is an alternative treatment to ligation, which is a less invasive treatment [11, 12]. In our cases (cases 1 and 5), the aneurysms were located in the distal part of the PFAA and their large size made it difficult to perform reconstruction. Furthermore, both patients had patent SFAs, and we therefore performed aneurysmectomy without graft replacement, which did not lead to ischemic complications.

In conclusion, we herein reported a case series of PFAAs treated surgically with aneurysmectomy with or without graft replacement. Providing an early diagnosis and surgical treatment is necessary to prevent complications, and reconstruction of the PFA is recommended, unless the SFA is patent and performing graft replacement is technically difficult.

References

[1] C. Harbuzariu, A. A. Duncan, T. C. Bower, M. Kalra, and P. Gloviczki, "Profunda femoris artery aneurysms: association with aneurysmal disease and limb ischemia," *Journal of Vascular Surgery*, vol. 47, no. 1, pp. 31–35, 2008.

[2] S. R. Posner, J. Wilensky, J. Dimick, and P. K. Henke, "A true aneurysm of the profunda femoris artery: a case report and review of the english language literature," *Annals of Vascular Surgery*, vol. 18, no. 6, pp. 740–746, 2004.

[3] G. Gemayel, D. Mugnai, E. Khabiri, J. Sierra, N. Murith, and A. Kalangos, "Isolated bilateral profunda femoris artery aneurysm," *Annals of Vascular Surgery*, vol. 24, no. 6, pp. 824.e11–824.e13, 2010.

[4] T. Shintani, T. Norimatsu, K. Atsuta, T. Saitou, S. Higashi, and H. Mitsuoka, "Initial experience with proximal ligation for profunda femoris artery aneurysms: report of three cases," *Surgery Today*, vol. 44, no. 4, pp. 748–752, 2014.

[5] C. A. Johnson, J. M. Goff, S. T. Rehrig, and N. C. Hadro, "Asymptomatic profunda femoris artery aneurysm: diagnosis and rationale for management," *European Journal of Vascular and Endovascular Surgery*, vol. 24, no. 1, pp. 91–92, 2002.

[6] B. S. Cutler and R. C. Darling, "Surgical management of arteriosclerotic femoral aneurysms," *Surgery*, vol. 74, no. 5, pp. 764–773, 1973.

[7] F. Milotic, I. Milotic, and V. Flis, "Isolated atherosclerotic aneurysm of the profunda femoris artery," *Annals of Vascular Surgery*, vol. 24, no. 4, pp. 552.e1–552.e3, 2010.

[8] G. Piffaretti, G. Mariscalco, M. Tozzi, N. Rivolta, M. Annoni, and P. Castelli, "Twenty-year experience of femoral artery aneurysms," *Journal of Vascular Surgery*, vol. 53, no. 5, pp. 1230–1236, 2011.

[9] P. F. Lawrence, M. P. Harlander-Locke, G. S. Oderich et al., "The current management of isolated degenerative femoral artery aneurysms is too aggressive for their natural history," *Journal of Vascular Surgery*, vol. 59, no. 2, pp. 343–349, 2014.

[10] A. Idetsu, M. Sugimoto, M. Matsushita, and T. Ikezawa, "Solitary profunda femoris artery aneurysm," *Annals of Vascular Surgery*, vol. 25, no. 4, pp. 558.e13–558.e15, 2011.

[11] C. Klonaris, J. K. Bellos, A. Katsargyris, E. D. Avgerinos, M. Moschou, and C. Verikokos, "Endovascular repair of two tandem profunda femoris artery aneurysms," *Journal of Vascular and Interventional Radiology*, vol. 20, no. 9, pp. 1253–1254, 2009.

[12] G. Brancaccio, G. M. Celoria, T. Stefanini, R. Lombardi, and E. Falco, "Endovascular repair of a profunda femoris artery aneurysm," *Annals of Vascular Surgery*, vol. 25, no. 7, pp. 980.e11–980.e13, 2011.

Successful Obliteration of a Pseudoaneurysm from Post-CEA Repair Secondary to a Pruitt-Inahara Shunt Using a Stent Graft

Vishal Dahya and Prasad Chalasani

Florida State University College of Medicine, 1115 West Call Street, Tallahassee, FL 32306-4300, USA

Correspondence should be addressed to Prasad Chalasani; pchalasani@hotmail.com

Academic Editors: M. Reinhard and S. Yamashiro

Pseudoaneurysms of the carotid artery are very uncommon complications following carotid endarterectomy. Pseudoaneurysms are usually caused by any kind of blunt injury or trauma during carotid artery surgery. CEA has become an increasingly more common vascular surgery performed in the United States. The standard of treatment for a carotid PA has been open surgical repair with excision of the defect and then a graft reconstruction of the artery. Advancements in endovascular intervention have helped to make it a more popular choice in treatment because of the positive results and less invasive approach. This case report describes the successful obliteration of a large post-CEA PA using a stent graft. The PA was likely secondary to the use of a Pruitt-Inahara Shunt because it was found to be distal to the endarterectomized area of the carotid artery which means that the defect was likely caused by the balloon portion of the shunt. This case demonstrates the feasibility of using endovascular interventional techniques to treat a PA using a stent graft.

1. Introduction

Pseudoaneurysms (PAs) of the carotid artery are very uncommon complications following carotid endarterectomy (CEA) [1, 2]. PAs are usually caused by any kind of blunt injury or trauma during carotid artery surgery [3]. CEA has become an increasingly more common vascular surgery performed in the United States. More common complications of this type of surgery include hematoma formation, stroke, myocardial infarction, and cranial nerve injury [2]. The incidence of a post-CEA PA is estimated to be around 0.3%, and it has been suggested by various researchers that the risk of this complication is increased by the use of patch closure [4–6]. The standard of treatment for a carotid PA has been open surgical repair with excision of the defect and then a graft reconstruction of the artery. Advancements in endovascular intervention have helped to make it a more popular choice in treatment because of the positive results and less invasive approach [7, 8]. This case report describes the successful obliteration of a large post-CEA PA using a stent graft. The PA was likely secondary to the use of a Pruitt-Inahara Shunt because it was found to be distal to the endarterectomized area of the carotid artery which means that the defect was likely caused by the balloon portion of the shunt. This case demonstrates the feasibility of using endovascular interventional techniques to treat a PA using a stent graft.

2. Case Report

An 86-year-old man presented with a headache and blurred vision. His surgical history was significant for an uneventful left sided CEA with a Vascular Patch (Synovis VG-0106N) and utilizing a Pruitt-Inahara Shunt during the procedure. This surgery was performed 2 months ago for high grade left internal carotid stenosis (90%). Patient was having no other associated symptoms and had no clinical signs of infection. Computed tomography (CT) angiography of the head and neck was then performed, revealing a 1.2 × 2.0 cm pseudoaneurysm with a small amount of surrounding thrombus within the distal left cervical internal carotid artery just proximal to the petrous portion (Figure 1). The PA was found to be distal to the endarterectomized area of the carotid artery which means that the defect was likely caused by the balloon portion of the shunt. A short segment of high grade

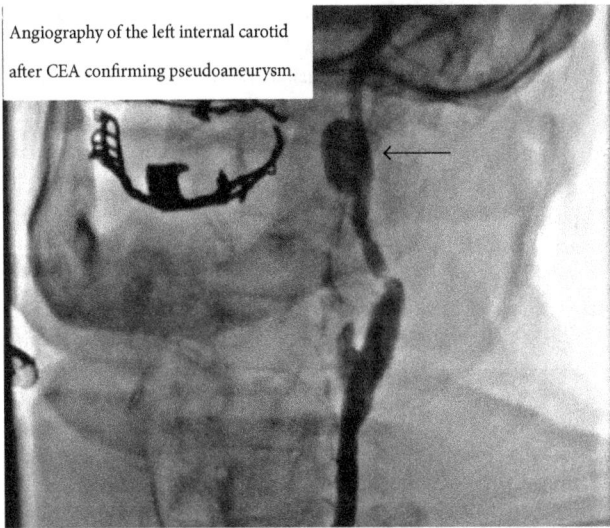

Angiography of the left internal carotid after CEA confirming pseudoaneurysm.

FIGURE 1: Computed tomography angiography of left internal carotid artery; pseudoaneurysm location is confirmed.

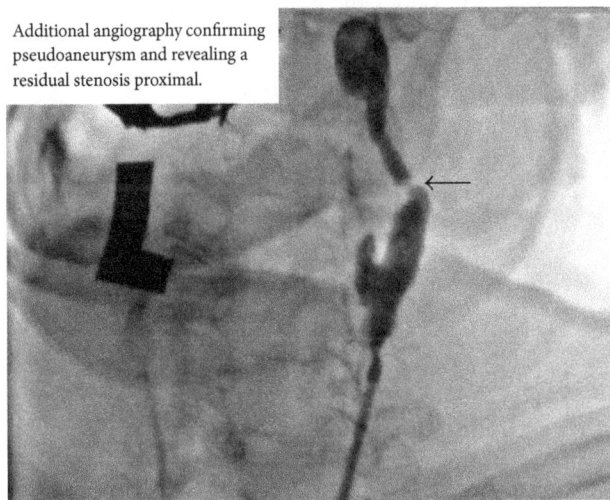

Additional angiography confirming pseudoaneurysm and revealing a residual stenosis proximal.

FIGURE 2: Additional angiography; residual stenosis is seen proximal to the pseudoaneurysm.

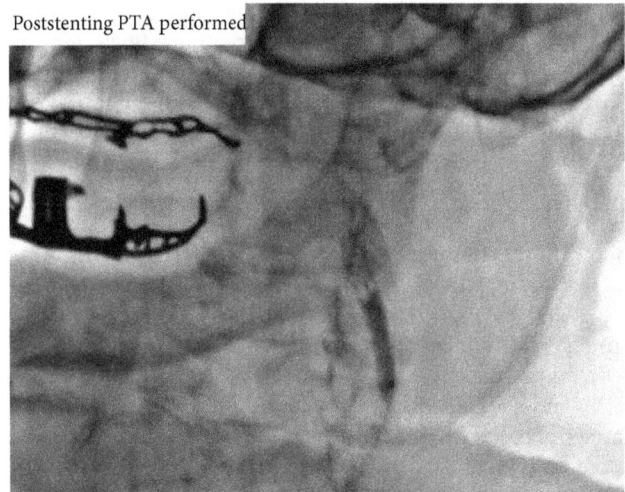

Poststenting PTA performed

FIGURE 3: Poststenting percutaneous transluminal angiography; stent graft placement is seen with angiography.

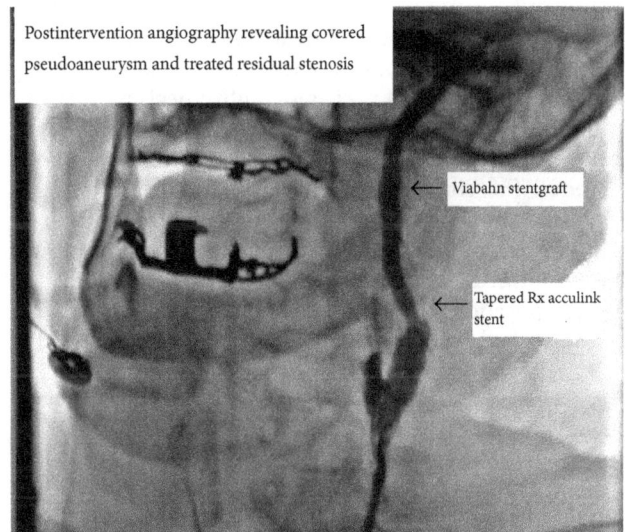

Postintervention angiography revealing covered pseudoaneurysm and treated residual stenosis

Viabahn stentgraft

Tapered Rx acculink stent

FIGURE 4: Postintervention angiography; pseudoaneurysm is successfully obliterated and residual stenosis has been treated.

stenosis (80%) was also revealed in the postbulbar region of the proximal left internal carotid artery (Figure 2). Patient was then taken to the catheterization lab for endovascular exclusion of the PA. The right groin was prepped, and a 6 French catheter was placed in the femoral artery. An internal mammary catheter was used and then selectively cannulated the internal mammary to gain access to the left carotid artery where angiography was performed. A 0.035 wire was then passed through, and a 7 French 9 cm long sheath was passed into the left common carotid artery where a repeat angiography was performed. Then a 0.014 BMW wire was passed across those lesions, and the position was confirmed. A 6 × 50 mm long covered Viabahn stent (W. L. Gore & Associates Inc., Flagstaff, AZ) was successfully deployed across the PA, but there were still the tight stenosis and 90-degree bend of the graft anastomosis of the endarterectomy

site. For the residual stenosis, a 7 × 10 stent (Nitinol Acculink) was successfully deployed and expanded using a 5 Balloon to 6 Atmospheres (Figure 3). After full expansion was noted, the balloon was withdrawn, and completion angiography was performed confirming complete obliteration of the PA (Figure 4). Patient recovered with no postoperative neurological symptoms and had no complications upon 3-year followup.

3. Discussion

Pseudoaneurysms are known to be a rare postoperative complication of CEA, but research is being done to identify the exact cause of these defects. Reported causes of post-CEA PAs include infection of prosthetic material, blunt injury, and suture failure [1, 2]. Not many cases have been reported of PAs being caused by the shunt used during the CEA procedure. The Pruitt Inahara Shunt is a device that allows for the maintenance of cerebral blood flow during carotid surgery. This shunt is placed into the vessel and uses balloons to keep the artery patent as the plaque is being removed [9]. Since the PA in our case was located distal to the vascular patch site or the endarterectomized area of the carotid artery, we concluded that the balloon portion of the shunt likely caused blunt trauma to the artery. This blunt trauma allowed for the formation of the left internal carotid PA [10]. The standard treatment of PAs for many years has been open carotid surgery, but endovascular intervention has made progress which has enabled it to gain more popularity [7, 8]. In our case, endovascular intervention was chosen because of the large size of the PA and the history of prior CEA which would increase the difficulty of an open repair. A self-expanding stent graft was also chosen to allow for complete obliteration of the PA and improve the carotid blood flow.

4. Conclusion

In conclusion, endovascular treatment of a post-CEA PA with a stent graft has shown encouraging results, but long term data is needed to make a definitive decision that this is the therapy of choice. A similar case was described by the Department of Vascular Surgery at the University of Florence. This study concluded with the similar notion that PA formation can be seen with overinflation of the balloon [11]. We cannot be certain of the exact mechanism of how the PA formed, and more studies must be done to identify the complications of shunt induced blunt trauma. A larger case series is also needed on post-CEA PAs to understand the exact genesis and formation of the PA.

References

[1] N. S. Ilijevski, P. Gajin, V. Neskovic, J. Kolar, and D. Radak, "Postendarterectomy common carotid artery pseudoaneurysm," Vascular, vol. 14, no. 3, pp. 177–180, 2006.

[2] R. A. Litwinski, K. Wright, and P. Pons, "Pseudoaneurysm formation following carotid endarterectomy: two case reports and a literature review," Annals of Vascular Surgery, vol. 20, no. 5, pp. 678–680, 2006.

[3] T. H. Cogbill, E. E. Moore, M. Meissner et al., "The spectrum of blunt injury to the carotid artery: a multicenter perspective," Journal of Trauma, vol. 37, no. 3, pp. 473–479, 1994.

[4] B. R. Grimsley, J. K. Wells, G. J. Pearl et al., "Bovine pericardial patch angioplasty in carotid endarterectomy," American Surgeon, vol. 67, no. 9, pp. 890–895, 2001.

[5] J. May, G. H. White, R. Waugh, and J. Brennan, "Endoluminal repair of internal carotid artery aneurysm: a feasible but hazardous procedure," Journal of Vascular Surgery, vol. 26, no. 6, pp. 1055–1060, 1997.

[6] N. D. Martin, R. A. Carabasi, J. Bonn, J. Lombardi, and P. DiMuzio, "Endovascular repair of carotid artery aneurysms following carotid endarterectomy," Annals of Vascular Surgery, vol. 19, no. 6, pp. 913–916, 2005.

[7] R. L. Bush, P. H. Lin, and T. F. Dodson, "Endoluminal stent placement and coil embolization for the management of carotid artery pseudoaneurysms," Journal of Endovascular Therapy, vol. 8, no. 1, pp. 53–561, 2001.

[8] K. Singh, D. Yakoub, J. Schor, J. Deitch, J. Scheiner, and C. Dossa, "Endovascular treatment of shunt induced carotid pseudoaneurysm: less invasive but still a big risk," Journal of Vascular Surgery, vol. 56, no. 3, p. 894, 2012.

[9] P. D. Hayes, T. Vainas, S. Hartley et al., "The Pruitt-Inahara shunt maintains mean middle cerebral artery velocities within 10% of preoperative values during carotid endarterectomy," Journal of Vascular Surgery, vol. 32, no. 2, pp. 299–306, 2000.

[10] K. Gupta, K. Dougherty, H. Hermman, and Z. Krajcer, "Endovascular repair of a giant carotid pseudoaneurysm with the use of Viabahn stent graft," Catheterization and Cardiovascular Interventions, vol. 62, no. 1, pp. 64–68, 2004.

[11] N. Troisi, W. Dorigo, R. Pulli, and C. Pratesi, "A case of traumatic internal carotid artery aneurysm secondary to carotid shunting," Journal of Vascular Surgery, vol. 51, no. 1, pp. 225–227, 2010.

Exercise Induced Left Bundle Branch Block Treated with Cardiac Rehabilitation

Nathan S. Anderson, Alexies Ramirez, Ahmad Slim, and Jamil Malik

Cardiology Service, Brooke Army Medical Center, 3551 Roger Brooke Drive, San Antonio, TX 78234-6200, USA

Correspondence should be addressed to Jamil Malik; jamil.a.malik.mil@mail.mil

Academic Editors: J.-W. Chen, N. Espinola-Zavaleta, and A. Iyisoy

Exercise induced bundle branch block is a rare observation in exercise testing, accounting for 0.5 percent of exercise tests. The best treatment of this condition and its association with coronary disease remain unclear. We describe a case associated with normal coronary arteries which was successfully treated with exercise training. While this treatment has been used previously, our case has a longer followup than previously reported and demonstrates that the treatment is not durable in the absence of continued exercise.

1. Introduction

The patient was a 42-year-old woman who presented with exertional chest pain, palpitations, and dyspnea that resolved with rest. She had a normal physical exam and her only medication was an oral contraceptive. 12-lead electrocardiogram was normal with the following intervals: PR interval was 154 millisecond (msec), QRS was narrow at 82 msec, and QT interval was normal at 392 msec, corrected QT (QTc) using Bazett's formula was 431 msec (Figure 1). Laboratory tests including hemoglobin and cardiac troponin T were normal.

She was referred for exercise stress testing using the Bruce protocol during which she developed a left bundle branch block (LBBB) with a QRS duration of 120 msec at a heart rate of 112 beats per minute (bpm) (Figure 2). During the aberrant conduction and at peak exercise, her symptoms of chest pain and palpitations returned. She was able to exercise through her discomfort, reaching a peak heart rate of 171 bpm and 10.4 metabolic equivalent (MET) at 9 : 11 min of exercise. The test was stopped due to limiting chest discomfort that persisted until her heart rate returned to 100 bpm at 2 : 30 min of recovery and normal conduction was restored. An echocardiogram was performed and revealed no structural abnormalities other than a small patent foramen ovale (PFO). Concerns

regarding ischemia as the etiology for her conduction abnormalities prompted coronary angiography that demonstrated normal coronary arteries with no evidence of atherosclerosis.

The patient was a military service member on active duty status, which would require passing a physical fitness test, something her symptoms had not permitted. In the absence of structural heart disease leading to her conduction abnormality at peak exercise, patient was prescribed an exercise program in an attempt to improve symptoms with physiologic conditioning and left ventricular remodeling. Patient underwent cardiac rehabilitation exercise prescription with five times weekly 30-minute submaximal aerobic exercise. As previously reported by Heinsimer et al. [1], cardiac rehabilitation exercise training has been used to treat rate-related left bundle branch block with noted improvement in symptoms.

After three months of regular exercise training with 30-minute sessions per day for five days a week, the patient's symptoms improved with development of LBBB and chest pain at a considerably higher heart rate of 150 bpm (Figure 3). The morphology of the LBBB remained the same. Notably, offset of aberrancy remained unchanged, with her last stress test demonstrating return to normal conduction at 108 bpm. With her symptoms improving, she became much less consistent in her attendance at cardiac rehabilitation

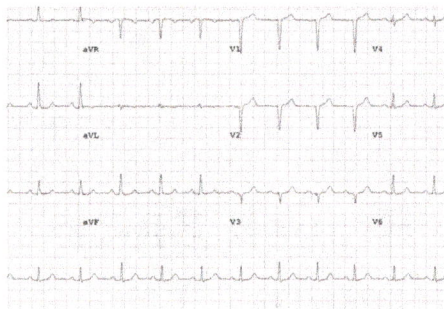

FIGURE 1: Baseline electrocardiogram demonstrating normal baseline conduction.

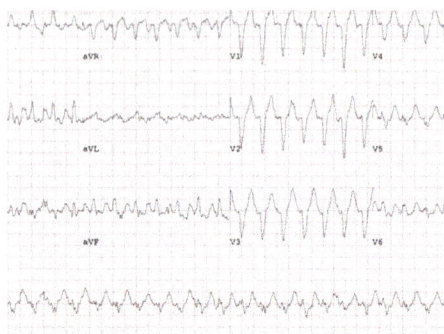

FIGURE 2: Electrocardiogram at peak exertion demonstrating left bundle branch block morphology.

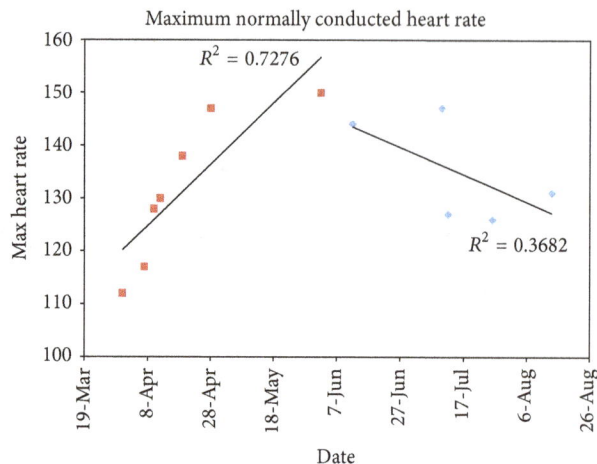

FIGURE 3: Plot of maximum normally conducted heart rates over time, demonstrating an increase in maximum rate with regular exercise training (red) and a decrease with nonadherence to regular training (blue).

sessions. As she became more noncompliant with her attendance, her heart rate threshold for development of symptoms with aberrancy dropped again to 120–130 bpm, a marginal improvement from her baseline.

2. Discussion

Symptomatic exertional rate-related left bundle branch block associated with symptoms of chest pain and palpitation was first described by Eichert in 1946 with subsequent reports by multiple other authors [1–5]. However, the prognosis and best treatment course have not been well established. Seven small case series have reported populations of rate-related left bundle branch block, and two have attempted to provide prognostic data [2, 5–10].

Virtanen et al. reported a series of seven patients with exertional chest pain and exercise induced LBB, who in the process of evaluating the cause of chest pain were found to have normal coronary arteriogram despite the persistence of the exertional chest pain associated with LBBB at peak exercise [11]. On the other hand, in a different case series of 11 patients with left bundle branch block induced with exercise treadmill testing, drawn from 4100 consecutive exercise tests at their institution, the incidence of obstructive coronary disease was found to be 63% (7 out of 11 patients) on left heart catheterization. These results lead the authors to conclude that exercise induced LBBB is almost always associated with coronary disease [6].

In a different study aimed at identifying the heart rate parameters during exercise at which LBBB is induced, in 2,584 consecutive patients who underwent treadmill testing, the incidence of exercise induced LBBB was 1.1% (occurred at range of 60 to 163 bpm). Of these 28 patients, 19 (68%) had no obstructive coronary disease on subsequent catheterization. Authors further demonstrated the rate at which the LBBB developed was important for determining prognosis. None of the patients in this study with exercise induced LBBB at heart rates over 125 bpm had coronary disease [5].

Williams et al. [8] published a case control series of 70 patients with exercise induced LBBB, drawn from a series of 17,277 consecutive treadmill tests. The control patients were matched according to the variables of sex, hypertension, diabetes, smoking, beta-blocker use, and history of coronary disease. Not every patient in this cohort underwent coronary angiography, but outcomes were followed for a mean of 3.7 years. A composite endpoint of all-cause mortality, revascularization (percutaneous or surgical), nonfatal myocardial infarction, or need for an implanted pacemaker or defibrillator was used. At four years of followup, the composite endpoint occurred in 10% of the control cohort, and in 19% of the case cohort. Significantly, this endpoint was independent of documented coronary disease, with an adjusted relative risk of 2.73 (see Table 1). Note that not every patient underwent diagnostic angiography.

The above studies demonstrate that exercise induced LBBB is a rare condition, occurring in less than one percent of exercise treadmill tests. The incidence of coronary disease in this population remains unclear. There exist no trials of therapy for these patients, and, despite the fact that several authors [1, 3, 10, 13] describe significant symptoms with this condition, discussions of treatment are limited to case reports. Pharmacologic therapy has been discussed, with nitroglycerin administration terminating the aberrant conduction in one patient [4]. Beta-blockers have been used to decrease the heart rate response to exercise and therefore

TABLE 1: All published case series of patients with exercise induced LBBB, with incidence and prevalence of coronary artery disease.

	Authors/date							
	Virtanen et al., 1982 [11]	Wayne et al., 1983 [7]	Vasey et al., 1985 [6]	Heinsimer et al., 1987 [10]	Williams et al., 1988 [8]	Moran et al., 1992 [12]	Hertzeanu et al., 1992 [3]	Grady et al., 1998 [9]
Number of patients	7	11	28	15	37	29	11	70
Mean age in years	44.6	57	53	52	61	63	48	68
Normal perfusion imaging	Not reported	Not reported	Not reported	Not reported	Not reported	17	Not reported	Not reported
Abnormal perfusion imaging	Not reported	Not reported	Not reported	Not reported	Not reported	20	Not reported	Not reported
Normal coronary angiography	7	4	19	7	11	4	7	8
Abnormal coronary angiography	0	7	9	8	26	14	3	35
HR onset with no associated CAD	106 ± 30	94 ± 34	Not reported	124 ± 15	118	129 ± 32	85 ± 25	Not reported
HR onset with associated CAD	Not reported	104 ± 47	Not reported	124 ± 22	Not reported	114 ± 29	126 ± 25	Not reported

avoid the development of the aberrancy. But only one study to date has demonstrated nonpharmacologic therapy through exercise training [2]. This study formed the basis of our treatment plan; however, we report a longer period of followup, which demonstrated that continued exercise is necessary to maintain the beneficial effects.

Vasey et al. [6] have proposed a mechanism for this aberrant conduction. The primary cause is delayed recovery, with one bundle branch having a block in phase 3 of the action potential, which can vary in length. With the increase in heart rate associated with exercise, eventually stimuli arrive from the proximal portion of the conduction system before the fascicle has repolarized and block occurs. This is generally coupled, in their model, with phase 4 hypopolarization, which causes bradycardia related LBBB; however, exploring this possibility would require an electrophysiological study, which was not performed in our patient. Critical to relating this experimental finding to our patient, however, is the observation that exercise induces upregulation of the potassium channels responsible for phase 3 of the action potential, with concomitant shortening of this phase. It seems reasonable to assume therefore that exercise training allows a shortening of phase 3 of the action potential and the increase in rate at which LBBB occurs. Deconditioning could reasonably be assumed to have the opposite effect, with the associated decrease in critical rate noted in our patient. It is worth noting that in one previous study, repeat testing years after the first evidence of exercise induced LBBB showed patients were developing the condition at lower heart rates and presumably developing symptoms with less activity [2].

In either case, treating the symptoms, allowing the patient to participate in more strenuous exercise, should have a morbidity benefit, as well as the mortality benefit which accrues from aerobic exercise.

3. Summary

Exercise-induced bundle branch block in the absence of coronary disease remains a rare condition in the United States. Though no treatment has yet been demonstrated to be effective in reducing mortality, treatment of this condition through the relatively simple intervention of cardiac rehabilitation proved an effective intervention to decrease symptoms. With regular exercise training, our patient was able to increase the rate at which she developed aberrant conduction and symptoms of chest pain and palpitations.

Disclosure

The opinions or assertions contained herein are the private views of the authors and are not to be construed as reflecting the views of the Department of the Army or the Department of Defense. This research received no specific grant from any funding agency in the public, commercial, or not-for-profit sectors.

References

[1] J. A. Heinsimer, T. N. Skelton, and R. M. Califf, "Rate-related left bundle branch block with chest pain and normal coronary arteriograms treated by exercise training," *American Journal of the Medical Sciences*, vol. 292, no. 5, pp. 317–319, 1986.

[2] H. Eichert, "Transient bundle branch block associated with tachycardia," *American Heart Journal*, vol. 31, no. 4, pp. 511–518, 1946.

[3] H. Hertzeanu, L. Aron, R. J. Shiner, and J. Kellermann, "Exercise dependent complete left bundle branch block," *European Heart Journal*, vol. 13, no. 11, pp. 1447–1451, 1992.

[4] E. Perin, F. Petersen, and A. Massumi, "Rate-related left bundle branch block as a cause of non-ischemic chest pain," *Catheterization and Cardiovascular Diagnosis*, vol. 22, no. 1, pp. 45–46, 1991.

[5] L. A. Sechi, S. De Carli, L. Zingaro, and E. Bartoli, "Resolution of rate-related left bundle branch block after nitrate therapy," *European Heart Journal*, vol. 17, no. 1, pp. 150–151, 1996.

[6] C. Vasey, J. O'Donnell, S. Morris, and P. McHenry, "Exercise-induced left bundle branch block and its relation to coronary artery disease," *American Journal of Cardiology*, vol. 56, no. 13, pp. 892–895, 1985.

[7] V. S. Wayne, R. L. Bishop, L. Cook, and D. H. Spodick, "Exercise-induced bundle branch block," *American Journal of Cardiology*, vol. 52, no. 3, pp. 283–286, 1983.

[8] M. A. Williams, D. J. Esterbrooks, C. K. Nair, M. M. Sailors, and M. H. Sketch, "Clinical significance of exercise-induced bundle branch block," *American Journal of Cardiology*, vol. 61, no. 4, pp. 346–348, 1988.

[9] T. A. Grady, A. C. Chiu, C. E. Snader et al., "Prognostic significance of exercise-induced left bundle-branch block," *The Journal of the American Medical Association*, vol. 279, no. 2, pp. 153–156, 1998.

[10] J. A. Heinsimer, J. M. Irwin, and L. L. Basnight, "Influence of underlying coronary artery disease on the natural history and prognosis of exercise-induced left bundle branch block," *American Journal of Cardiology*, vol. 60, no. 13, pp. 1065–1067, 1987.

[11] K. S. Virtanen, J. Heikkila, R. Kala, and P. Siltanen, "Chest pain and rate-dependent left bundle branch block in patients with normal coronary arteriograms," *Chest*, vol. 81, no. 3, pp. 326–331, 1982.

[12] J. F. Moran, B. Scurlock, R. Henkin, and P. J. Scanlon, "The clinical significance of exercise-induced left bundle-branch block," *Journal of Electrocardiology*, vol. 25, no. 3, pp. 229–235, 1992.

[13] A. P. Michaelides, A. N. Kartalis, M.-N. K. Aigyptiadou, and P. K. Toutouzas, "Exercise-induced left bundle branch block accompanied by chest pain: correlation with coronary artery disease," *Journal of Electrocardiology*, vol. 37, no. 4, pp. 325–328, 2004.

Anomalous Left Main Coronary Artery: Case Series of Different Courses

Adam T. Marler, Jamil A. Malik, and Ahmad M. Slim

Cardiology Service, San Antonio Military Medical Center, Fort Sam Houston, TX 78234, USA

Correspondence should be addressed to Ahmad M. Slim; ahmad.m.slim.mil@mail.mil

Academic Editors: H. Nakajima and Y.-J. Wu

Background. Congenital anomalies of the coronary arteries are a cause of sudden cardiac death. Of the known anatomic variants, anomalous origination of a coronary artery from an opposite sinus of Valsalva (ACAOS) remains the main focus of debate. *Case Series*. We present three cases, all presenting to our facility within one week's time, of patients with newly discovered anomalous origination of the left coronary artery from the right sinus of Valsalva (L-ACAOS). All patients underwent cardiac computed tomography for evaluation of coronary anatomy along with other forms of functional testing. Despite the high risk nature of two of the anomalies, the patients are being treated medically without recurrence of symptoms. *Summary*. After review of the literature, we have found that the risk of sudden cardiac death in patients with congenital coronary anomalies, even among variants considered the highest risk, may be overestimated. In addition, the exact prevalence of coronary anomalies in the general population is currently underestimated. A national coronary artery anomaly registry based on cardiac computed tomography and invasive coronary angiography data would be helpful in advancing our understanding of these cardiac peculiarities. The true prevalence of congenital coronary anomalies and overall risk of sudden cardiac death in this population are not well known. Surgical intervention remains the mainstay of therapy in certain patients though recent investigations into the pathophysiology of these abnormalities have shown that the risk of surgery may outweigh the minimal reduction in risk of sudden cardiac death.

1. Background

Coronary artery anomalies remain an important cause of debilitating cardiac symptoms and in some instances sudden cardiac death. Anomalies are most often classified into abnormalities of origin, distribution, and association with fistulae when present. The precise prevalence of coronary artery anomalies is not well defined. A study completed by Yamanaka and Hobbs in 1990 found the overall incidence of coronary artery anomalies in more than 120,000 patients undergoing coronary angiography to be 1.3% [1]. In a retrospective review of the Department of Defense data from 1977 to 2001, nontraumatic sudden death occurred in 126 military recruits out of over 6 million cases reviewed. Of these patients, the cause of death was identified as a coronary artery anomaly in 39 patients with 21 of those having an anomalous coronary artery origin. All 21 of these patients were found to have an anomalous origination of the left coronary artery from the right sinus of Valsalva (L-ACAOS) with an interarterial course between the pulmonary artery and aorta [2, 3].

Anomalous origin of the left coronary artery from the right sinus of Valsalva may be further separated into four separate subtypes. (1) The left main coronary artery courses between the aorta and the pulmonary artery. (2) The left main coronary artery tracks anteriorly over the right ventricular outflow tract. (3) The left main coronary artery takes an intramyocardial course before resurfacing at the proximal portion of the interventricular groove. (4) The left main coronary artery passes posteriorly around the aortic root [4]. Of these, the first anomalous configuration is classically considered the most dangerous placing patients at the highest risk of sudden cardiac death [5]. In this paper, we share examples of three of the four subtypes of anomalous origin of the left coronary artery from the right sinus of Valsalva.

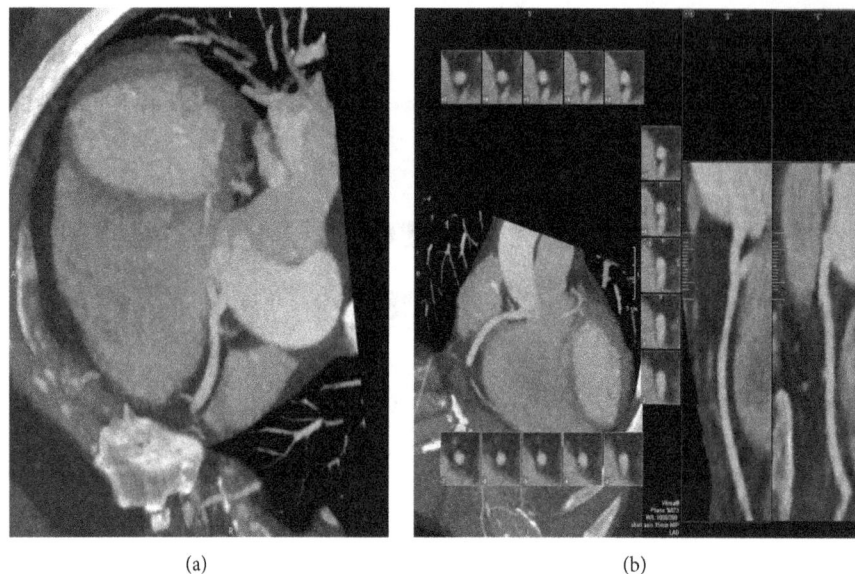

(a)

(b)

FIGURE 1: Cardiac computed tomography showing anomalous left main off of the right sinus of Valsalva and subsequent intraseptal course.

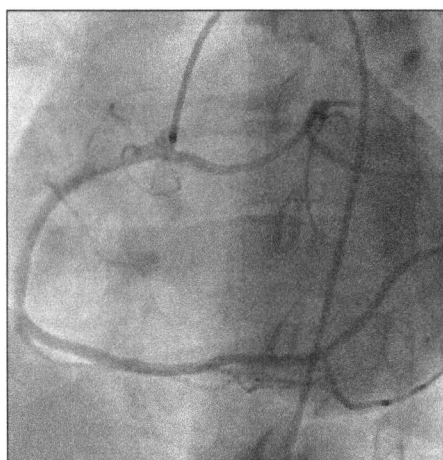

FIGURE 2: Left anterior oblique view of left main coronary artery with an anomalous origin off the right sinus of Valsalva with intraseptal course.

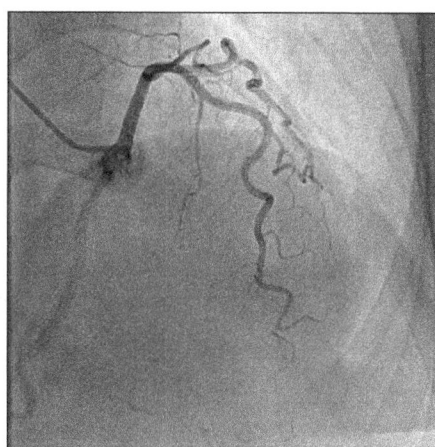

FIGURE 3: Right anterior oblique-cranial view of left main coronary artery with an anomalous origin off the right sinus of Valsalva with interarterial course.

2. Case Series

Case 1. A 42-year-old female with hypertension and hyperlipidemia was admitted to our facility for atypical chest pain. There was no reported history of syncope. Serial cardiac biomarkers were normal and the patient underwent coronary CT angiogram for assessment of coronary anatomy. Cardiac CT revealed no significant coronary artery disease but did show a left main coronary artery with an anomalous origin off of the right sinus of Valsalva with subsequent intraseptal course (Figure 1). Invasive coronary angiography (Figure 2) was completed with normal fractional flow reserve measurements in the proximal left anterior descending with adenosine infusion. The patient is currently doing well without further symptoms on optimal medical therapy alone.

Case 2. A 72-year-old female with hypertension and hyperlipidemia was admitted to the chest pain unit for evaluation of atypical chest pain. There was no reported history of lightheadedness, dizziness, or syncope. The patient underwent a stress echocardiography with no ischemic changes on electrocardiogram and no angina with evidence of mid anteroseptal wall hypokinesis at peak exercise. The patient underwent invasive coronary angiography (Figure 3) showing no significant coronary artery disease and a left main coronary artery with an anomalous takeoff from the right coronary cusp. The myocardial course of the left main was unable to be definitively determined by invasive coronary angiography and cardiac CT was completed. Cardiac CT showed the left main to have an anomalous takeoff from the right coronary cusp with a course between the great vessels (Figures 4 and 5).

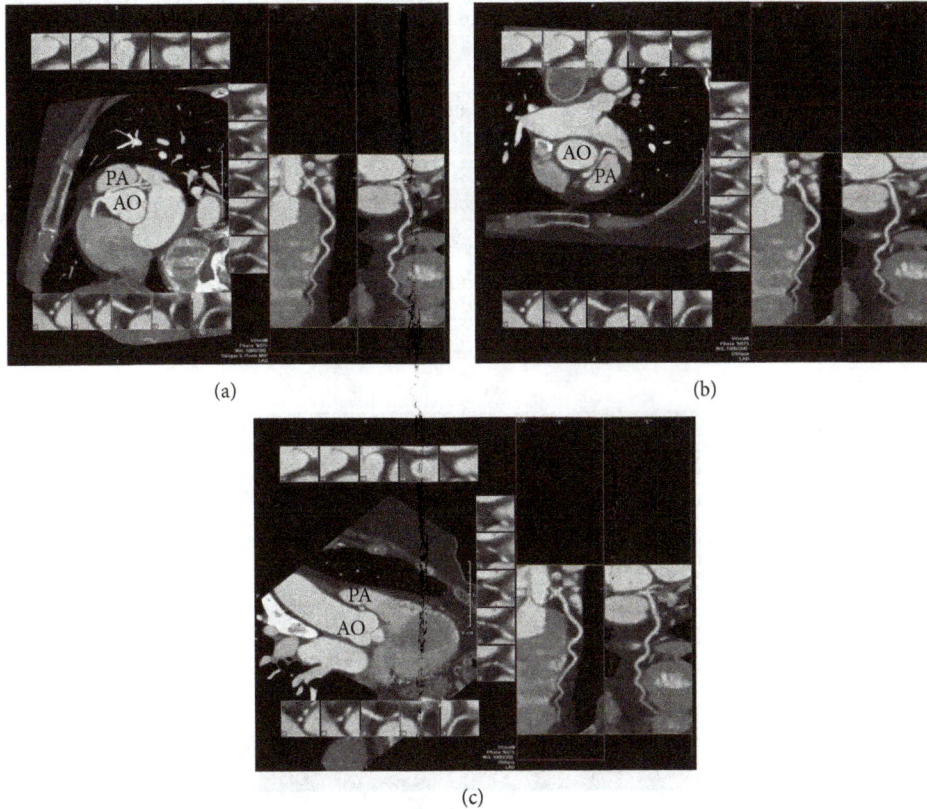

(a)

(b)

(c)

FIGURE 4: Cardiac computed tomography images of anomalous left main coronary artery off of the right sinus of Valsalva with a course between the pulmonary artery (PA) and aorta (AO).

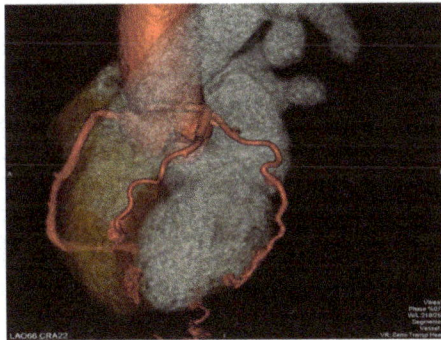

FIGURE 5: Three dimensional reconstruction exhibiting the interarterial course of the left main coronary artery as presented in Case 2.

The patient is currently asymptomatic on maximal medical therapy.

Case 3. This is a 21-year-old case of a male with exercise limiting chest pain and no reported history of syncope. The patient reported intermittent chest pain since the age of 16 which had become worse since the beginning of the military training. The patient underwent coronary CT angiogram showing a left main coronary artery with an anomalous takeoff from the right coronary cusp. The left main coronary artery (LMCA) was seen to take a posterior course behind the ascending aorta before bifurcating into the left anterior descending and left circumflex arteries (Figure 6). Exercise stress testing was completed with myocardial perfusion imaging during which the patient exercised for 14 minutes and 35 seconds (14.4 METS) with no ischemic EKG changes and no angina. Myocardial perfusion images showed no evidence for ischemia, normal left ventricular ejection fraction, and normal wall motion. The patient was started on no additional medical therapy and continues to experience some symptoms with heavy exertion.

3. Discussion

Coronary artery anomalies represent a life-threatening form of congenital cardiac pathology. The underlying cause of sudden cardiac death in patients with congenital coronary abnormalities is the source of some debate with multiple competing theories. Death may result from contortion of the vessel's slit-like, tangential origin during exercise leading to ischemia and resultant arrhythmia. Another theory purports that compression of the anomalous coronary occurs with dilation of the aorta and pulmonary artery during exercise. It is also possible that frequent episodes of myocardial ischemia lead to myocardial fibrosis and potential nidus for a deadly arrhythmia [3, 6]. Finally, Anjelini and associates evaluated three patients with L-ACAOS by intravascular ultrasound both at rest and after pharmacologic challenge with

(a)

(b)

(c)

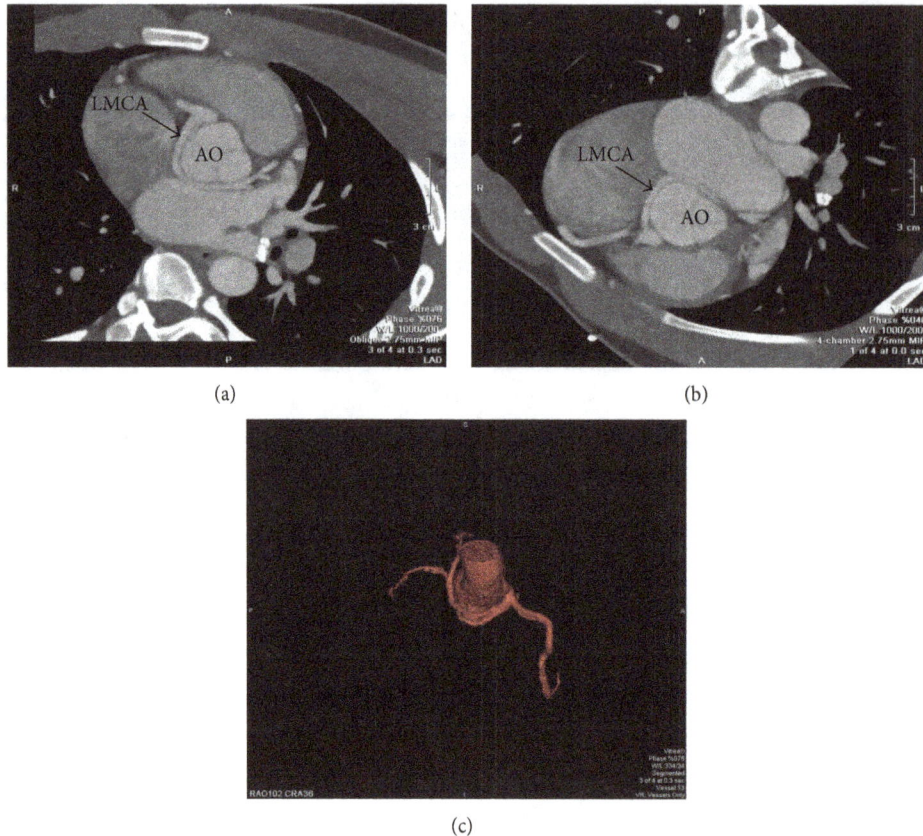

FIGURE 6: Cardiac computed tomography and three dimensional reconstruction showing an anomalous left main coronary artery (LMCA) off of the right sinus of Valsalva assuming a posterior course around the aorta (AO).

saline/atropine/dobutamine ("SAD" test). The group discovered the severity of ischemia to be related to degree of coronary intussusception, level of intramural hypoplasia, and lateral compression of the vessel by expansion of the aorta [2, 5, 6]. The true cause of death is likely an aggregate form of the currently proposed theories.

In addition to contention over the true mechanism of death related to coronary artery anomalies, the true prevalence of disease within the general population has remained a mystery. Congenital coronary anomalies are likely under-recognized as completing an anatomic assessment in a very large portion of the population would seem unfeasible. As mentioned above, the angiographic study completed by Yamanaka and Hobbs found the overall incidence of coronary artery anomalies in a population of more than 120,000 patients to be 1.3%. In this same study, "benign" coronary anomalies were the most frequently discovered with an incidence of 1.07%. L-ACAOS was found in only 22 patients comprising a fairly small portion of abnormalities considered potentially serious [1]. If these same statistics were theoretically applied to the 6.3 million military recruits reviewed by Eckart et al., the overall number of the expected coronary artery anomalies would be 81,900. In the same study, the expected number of military recruits with L-ACAOS would be 1,071. In total, the review found only 21 deaths attributable to an anomalous coronary artery origin, all of which were

the L-ACAOS variant. This suggests that the prevalence of congenital coronary anomalies in the general population is much higher than previously predicted. Also, it is very likely that the overall risk of sudden cardiac death in patients with congenital coronary anomalies is much less than previously reported [3, 6]. In fact, this has been suggested by a group from the New York University School of Medicine in reviews published in 2005 as well as in 2012 [6, 7].

All three patients presented in this case series were found to have a different anatomic configuration of the L-ACAOS variant. Cases included one with an interarterial course, one with an intramural course, and one with a posterior course. Two of the three patients have remained symptom free since the initial presentation. None of the patients underwent surgical correction of their unique coronary anomaly as the risk of surgery outweighed the potential benefit of correction based on completed functional studies. None of the patients were evaluated by intravascular ultrasound as completed by Angelini's group in 2006 [2]. Of interest is the fact that the patient with the reportedly most benign variant, LMCA with a posterior course, developed the most severe symptoms likely related to his high level of activity as a military member. In contrast, the patient with an interarterial course, considered to be the most insidious variant, developed symptoms in the eighth decade of life potentially due to prolonged hypertension and associated changes in aortic morphology.

4. Conclusion

In conclusion, congenital coronary artery anomalies remain as a cause of sudden cardiac death though it appears that the risk is lower than previously thought. The true prevalence of coronary artery anomalies in the general population is unknown. In addition, the absolute risk of sudden cardiac death is difficult to predict and hinges upon multiple variables. Treatment of coronary artery anomalies is controversial and dependent on the discovered anatomy. Surgery is the mainstay of treatment though beta blockers and calcium channel blockers have been utilized to lessen ischemic symptoms. In the current case series, we present three patients of three different generations with three different variants of left coronary artery from the right sinus of Valsalva. Two of the three patients are currently being treated medically and continue to remain symptom free. As imaging with cardiac computed tomography continues, maintenance of a congenital coronary anomaly registry would help to broaden our medical knowledge and improve diagnostic and therapeutic modalities for future generations.

References

[1] O. Yamanaka and R. E. Hobbs, "Coronary artery anomalies in 126,595 patients undergoing coronary arteriography," *Catheterization and Cardiovascular Diagnosis*, vol. 21, no. 1, pp. 28–40, 1990.

[2] P. Angelini, R. P. Walmsley, A. Libreros, and D. A. Ott, "Symptomatic anomalous origination of the left coronary artery from the opposite sinus of valsalva: clinical presentations, diagnosis, and surgical repair," *Texas Heart Institute Journal*, vol. 33, no. 2, pp. 171–179, 2006.

[3] R. E. Eckart, S. L. Scoville, C. L. Campbell et al., "Sudden death in young adults: a 25-year review of autopsies in military recruits," *Annals of Internal Medicine*, vol. 141, no. 11, pp. 829–834, 2004.

[4] M. Hauser, "Congenital anomalies of the coronary arteries," *Heart*, vol. 91, no. 9, pp. 1240–1245, 2005.

[5] P. Angelini, "Anomalous origin of the left coronary artery from the opposite sinus of valsalva: typical and atypical features," *Texas Heart Institute Journal*, vol. 36, no. 4, pp. 313–315, 2009.

[6] J. M. Peñalver, R. S. Mosca, D. Weitz, and C. K. Phoon, "Anomalous aortic origin of coronary arteries from the opposite sinus: a critical appraisal of risk," *BMC Cardiovascular Disorders*, vol. 12, p. 83, 2012.

[7] S. Mirchandani and C. K. L. Phoon, "Management of anomalous coronary arteries from the contralateral sinus," *International Journal of Cardiology*, vol. 102, no. 3, pp. 383–389, 2005.

8

Modification of the No-Touch Technique during Renal Artery Stenting

John A. Stathopoulos

Columbia University, 30-10 38th Street, 2nd Floor, Astoria, NY 11103, USA

Correspondence should be addressed to John A. Stathopoulos; jastathopoulos@hotmail.com

Academic Editors: B. S. Brooke, N. Espinola-Zavaleta, L. Masotti, E. Minar, and N. Papanas

Renal artery stenting has been established as the primary form of renal artery stenosis revascularization procedure. The no-touch technique is proposed in order to avoid renal artery injury and atheroembolism during renal artery stenting. We describe a modification of the no-touch technique by using an over-the-wire (OTW) balloon or a Quickcross 0.014″ catheter with a 0.014″ coronary wire inside, instead of the rigid 0.035″ J wire. The reported technique, while it prevents direct contact of the guiding catheter with the aortic wall, at the same time it allows for a closer contact with the renal arterial ostium and a more favorable guiding catheter orientation, compared to what is achieved with the use of the more rigid 0.035″ J wire, thus improving visualization, reducing the amount of contrast required, and potentially decreasing complications.

1. Introduction

Renal artery stenting has been widely used for the treatment of renal artery stenosis. The technical aspects of stenting have improved over the last years, and procedural safety is recognized as of paramount importance. Two invasive techniques are proposed in order to avoid renal artery injury and atheroembolism during renal artery stenting [1]: the catheter-in-catheter and the so-called no-touch technique.

The no-touch technique [2] uses a 0.035″ J wire inside the guiding catheter, to lift the tip off the aortic wall. With the 0.035″ wire in place, the guiding catheter is aligned with the renal artery, and a 0.014″ guidewire is used to cross the stenosis. The 0.035″ wire is then removed, and the guiding catheter is advanced over the 0.014″ wire to engage the renal artery.

We report a modification of the no-touch technique by using an over-the-wire (OTW) balloon or a Quickcross 0.014″ catheter (Spectranetics) with a 0.014″ coronary wire inside, instead of the rigid 0.035″ J wire.

2. Case 1

A 67-year-old lady, with uncontrolled severe hypertension despite therapy, peripheral arterial disease (PAD), and left ventricular hypertrophy was diagnosed with right renal artery stenosis and referred for renal angiography.

An abdominal aortogram confirmed the presence of significant right renal artery stenosis. Renal percutaneous transluminal angioplasty (PTA) was then undertaken.

The procedural steps were as follows.

(1) A 6F internal mammary artery (IMA) guiding catheter (Launcher, Medtronic) was introduced and was placed at the level of the right renal artery but pointed away of the right renal artery ostium, without touching the aortic wall.

(2) A 0.014″ Balance (Abbott) coronary wire in a 0.014″ Quickcross catheter (Spectranetics) was introduced in the 6F guiding catheter with the tip of the wire protruding about one inch outside the Quickcross catheter (Spectranetics) and was advanced outside and above the tip of the guiding catheter towards the

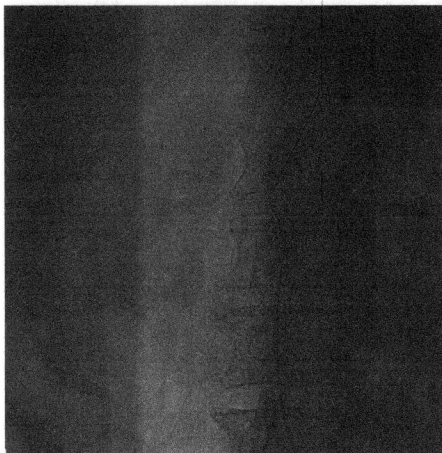

FIGURE 1

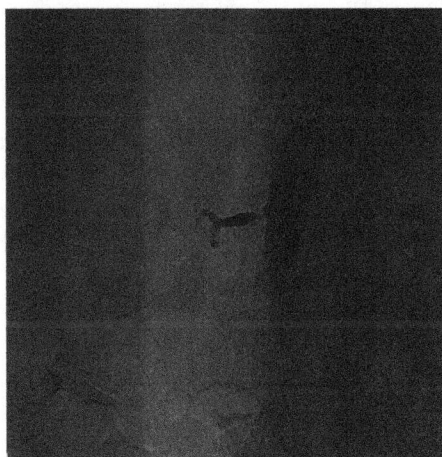

FIGURE 2

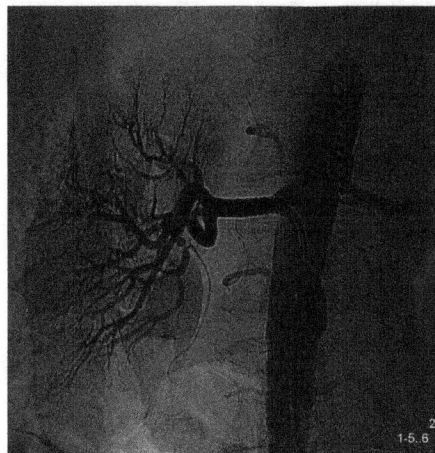

FIGURE 3

slowly inside the IMA guiding catheter allowing for the gentle cannulation of the right renal artery ostium. In that way, scraping of the aortic plaque from the guiding catheter manipulations during renal artery ostium cannulation was minimal.

(7) Then, the Balance wire (Abbott) was advanced across the lesion into the distal renal artery.

(8) The Balance wire (Abbott) was exchanged through the Quickcross catheter (Spectranetics) for a Sta-biliser Plus 0.014$''$ wire (Cordis), and the lesion was predilated with a 3.5 × 12 mm Trek RX balloon (Abbott).

(9) A 5.0 × 15 mm Herculink Elite RX stent (Abbott) was then deployed across the lesion and flaring postdilatation performed with the stent balloon. Subsequent angiography revealed optimal stent deployment and absence of peripheral embolization, dissection, or perforation (Figure 3).

Three days after the procedure, the patient experienced generalized rash attributed to clopidogrel, and prasugrel was started instead. Repeat blood pressure at the office was only mildly elevated despite the fact that the patient had stopped taking the prescribed antihypertensive medications.

3. Case 2

An 83-year-old gentleman, with chronic renal insufficiency, coronary artery disease and PAD, resistant hypertension, and intolerance to angiotensin converting enzyme (ACE) inhibitors, was diagnosed with severe left renal artery stenosis by magnetic resonance angiography (MRA) (Figure 4). Selective angiography of the left renal artery was performed revealing eccentric subtotal 98% occlusion (Figure 5).

Renal artery angioplasty was decided, and the same procedural steps were performed as described in Case 1, but instead of a 0.014$''$ Quickcross catheter (Spectranetics), we used an OTW Sprinter (Medtronic) 2.5 × 12 mm balloon.

more proximal abdominal aorta (at a higher level than the ostium of the renal artery).

(3) With the Balance wire (Abbott) and Quickcross catheter (Spectranetics) protruding about two inches outside the guiding catheter, the guiding catheter was manipulated and oriented towards the ostium of the right renal artery (Figure 1). The guiding catheter was cleared of blood and possible debris.

(4) The ostium of the right renal artery was identified by injecting small puffs of contrast without direct contact of the angulated tip of the IMA guiding catheter with the aortic wall.

(5) While in front of the ostium and despite the fact that the guiding catheter was not engaged, not touching the ostium of the artery, selective angiography of the right renal artery was performed revealing 85% stenosis (Figure 2).

(6) Subsequently, first, the Balance wire (Abbott) was retracted inside the Quickcross catheter (Spectranetics), protecting the tip of the wire, and then, second, the Quickcross catheter (Spectranetics) was retracted

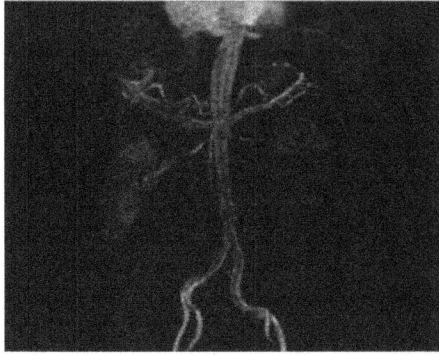

FIGURE 4

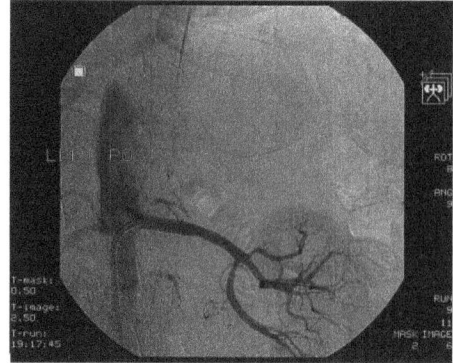

FIGURE 6

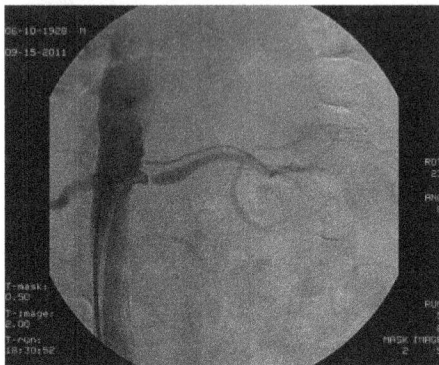

FIGURE 5

A 6.0 × 15 mm Herculink Elite RX stent (Abbott) was deployed across the lesion. Subsequent angiography revealed optimal stent deployment and absence of complications (Figure 6). Overall, less than 15 cc of contrast was used for the renal angioplasty. Three weeks after the procedure, creatinine was stable and blood pressure was 130/90 mmHg on two antihypertensive medications (decreased from three prior to procedure).

4. Discussion

Renal artery stenting has been established as the primary form of renal artery stenosis revascularization procedure. Although, the renal vascular bed is considered more forgiving than other vascular beds to potential complications during renal artery stenting, the no-touch technique [2] is proposed in order to avoid renal artery injury and atheroembolism [1]. The no-touch technique [2] uses a $0.035''$ J wire inside the guiding catheter, to lift the tip off the aortic wall. With the $0.035''$ wire in place, the guiding catheter is aligned with the renal artery, and a $0.014''$ guidewire is used to cross the stenosis. The $0.035''$ wire is then removed, and the guiding catheter is advanced over the $0.014''$ wire to engage the renal artery.

We describe our experience by using either an OTW balloon or a $0.014''$ Quickcross (Spectranetics) support catheter

with a $0.014''$ coronary wire inside in order to reduce direct contact with the aortic wall. While this prevents direct contact with the aortic wall, at the same time it allows for a closer contact with the ostium and a more favorable guiding catheter orientation towards the renal artery ostium—especially with angulated oriented ostia, compared to what is achieved with the rigid $0.035''$ J wire. This allows for a better visualization of the ostium with injection of even small contrast puffs. Furthermore, the use of the described modified no-touch technique may reduce the theoretical higher risk of aortic injury by the use of the $0.035''$ rigid J wire.

Alternatively, the described modified no-touch technique can be also performed with the use of a 5F guiding catheter ($0.058''$ inner diameter).

In conclusion, the reported technique by using an OTW balloon or the Quickcross catheter (Spectranetics) with a $0.014''$ coronary wire inside, while it prevents direct contact of the guiding catheter with the aortic wall, at the same time it allows for a closer contact with the arterial ostium and a more favorable guiding catheter orientation, compared to what is achieved with the use of the more rigid $0.035''$ J wire, thus improving visualization, reducing the amount of contrast required, and potentially decreasing complications.

References

[1] R. D. Safian and R. D. Madder, "Refining the approach to renal artery revascularization," *Journal of the American College of Cardiology*, vol. 2, no. 3, pp. 161–174, 2009.

[2] R. L. Feldman, T. J. Wargovich, and J. A. Bittl, "No-touch technique for reducing aortic wall trauma during renal artery stenting," *Catheterization and Cardiovascular Interventions*, vol. 46, no. 2, pp. 245–248, 1999.

9

Successful Use of the MYNXGRIP Closure Device during Repeated Transbrachial Percutaneous Peripheral Intervention

Klaus Hertting and Werner Raut

Department of Cardiology and Angiology, Krankenhaus Buchholz, 21244 Buchholz in der Nordheide, Germany

Correspondence should be addressed to Klaus Hertting; hertting@hotmail.com

Academic Editor: Antonio Silvestro

The use of closure devices after transbrachial arterial puncture is still controversial. Here we report on a case where the MYNXGRIP (AccessClosure Inc., Santa Clara, CA, USA) could be used successfully in a patient, who underwent percutaneous peripheral arterial intervention twice via transbrachial access.

1. Introduction

Percutaneous vascular interventions via the brachial artery (BA) represent a commonly used vascular access. Today, manual compression is the most widely used way to close the arterial puncture [1, 2]. The local complication rate of brachial access route is up to seven percent (older studies report even higher event rates), mostly comprising large hematomas, false aneurysms, thrombotic occlusions, or nerve injuries with subsequent dysfunction of the forearm [1, 2].

Dedicated closure devices in the femoral artery were tested in a series of studies and registries [3, 4]. In a small retrospective study, Mirza et al. reported no significant difference regarding vascular complications after the use of closure devices or manual compression for closure of BA puncture [5].

Here, we report the repeated use of the MYNXGRIP closure device (AccessClosure Inc., Santa Clara, CA, USA) in a patient who required a staged revascularization for bilateral critical limb ischemia. The device uses a biodegradable polyethylene-glycol sealant attaching to the outer layer of the vessel wall. The sealant is administered through the sheath while an inflated balloon inside the vessel provides temporary hemostasis and prevents protrusion of the sealant into the lumen [6]. The patient gave informed consent for the publication.

2. Case Presentation

We report on a 69-year-old lady who presented with bilateral critical limb ischemia (Rutherford V) caused by a high grade stenosis of the left and an occlusion of the right common femoral artery (CFA). As the patient had significant comorbidities (mild dementia, liver cirrhosis, and reduced kidney function) and has had surgery of both CFA previously, it was decided to try an interventional revascularization of both CFA. A transbrachial access route with the use of a closure device was considered as appropriate in this situation. Preprocedural ultrasound revealed a left BA without relevant atherosclerosis and a diameter of 3.4 mm. The patient was pretreated with 100 mg aspirin daily.

After puncturing the low brachial artery (using a 21-gauge needle and ultrasound guidance) and administration of 5000 units of heparin, a 90 cm 6F sheath was introduced and angioplasty with stent implantation into the left external iliac and CFA could be performed with good angiographic result. The occlusion of the right CFA was scheduled for another intervention.

The 90 cm sheath was then exchanged for a 10 cm 6F sheath. Subsequently, an angiography has been performed after intra-arterial application of 200 μg nitroglycerin [Figure 1]. The balloon of the MYNXGRIP was prepared using a mixture of contrast-dye and saline to allow visualization during the placement. The device was inserted into

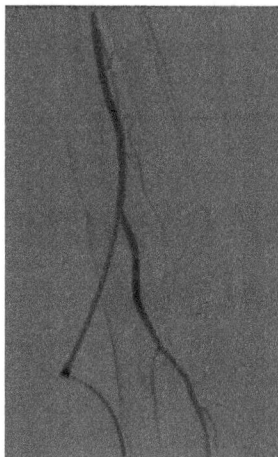

FIGURE 1: Angiography of the left brachial artery at the end of the first procedure after placement of a 6F-10 cm sheath.

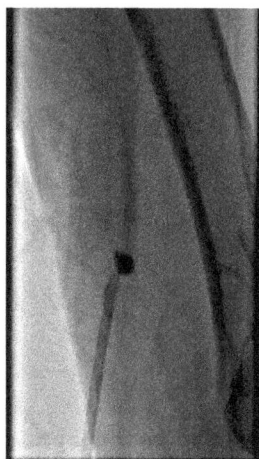

FIGURE 2: Retrieval of the inner blocking balloon of the MYNXGRIP and of the sheath towards the puncture site. Note the slight shift between the sheath and the blocking balloon indicating appropriate wall contact.

the sheath and the balloon inflated and slowly withdrew towards the puncture site under fluoroscopic surveillance [Figure 2]. After confirming appropriate wall contact the MYNXGRIP sealant was applied according to the instructions for use. Finally, after confirmation of hemostasis, the puncture site was covered by a small dressing avoiding extensive compression of the artery. Radial and ulnar pulse proved to be strongly palpable. After procedure the patient received a loading dose of 600 mg clopidogrel and then 75 mg daily.

Duplex ultrasound control the day after the procedure showed an echolucent area at the puncture site, representing the MYNXGRIP sealant and patent brachial, radial, and ulnar arteries [Figure 3].

Two days later, a repeated puncture about 1 cm central to the previous puncture site was performed again under ultrasound guidance. Recanalization and stenting of the right CFA could be performed. Angiography of the BA at the end

of the procedure showed a patent BA with preserved flow into the forearm. After exchanging for a 6F 10 cm sheath a MYNXGRIP device could be placed without problems.

Duplex ultrasound the day after the second procedure revealed a mild diffuse subcutaneous hematoma without signs of false aneurysm, av-fistula, dissection, or thrombosis but with regular flow in the BA and into the radial and ulnar arteries. This result could be confirmed after 7 days prior to patients discharge. No relevant clinical impairments of the left arm occurred.

3. Discussion

Here we report on the repeated use of the MYNXGRIP closure device in the left brachial artery (BA) for peripheral intervention. To our knowledge, this is the first report of usage in this setting.

Puncturing the BA is somewhat different in comparison to the common femoral artery (CFA). First, the diameter of the adult BA ranges from 3 to 6 mm, whereas the CFA usually provides a larger diameter [7, 8]. Second, the BA is more susceptible for vascular spasm [1]. Third, the amount of subcutaneous tissue is less in the BA than in the CFA area [1]. Fourth, the puncture site of the BA is less well defined than that of the CFA. The range of anatomic variabilities of the BA comprises variable origins of the forearm arteries, variable courses of the BA, a highly variable deep venous system, and so forth [1]. Thus, puncturing the BA sometimes is more difficult and eventually requires more dedicated techniques (e.g., ultrasound guidance).

So far, the use of different closure devices in the BA has been published. The largest series comes from Lupattelli et al., reporting on 159 patients where an Angio-Seal (St. Jude Medical, St. Paul, MN, USA) closure device had been used with high success and low complication-rates, but also smaller registries exist [9, 10]. Of note, in the registry of Lupattelli in 79 of the 238 patients (33%) with brachial access a closure device had not been implanted, mostly because the diameter of the artery appeared too small [9]. Other reports describe the use of different closure devices, such as nitinol clips or suture closures also with high safety and success rates [11, 12].

The main differences of the MYNXGRIP-system are the fact that theoretically it leaves no material (neither permanent nor degradable) inside the vessel lumen and additionally leaves no permanent material in or directly adjacent to the vessel wall, as done by other devices [6]. Nevertheless, some authors report a relevant rate of intraluminal migration of the sealant material (18%) or formation of false aneurysm (11%) [13–15]. Grandhi et al. reported in their analysis on the use of the MYNX device in transfemoral cerebrovascular interventions an association of lower body-mass index and complication rate [16]. Whether the safety and efficacy of the device are comparable to other systems still remains unclear so far [17–19]. However, patient comfort may be higher with the use of the MYNXGRIP compared to the Angio-Seal [14]. Garasic et al. investigated the successful use

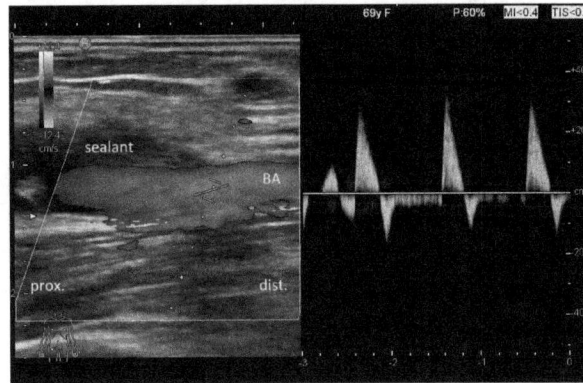

FIGURE 3: Ultrasound study of the left brachial artery the day after the first procedure (BA, brachial artery).

of the MYNXGRIP device in repeated arterial puncture in a sheep model [20].

Possible problems with the use of the MYNXGRIP-device in the BA are (1) the development of significant spasm precluding the inner balloon to get in appropriate contact with the vessel wall at the puncture site, (2) dislodgement of the MYNX sealant into the arterial lumen causing a thrombotic occlusion, (3) venous thrombosis due to placement of the MYNX sealant after accidentally puncturing the artery through an adjacent vein, (4) protrusion of MYNX sealant above the level of epidermis because of a shorter puncturing channel in comparison to CFA puncture, (5) secondary infections, and (6) failure of the device to achieve adequate hemostasis.

To avoid these pitfalls we recommend the use of duplex ultrasound for a guided puncture. This might help to identify an appropriate puncture site and to reduce the number of misplaced punctures (including venous punctures). Before placing the closure device an angiography of the puncture site should be performed after the administration of vasodilators (e.g., nitroglycerin or verapamil) if possible. The inner balloon of the MYNXGRIP should be filled with diluted contrast-dye and the placement should be performed under radiographic control in order to ensure appropriate placement of the inner closure balloon. If the MYNX sealant protrudes close or even outside the skin level it is recommended to moisten it once with water or saline to prevent local skin irritations or even infections.

4. Summary

The safe and successful use of the MYNXGRIP closure device after repeated puncture of the brachial artery could be demonstrated in this case.

Disclosure

Klaus Hertting received consulting salaries from BIOSENSORS.

References

[1] J. A. Alvarez-Tostado, M. A. Moise, J. F. Bena et al., "The brachial artery: a critical access for endovascular procedures," *Journal of Vascular Surgery*, vol. 49, no. 2, pp. 378–385, 2009.

[2] C. L. Juscafresa, L. C. Pont, and C. A. Velasco, "CUSUM analysis of brachial artery access for peripheral endovascular interventions," *International Angiology*, vol. 33, no. 5, pp. 441–445, 2014.

[3] J. A. Reekers, S. Müller-Hülsbeck, M. Libicher et al., "CIRSE vascular closure device registry," *CardioVascular and Interventional Radiology*, vol. 34, no. 1, pp. 50–53, 2011.

[4] F. Biancari, V. D'Andrea, C. Di Marco, G. Savino, V. Tiozzo, and A. Catania, "Meta-analysis of randomized trials on the efficacy of vascular closure devices after diagnostic angiography and angioplasty," *The American Heart Journal*, vol. 159, no. 4, pp. 518–531, 2010.

[5] A. K. Mirza, S. N. Steerman, S. S. Ahanchi, J. A. Higgins, S. Mushti, and J. M. Panneton, "Analysis of vascular closure devices after trans brachial artery access," *Vascular and Endovascular Surgery*, vol. 48, no. 7-8, pp. 466–469, 2014.

[6] D. Scheinert, H. Sievert, M. A. Turco et al., "The safety and efficacy of an extravascular, water-soluble sealant for vascular closure: initial clinical results for Mynx," *Catheterization and Cardiovascular Interventions*, vol. 70, no. 5, pp. 627–633, 2007.

[7] J. D. Ostrem, D. R. Dengel, K. L. Marlatt, and J. Steinberger, "Comparison of baseline brachial artery measurements and effect on peak flow-mediated dilation," *Clinical Physiology and Functional Imaging*, vol. 35, no. 1, pp. 34–40, 2015.

[8] Y.-Y. Lin, R.-F. Shie, K.-S. Liu et al., "Diameter change of common femoral arteries after percutaneous endovascular aortic repair with the use of the preclose technique," *Journal of Vascular Surgery*, vol. 60, no. 1, pp. 50–56, 2014.

[9] T. Lupattelli, J. Clerissi, G. Clerici et al., "The efficacy and safety of closure of brachial access using the AngioSeal closure device: experience with 161 interventions in diabetic patients with critical limb ischemia," *Journal of Vascular Surgery*, vol. 47, no. 4, pp. 782–788, 2008.

[10] A. Belenky, D. Aranovich, F. Greif, G. Bachar, G. Bartal, and E. Atar, "Use of a collagen-based device for closure of low brachial artery punctures," *CardioVascular and Interventional Radiology*, vol. 30, no. 2, pp. 273–275, 2007.

[11] A. Puggioni, E. Boesmans, K. Deloose, P. Peeters, and M. Bosiers, "Use of StarClose for brachial artery closure after percutaneous endovascular interventions," *Vascular*, vol. 16, no. 2, pp. 85–90, 2008.

[12] A. Kim, B. Fusman, N. Jolly, and T. Feldman, "Percutaneous suture closure for brachial artery puncture," *Journal of Interventional Cardiology*, vol. 15, no. 4, pp. 277–280, 2002.

[13] M. A. Islam, A. K. George, and M. Norris, "Popliteal artery embolization with the Mynx closure device," *Catheterization and Cardiovascular Interventions*, vol. 75, no. 1, pp. 35–37, 2010.

[14] K. M. Fargen, G. J. Velat, M. F. Lawson et al., "Occurrence of angiographic femoral artery complications after vascular closure with Mynx and AngioSeal," *Journal of NeuroInterventional Surgery*, vol. 5, no. 2, pp. 161–164, 2013.

[15] J. D. Fields, K. C. Liu, D. S. Lee et al., "Femoral artery complications associated with the Mynx closure device," *American Journal of Neuroradiology*, vol. 31, no. 9, pp. 1737–1740, 2010.

[16] R. Grandhi, H. Kanaan, A. Shah et al., "Safety and efficacy of percutaneous femoral artery access followed by Mynx closure in cerebral neurovascular procedures: a single center analysis," *Journal of NeuroInterventional Surgery*, vol. 6, no. 6, pp. 445–450, 2014.

[17] S. Azmoon, A. L. Pucillo, W. S. Aronow et al., "Vascular complications after percutaneous coronary intervention following hemostasis with the Mynx vascular closure device versus the AngioSeal vascular closure device," *Journal of Invasive Cardiology*, vol. 22, no. 4, pp. 175–178, 2010.

[18] S. Bangalore, N. Arora, and F. S. Resnic, "Vascular closure device failure: frequency and implications: a propensity-matched analysis," *Circulation: Cardiovascular Interventions*, vol. 2, no. 6, pp. 549–556, 2009.

[19] S. Noor, S. Meyers, and R. Curl, "Successful reduction of surgeries secondary to arterial access site complications: a retrospective review at a single center with an extravascular closure device," *Vascular and Endovascular Surgery*, vol. 44, no. 5, pp. 345–349, 2010.

[20] J. M. Garasic, L. Marin, and R. D. Anderson, "Acute evaluation of the Mynx vascular closure device during arterial re-puncture in an ovine model," *Journal of Invasive Cardiology*, vol. 21, no. 6, pp. 283–285, 2009.

Concomitant Deep Venous Thrombosis, Femoral Artery Thrombosis, and Pulmonary Embolism after Air Travel

Salim Abunnaja, Marshall Clyde, Andrea Cuviello, Robert A. Brenes, and Giuseppe Tripodi

The Stanley J. Dudrick Department of Surgery, Saint Mary's Hospital, 56 Franklin Street, Waterbury, CT 06706, USA

Correspondence should be addressed to Salim Abunnaja; salim.abunnaja@stmh.org

Academic Editor: Andreas Zirlik

The association between air travel and deep venous thrombosis and/or pulmonary embolism "economy-class syndrome" is well described. However, this syndrome does not describe any association between long duration travel and arterial thrombosis or coexistence of venous and arterial thrombosis. We present a case of concomitant deep venous thrombosis, acute femoral artery thrombosis, and bilateral pulmonary embolisms in a patient following commercial air travel. Echocardiogram did not reveal an intracardiac shunt that may have contributed to the acute arterial occlusion from a paradoxical embolus. To our knowledge, this is the first report in the literature that associates air traveling with both arterial and venous thrombosis.

1. Introduction

The association between air travel and deep venous thrombosis/pulmonary embolism was first reported in 1954 [1]. Soon after, the phrase "economy-class syndrome" [2, 3] was used to describe this problem, with several more published case series appearing in the literature [4–6]. The mechanism behind the increased risk for clotting complications was proposed to include blood stasis, along with one or more of the following: lower extremity fluid retention, hemoconcentration of clotting factors, and possible activation of the coagulation cascade [7–9]. A few authors have also related this condition to long duration travel by car and train [10–12]. This syndrome, however, does not describe an association between long duration travel and arterial thrombosis or the coexistence of venous and arterial thrombosis simultaneously. We report a case of concomitant deep venous thrombosis and acute femoral artery thrombosis along with bilateral pulmonary embolism after a long overseas flight.

2. Case Report

A 50-year-old woman from Montenegro presented to our institution with shortness of breath that was associated with pleuritic chest pain. Her symptoms began during a long overseas flight and progressively worsened after disembarking the plane.

She also complained of left leg pain and swelling. The patient's past medical history was significant for hypertension and diabetes mellitus. She never smoked and was not on any hormonal treatments. On physical exam, heart rate was 115, respiratory rate was 32, and she appeared to be in mild distress. Bilateral breath sounds were clear to auscultation. Of note, the patient had swelling of the left lower extremity and foot with some dark discoloration, absence of distal pulses, and impaired sensation. Initial laboratory tests revealed respiratory alkalosis (pH 7.45, pCO2 28, paO2 111, and HCO3 22.5), a normal coagulation profile, and a D-dimer of 1300 ug/L. Cardiac enzymes were within normal limits. EKG showed sinus tachycardia. A CT scan of the chest revealed bilateral pulmonary embolisms (Figure 1). Arterial and venous Doppler imaging of both lower extremities showed an occlusive left popliteal vein thrombus and an occlusive left common femoral artery thrombosis.

A heparin drip was initiated immediately and the patient was admitted to the intensive care unit with a low threshold to proceed to the operating room for either thrombectomy or catheter-based thrombolysis. Fortunately, few hours following the initiation of treatment a significant improvement was noticed in the patient's shortness of breath and chest pain.

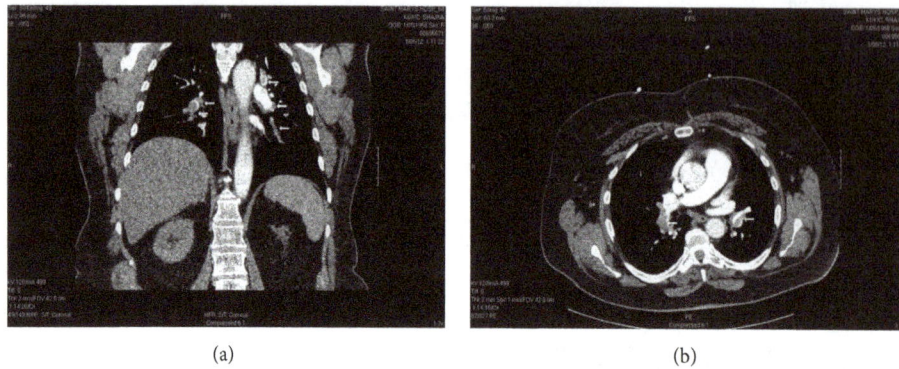

(a)

(b)

FIGURE 1: CT scan of chest, coronal view. White arrows point to bilateral pulmonary emboli.

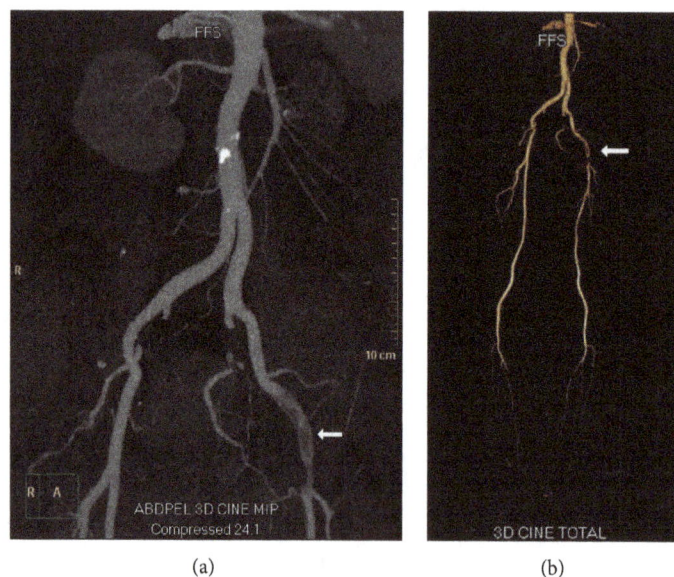

(a)

(b)

FIGURE 2: CTA of bilateral lower extremities. White arrow points to filling defect of left external iliac artery.

Additionally, her left leg swelling and skin discoloration were markedly improved as well; however, she continued to have a dull aching pain in her left foot with weak, monophasic, dopplerable distal pulses. The patient underwent a CTA of her left lower extremity with distal runoff, which demonstrated a subocclusive filling defect extending from the origin of the left common femoral artery to the distal superficial femoral artery, with normal popliteal and three-vessel runoff to the ankle (Figure 2). With an unclear source of this arterial thrombosis, an echocardiogram was obtained to rule out a cardiac source of an acute embolus, as well as a paradoxical systemic arterial embolism through a patent foramen ovale (PFO). The transthoracic echocardiogram was normal with no evidence of an intracardiac shunt, right heart strain, or mural thrombus. Given the acute nature of the patient's condition and her only partial response to nonoperative management, the patient was taken to the operating room. An open mechanical left iliofemoral arterial thrombectomy was

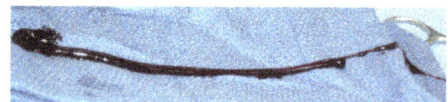

FIGURE 3: Large blood clot removed from the left iliofemoral artery intraoperatively. CTA of bilateral lower extremities. White arrow points to filling defect of left external iliac artery.

performed using a Fogarty catheter. A large clot was retrieved from both the superficial femoral and external iliac arteries (Figure 3). Postoperatively the patient's symptoms dramatically improved and her physical exam revealed palpable distal pulses in her left foot with mild reperfusion symptoms.

Although the initial results for hypercoagulation workup such as protein C, protein S factor II assay, and ANA screen were all within normal limits, these results are difficult to interpret in the setting of acute thrombosis and anticoagulant medication therapy. She was discharged on Warfarin with a plan for full hypercoagulation workup after discontinuing the Warfarin in 6 months with a potential need for long life anticoagulation pending the workup. After discharge, the patient traveled back to her homeland and was unfortunately lost for followup.

3. Discussion

Stasis caused by sitting and immobility during prolonged journeys (>5 hours) is considered a risk factor for deep venous thrombosis and pulmonary embolism. Rudolf Virchow described a triad that predisposes an individual to thrombosis, which includes immobility, endothelial damage, and hypercoagulability. This case report hones in on the immobility aspect experienced by long distance travelers but can also include patients who are immobile due to disabilities or recent major surgery. Endothelial damage can be caused by a number of variables including smoking, atherosclerosis, trauma, and even prolonged immobility [7, 13, 14]. A hypercoagulable state can be induced, as with patients with cancer, or inherited, like those individuals with factor 5 Leiden or protein C/S deficiencies [14]. What is remarkable is that over the last twenty years, greater than 200 cases of pulmonary embolism have been reported in association with "economy-class syndrome" [2, 7, 11, 13, 15]. Landgraf et al. proposed the mechanism mentioned previously of blood stasis in association with immobility effects such as fluid retention in the legs [9], reduction of oxygen in the cabin [16], hemoconcentration secondary to dehydration [14], and activation of coagulation [17]. It should be noted that this syndrome has also been described in first class or business class passengers and even in prolonged overland journeys like those via train, car, or coach [10–12]. For this reason, the syndrome has been referred to by some as "travelers' syndrome" [18]. In March 2001, the World Health Organization (WHO) accepted that there was a probable risk of presenting with pulmonary embolism after prolonged flights despite the low incidence and the presence of other risk factors in most of the passengers affected.

Acute arterial thrombosis on the other hand is traditionally regarded as a different disease with respect to pathophysiology, epidemiology, and treatment strategies when compared to venous thrombosis. To our knowledge, this is the first report in the literature that associates air travel with both acute venous and arterial thrombosis. Arterial thrombi tend to occur at places where plaques are formed and where shear stress is high, which results in platelet rich "white thrombi" [19]. In contrast, with venous thrombotic disease, thrombi tend to occur at sites where the vein wall is undamaged and blood flow and shear stress are low, resulting in red cell-rich "red thrombi" [19]. Stasis caused by sitting and immobility during prolonged traveling is therefore not considered a risk factor for acute arterial thrombosis. Nevertheless, it appears that venous thrombosis and arterial thrombosis are not completely separate entities. Becattini et al. demonstrated a 40% decrease in DVT recurrence rate by initiating antiplatelet therapy after cessation of warfarin therapy for DVT [20].

Recent research has shown a 40 to 50% risk reduction for venous thrombosis occurrence in patients taking statins for arterial diseases [21]. On the other hand, there is also a 1.5- to 3-fold increased venous thrombotic risk in individuals who have been exposed to traditional arterial thrombotic risk factors like diabetes, hypertension, and dyslipidemia [21, 22]. Furthermore, it appears from the literature that patients with arterial thrombosis have from 1.2-fold to more than 4-fold increased risk of developing subsequent venous thrombosis [23]. Despite these associations, acute cases of simultaneous arterial and venous thromboses are rarely seen in clinical practice, and there have only been a few cases reported in the literature [24–27], none of which have been linked to air travel.

It is important not to forget about a possible PFO in patients presenting with the coexistence of pulmonary and paradoxical systemic arterial embolism [28]. A small PFO is usually hemodynamically insignificant, while large-diameter PFOs may act as a pathway for the passage of thrombi, air, fat, vegetations, or vasoactive substances from the venous to the arterial circulation, potentially causing paradoxical emboli and stroke [29]. In our case, a normal echocardiogram excluded PFO as a possible cause of this unusual coexistence of pulmonary and systemic thrombosis.

Regardless of patient history or risk factors, as some patients may carry a coagulation disorder that has thus far been silent, there are certain precautions that those embarking on a long, sedentary journey can take to avoid coagulation complications such as deep venous thrombosis and pulmonary embolism. These recommendations include avoiding sitting with crossed legs, attempting to stand or move about every two hours for a couple of minutes, and engaging in flexion-extension exercises while seated. The avoidance of dehydration, excessive alcoholic intake, and tight clothing can assist in decreasing the risk for vasoocclusive complications during long journeys.

In this case, long-duration air travel in a seated position likely caused venous stasis leading to deep vein thrombosis, and we speculate it may have caused prolonged subtotal arterial compression which may have predisposed the patient to arterial thrombus formation. Due to the patient being lost to followup, we cannot investigate a possible hypercoagulable state which to this point has been unidentified. Case reports have attributed acute limb arterial thrombosis to a known hypercoagulable state (inherited [30] or acquired [31]) although the literature has not shown there be a statistical association between the two. In this case and similar cases, a hypercoagulable workup should include testing for Factor V Leiden and prothrombin 20210 mutations, deficiency of protein C, protein S, and antithrombin III; elevation of clotting factors VIII, IX, XI, and fibrinogen and homocysteine levels; and testing anticardiolipin antibodies. Most clinicians will elect to do the workup two to four weeks after stopping anticoagulation, because the results of some of these tests may potentially be affected by acute thrombosis and anticoagulation. The possibility of an unidentified cancer as a cause of the hypercoagulable state should also be kept in mind and investigated.

References

[1] J. Homans, "Thrombosis of the deep leg veins due to prolonged sitting," *The New England Journal of Medicine*, vol. 250, no. 4, pp. 148–149, 1954.

[2] I. S. Symington and B. H. R. Stack, "Pulmonary thromboembolism after travel," *The British Journal of Diseases of the Chest*, vol. 71, no. 2, pp. 138–140, 1977.

[3] J. M. Cruickshank, R. Gorlin, and B. Jennett, "Air travel and thrombotic episodes: the economy class syndrome," *The Lancet*, vol. 2, no. 8609, pp. 497–498, 1988.

[4] B. Eklof, R. L. Kistner, E. M. Masuda, B. V. Sonntag, and H. P. Wong, "Venous thromboembolism in association with prolonged air travel," *Dermatologic Surgery*, vol. 22, no. 7, pp. 637–641, 1996.

[5] A. Mercer and J. D. Brown, "Venous thromboembolism associated with air travel: a report of 33 patients," *Aviation Space and Environmental Medicine*, vol. 69, no. 2, pp. 154–157, 1998.

[6] R. Sarvesvaran, "Sudden natural deaths associated with commercial air travel," *Medicine, Science and the Law*, vol. 26, no. 1, pp. 35–38, 1986.

[7] R. A. Kraaijenhagen, D. Haverkamp, M. M. W. Koopman, P. Prandoni, F. Piovella, and H. R. Büller, "Travel and risk of venous thrombosis," *The Lancet*, vol. 356, no. 9240, pp. 1492–1493, 2000.

[8] H. P. Wright and S. B. Osborn, "Effect of posture on venous velocity, measured with 24NaCl," *British heart journal*, vol. 14, no. 3, pp. 325–330, 1952.

[9] H. Landgraf, B. Vanselow, D. Schulte-Huermann, M. V. Mulmann, and L. Bergau, "Economy class syndrome: rheology, fluid balance, and lower leg edema during a simulated 12-hour long distance flight," *Aviation Space and Environmental Medicine*, vol. 65, no. 10, pp. 930–935, 1994.

[10] B. Tardy, Y. Page, F. Zeni et al., "Phlebitis following travel," *Presse Médicale*, vol. 22, no. 17, pp. 811–814, 1993.

[11] E. Ferrari, T. Chevallier, A. Chapelier, and M. Baudouy, "Travel as a risk factor for venous thromboembolic disease: a case-control study," *Chest*, vol. 115, no. 2, pp. 440–444, 1999.

[12] S. K. Mittal, S. Chopra, and R. Calton, "Pulmonary embolism after long duration rail travel: economy class syndrome or rail coach syndrome," *Journal of Association of Physicians of India*, vol. 59, no. 7, pp. 458–459, 2011.

[13] P. L. J. Kesteven, "Traveller's thrombosis," *Thorax*, vol. 55, no. 1, pp. S32–S36, 2000.

[14] M. Ten Wolde, R. A. Kraaijenhagen, J. Schiereck et al., "Travel and the risk of symptomatic venous thromboembolism," *Thrombosis and Haemostasis*, vol. 89, no. 3, pp. 499–505, 2003.

[15] M. Bagshaw, R. Simons, and J. Krol, "Jet leg, pulmonary embolism, and hypoxia," *The Lancet*, vol. 348, no. 9024, pp. 415–416, 1996.

[16] M. Carruthers, A. E. Arguelles, and A. Mosovich, "Man in transit: biochemical and physiological changes during intercontinental flights," *The Lancet*, vol. 1, no. 7967, pp. 977–981, 1976.

[17] B. Bendz, M. Rostrup, K. Sevre, T. O. Andersen, and P. M. Sandset, "Association between acute hypobaric hypoxia and activation of coagulation in human beings," *The Lancet*, vol. 356, no. 9242, pp. 1657–1658, 2000.

[18] R. Benoit, "Travellar thromboembolic disease. The economy-class syndrome," *Journal des Maladies Vasculaires*, vol. 17, pp. 84–87, 1992.

[19] C. Jerjes-Sanchez, "Venous and arterial thrombosis: a continuous spectrum of the same disease?" *European Heart Journal*, vol. 26, no. 1, pp. 3–4, 2005.

[20] C. Becattini, G. Agnelli, A. Schenone et al., "Aspirin for preventing the recurrence of venous thromboembolism," *The New England Journal of Medicine*, vol. 366, no. 21, pp. 1959–1967, 2012.

[21] A. Squizzato, M. Galli, E. Romualdi et al., "Statins, fibrates, and venous thromboembolism: a meta-analysis," *European Heart Journal*, vol. 31, no. 10, pp. 1248–1256, 2010.

[22] W. Ageno, C. Becattini, T. Brighton, R. Selby, and P. W. Kamphuisen, "Cardiovascular risk factors and venous thromboembolism: a meta-analysis," *Circulation*, vol. 117, no. 1, pp. 93–102, 2008.

[23] H. T. Sørensen, E. Horvath-puho, K. K. Søgaard et al., "Arterial cardiovascular events, statins, low-dose aspirin and subsequent risk of venous thromboembolism: a population-based case-control study," *Journal of Thrombosis and Haemostasis*, vol. 7, no. 4, pp. 521–528, 2009.

[24] I. R. Khan, J. G. Reeves, P. J. Riesenman, and K. Kasirajan, "Simultaneous arterial and venous ultrasound-assisted thrombolysis for phlegmasia cerulea dolens," *Annals of Vascular Surgery*, vol. 25, no. 5, pp. 696.e7–696.e10, 2011.

[25] D. Nagaraja, A. B. Taly, and S. K. Shankar, "Simultaneous cerebral arterial and venous thrombosis.," *The Journal of the Association of Physicians of India*, vol. 38, no. 5, pp. 325–326, 1990.

[26] S. Juhl, K. Shorsh, H. Videbæk, and M. N. Binzer, "Concomitant arterial and venous thrombosis in a bodybuilder with severe hyperhomocysteinaemia and abuse of anabolic steroids," *Ugeskrift for Laeger*, vol. 166, no. 40, pp. 3508–3509, 2004.

[27] D. Gupta, P. Shukla, S. S. Bisht, M. L. B. Bhatt, M. C. Pant, and K. Srivastava, "Deep vein and artery thrombosis associated with cetuximab-based chemoradiotherapy," *Indian Journal of Pharmacology*, vol. 43, no. 4, pp. 478–480, 2011.

[28] S. Maffè, P. Dellavesa, A. Perucca, P. Paffoni, A. M. Paino, and M. Zanetta, "Pulmonary embolism associated with paradoxical arterial embolism in a patient with patent foramen ovale," *Giornale Italiano di Cardiologia*, vol. 9, no. 9, pp. 637–640, 2008.

[29] S. Buchholz, A. Shakil, G. A. Figtree, P. S. Hansen, and R. Bhindi, "Diagnosis and management of patent foramen ovale," *Postgraduate Medical Journal*, vol. 88, no. 1038, pp. 217–225, 2012.

[30] S. Pejkic, N. Savic, M. Paripovic, M. Sladojevic, P. Doric, and N. Ilic, "Vascular graft thrombosis secondary to activated protein C resistance: a case report and literature review," *Vascular*, vol. 22, no. 1, pp. 71–76, 2014.

[31] E. E. Rigdon, "Trousseau's syndrome and acute arterial thrombosis," *Cardiovascular Surgery*, vol. 8, no. 3, pp. 214–218, 2000.

Chimney-Graft as a Bail-Out Procedure for Endovascular Treatment of an Inflammatory Juxtarenal Abdominal Aortic Aneurysm

Francesca Fratesi, Ashok Handa, Raman Uberoi, and Ediri Sideso

Department of Vascular Surgery, Oxford University Hospitals NHS Trust, Oxford OX3 9DU, UK

Correspondence should be addressed to Francesca Fratesi; francesca.fratesi@gmail.com

Academic Editor: Konstantinos A. Filis

Inflammatory and juxtarenal Abdominal Aortic Aneurysm (j-iAAA) represents a technical challenge for open repair (OR) due to the peculiar anatomy, extensive perianeurysmal fibrosis, and dense adhesion to the surrounding tissues. A 68-year-old man with an 11 cm asymptomatic j-iAAA was successfully treated with elective EVAR and chimney-graft (ch-EVAR) without postprocedural complications. Target vessel patency and normal renal function are present at 24-month follow-up. The treatment of j-iAAA can be technically challenging. ch-EVAR is a feasible and safe bail-out method for elective j-iAAA with challenging anatomy.

1. Introduction

Inflammatory Abdominal Aortic Aneurysm (iAAA) is characterized by a thickened aortic wall and perianeurysmal fibrosis [1] with significant adhesions to the surrounding structures [2]. iAAAs are usually symptomatic and tend to present at a younger age with a triad of back pain, weight loss, and low grade fever. Elevated inflammatory markers with positivity of antinuclear antibody and elevation of IgG-4 plasma levels may be present [3]. Open repair (OR) remains the "gold standard" for treatment of iAAAs and juxtarenal aneurysms (jAAA), although there is an increased morbidity and mortality rate, longer operating time, and higher need for transfusions [4–7]. Endovascular repair (EVAR) offers an alternative as it obviates the need for extensive surgical dissection [4–6]. Fenestrated EVAR (f-EVAR) devices are used in jAAA to overcome the insufficient neck length resulting in inadequate sealing of standard endografts [8, 9]. Chimney-graft technique EVAR (ch-EVAR) was described to preserve the visceral aortic branches, deploying a stent parallel to the aortic endograft allowing the sealing in a healthier aortic zone [10]. A recent review of the ch-EVAR showed promising results in terms of morbidity, mortality, and durability at 6 and 12 months follow-up [11].

We present a unique case of a juxtarenal and inflammatory AAA (j-iAAA) successfully treated with ch-EVAR.

2. Case Presentation

A 68-year-old man presented with several months' history of abdominal and back pain associated with a pulsatile abdominal mass. His comorbidity included hypertension, being a current smoker, and previous lung empyema. CT-angiography (CTA) showed an 11 cm j-iAAA with periaortic inflammation (PAI) involving the body and the neck of the AAA extending to the level of the origin of the superior mesenteric artery (SMA). The preoperative CTA did not show any signs of hydronephrosis associated with the retroperitoneal fibrosis (Figure 1). OR with longitudinal xifopubic access was proposed as treatment of choice, but the intraoperative findings revealed a dense fibrotic tissue surrounding the aorta making the dissection hazardous (Figure 2) and for this reason the OR was abandoned being deemed too high a risk for complications. Postoperatively, the patient had a prolonged recovery period due to recurrent lung empyema and respiratory complications but was discharged home on day 11. Considering the size of the j-iAAA and the risk of rupture still present, an endovascular solution was

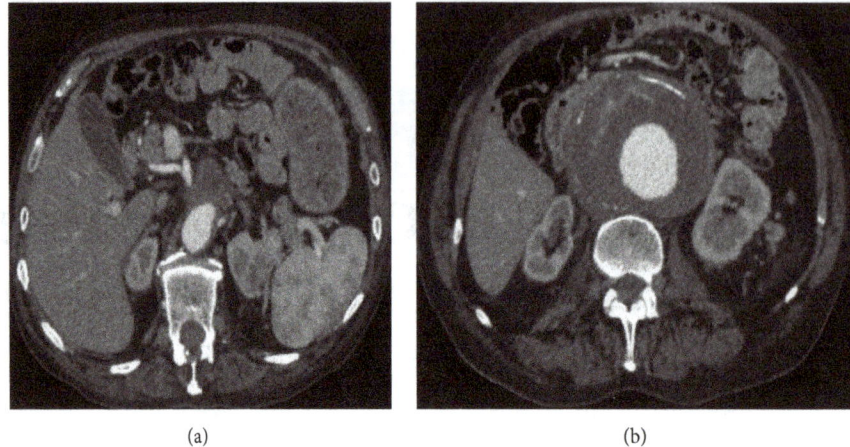

(a)   (b)

FIGURE 1: Preoperative CTA showing the extension of the AAA to the juxtarenal tract of the abdominal aorta (a) and the maximum diameter of the aneurysm (b). No signs of hydronephrosis were noted preoperatively.

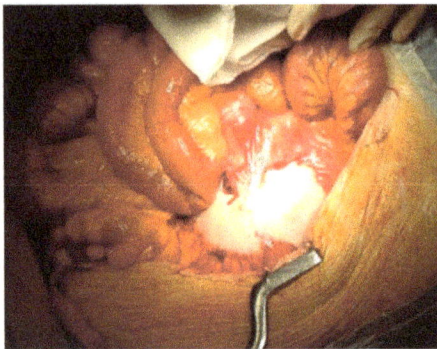

FIGURE 2: Intraoperative picture showing the thickened aortic wall and perianeurysmal fibrosis with significant adhesions to the surrounding structures encountered during the attempt of open repair.

sought. The anatomy of the j-iAAA was deemed not suitable for standard EVAR considering the length of the neck (<1 cm) and its angulation (α angle > 60 degrees). A custom-made f-EVAR was considered but deemed unsuitable due to the right renal artery small size (<3 mm in diameter). A MAG3-Renogram demonstrated the dominant renal function of the left kidney (37% versus 63%) and guided the decision to sacrifice the small right renal artery. Always considering the size of the j-iAAA and the risk of rupture and the length of time necessary to have a custom-made graft with only one vessel fenestration, EVAR with single left renal artery chimney-graft (ch-EVAR) was considered as the preferable option. The ch-EVAR was performed under general anaesthesia, with bilateral percutaneous femoral approach and left brachial artery open access. The left renal covered-stent (Advanta V12, Atrium, 5 × 29 mm) chimney-graft was released following the deployment of the main body of the stent-graft (Zenith Flex, Cook, main body 30 × 140 mm, oversize 15%) below the SMA. A bifurcated stent-graft was then completed. The chimney-graft was reinforced with a bare metal stent (Protégè EverFlex, Ev3, 6 × 60 mm). Completion angiogram showed

good position of the ch-EVAR with perfusion of the left kidney without any endoleaks. This was confirmed by CTA prior to discharge (Figure 3). Intraoperative blood loss was <500 mL. The patient was discharged on day 7 due to a recurrent lung empyema and need for a chest drain. No renal impairment was noted at the postoperative blood tests.

The follow-up was conducted with a Duplex Scan (DS) at 6 months which confirmed the patency of the ch-EVAR and the absence of endoleaks and the size of the j-iAAA was stable (11 cm). For this reason the follow-up CTA was conducted at one year, and it also confirmed the patency of the renal chimney-graft but it also revealed a late type 2 endoleak which was not present in the previous imaging. The CTA confirmed no aneurysm sac enlargement. The retroperitoneal periaortic inflammation (PAI) remained stable, without any signs of regression or progression noted at the CTA. The renal function was preserved at the blood test with also a maintenance of eGFR >90 mls/min/1.73 m^2. At the time of publication of this case report the patient completed the 24-month follow-up: the CTA confirmed a stable type 2 endoleak without any signs of sac enlargement. Also the PAI was stable without any signs of renal complications or involvement. The renal chimney stent-graft is still patent and there are no signs of in-stent stenosis or extrinsic compression. The follow-up will be conducted yearly thereafter considering the stability of the AAA and the type 2 endoleak will be managed conservatively unless a complication such as sac enlargement or symptoms related to the AAA will appear during the follow-up.

3. Discussion

Juxtarenal and inflammatory aneurysms present challenging OR management and EVAR offers an alternative, with good short and mid-term results. ch-EVAR has been described as a bail-out option, particularly in urgent or emergent situations or when a standard or custom-made EVAR is not possible [7–10]. A recent review on ch-EVAR for jAAA reported an overall mortality of 3.4% at 30-day and 7.9% at 1-year follow-up [11]. The authors highlight that, at 6 months, the patency

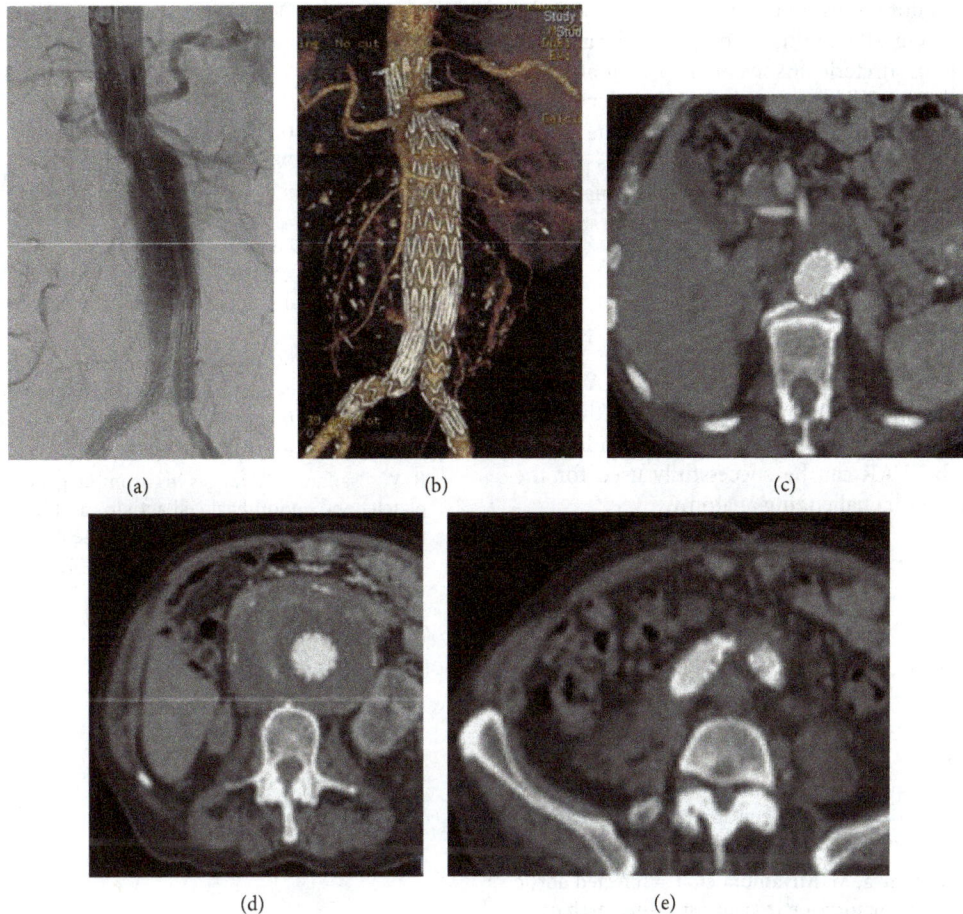

FIGURE 3: (a) Intraoperative completion angiography showing the good result of the ch-EVAR. (b) Reconstruction of postoperative CTA. Axial views of the postoperative CTA at the level of the origin of the left renal artery (c), mid-aneurysm (d), and bilateral common iliac arteries (e).

of the target vessels' chimney-grafts was 97.7%. Early type 1 endoleak was found in 7.4% of patients at completion of angiography and 10.2% at postoperative CTA; amongst this, 27.7% required treatment and 11.1% had a persistent type 1 endoleak [11]. Other authors reported a spontaneous regression of the leak in most cases (low-flow endoleak) at 12-month follow-up [12]. Late type 2 and type 3 endoleaks were present in 8.5% of the patients [11]. Good results of EVAR for iAAAs have been demonstrated in terms of short and mid-term morbidity and mortality, regression of PAI, and hydronephrosis [4, 12], but the benefit in the long term remains controversial. Paravastu et al. showed a trend for better outcome on mortality rate for EVAR compared to OR at 30 days (2% versus 6%, p = NS) and at 1 year (2% versus 14%, p = 0.01) [4]. Aneurysm related 1-year mortality was 0% for EVAR and 2% for OR (p = NS). In the subgroup of patients where hydronephrosis was analyzed, it was present in 48/85 (53%) of patients who underwent OR and 29/52 (56%) of patients who had EVAR; this regressed in 69% of OR and 38% of EVAR (p = 0.01), with progression observed in 9% and 21%, respectively (p = NS) [4]. At 1 year, PAI regressed in 73% of patients undergoing OR and 65% of patients treated with EVAR (p = 0.3) [4]. Stone et al. quantified the regression

in their series and noted a mean decrease in the thickness of the inflammatory rind of 50.8% (range 0% to 92.1%) [5]. It has been hypothesised that the exclusion of the iAAA can help with regression of PAI. This is supported by the observed regression of PAI in 65% of patients treated with EVAR [4]. There is a suggestion that the endograft results in an inflammatory reaction in the aorta and this can be considerable over time although this normalizes after 12 months [13]. In a retrospective review of the EUROSTAR database, PAI was related to a higher incidence of graft thrombosis and limb stenosis (3.9% versus 0.3%, p = 0.00059) [7], explained by the thick fibrotic tissue making ballooning and modeling after deployment more difficult [6].

This case is unique as it presents a combination of two challenging issues for EVAR. Elective chimney-graft was used due to the adverse anatomical features of the AAA and failure at open repair.

This is the first published case in the literature of a ch-EVAR used as the primary treatment of a juxtarenal and inflammatory aneurysm. Long-term patency of the chimney-graft and resolution of PAI are ongoing concerns. Limb stenosis may also be a concern, given the high incidence of limb stenosis/occlusion reported in the EUROSTAR registry [6].

In this case PAI has not regressed to date, but patency of the target vessel chimney-graft remains. Considering the absence of hydronephrosis or ureteric insolvent at presentation of the AAA or during the follow-up and also considering the presence of history of recurrent lung empyema, the use of corticosteroid in this case was not considered for this patient. Also the management of choice for the type 2 endoleak was conservative as the size of the aneurysm remained stable at 2-year follow-up and the AAA is still asymptomatic.

4. Conclusions

Treatment of both inflammatory and juxtarenal AAAs can be technically challenging. Open repair remains the gold standard, but EVAR is feasible with good early and mid-term results. Elective ch-EVAR can be successfully used for the treatment of iAAA with challenging anatomy.

References

[1] D. I. Walker, K. Bloor, G. Williams, and I. Gillie, "Inflammatory aneurysms of the abdominal aorta," *British Journal of Surgery*, vol. 59, no. 8, pp. 609–614, 1972.

[2] E. F. van Bommel, S. J. van der Veer, T. R. Hendriksz et al., "Persistent chronic peri- aortitis ('inflammatory a neurysm') after abdominal aortic a neurysm repair: systematic review of the litterature," *Vascular Medicine*, vol. 13, pp. 293–303, 2008.

[3] N. Ishizaka, K. Sohmiya, M. Miyamura et al., "Infected aortic aneurysm and inflammatory aortic aneurysm—in search of an optimal differential diagnosis," *Journal of Cardiology*, vol. 59, no. 2, pp. 123–131, 2012.

[4] S. C. V. Paravastu, J. Ghosh, D. Murray, F. G. Farquharson, F. Serracino-Inglott, and M. G. Walker, "A systematic review of open versus endovascular repair of inflammatory abdominal aortic aneurysms," *European Journal of Vascular and Endovascular Surgery*, vol. 38, no. 3, pp. 291–297, 2009.

[5] W. M. Stone, G. T. Fankhauser, T. C. Bower et al., "Comparison of open and endovascular repair of inflammatory aortic aneurysms," *Journal of Vascular Surgery*, vol. 56, no. 4, pp. 951–956, 2012.

[6] C. Lange, R. Hobo, L. J. Leurs, K. Daenens, J. Buth, and H. O. Myhre, "Results of endovascular repair of inflammatory abdominal aortic aneurysms. A report from the EUROSTAR database," *European Journal of Vascular and Endovascular Surgery*, vol. 29, no. 4, pp. 363–370, 2005.

[7] I. M. Nordon, R. J. Hinchliffe, P. J. Holt, I. M. Loftus, and M. M. Thompson, "Modern treatment of juxtarenal abominal aortic aneurysms with fenestrated endografting and open repair—a systematic review," *European Journal of Vascular and Endovascular Surgery*, vol. 38, no. 1, pp. 35–41, 2009.

[8] M. A. Qureshi and R. K. Greenberg, "New results with the Zenith graft in the treatment of the aortic aneurysms," *The Journal of Cardiovascular Surgery*, vol. 51, no. 4, pp. 503–514, 2010.

[9] N. Troisi, K. P. Donas, M. Austermann, J. Tessarek, T. Umscheid, and G. Torsello, "Secondary procedures after aortic aneurysm repair with fenestrated and branched endografts," *Journal of Endovascular Therapy*, vol. 18, no. 2, pp. 146–153, 2011.

[10] R. K. Greenberg, D. Clair, S. Srivastava et al., "Should patients with challenging anatomy be offered endovascular aneurysm repair?" *Journal of Vascular Surgery*, vol. 38, no. 5, pp. 990–996, 2003.

[11] A. Wilson, S. Zhou, P. Bachoo, and A. L. Tambyraja, "Systematic review of chimney and periscope grafts for endovascular aneurysm repair," *British Journal of Surgery*, vol. 100, no. 12, pp. 1557–1564, 2013.

[12] S. Puchner, R. A. Bucek, T. Rand et al., "Endovascular therapy of inflammatory aortic aneurysms: a meta-analysis," *Journal of Endovascular Therapy*, vol. 12, no. 5, pp. 560–567, 2005.

[13] M. F. Abdelhamid, R. S. M. Davies, D. J. Adam, R. K. Vohra, and R. W. Bradbury, "Changes in thrombin generation, fibrinolysis, platelet and endothelial cell activity, and inflammation following endovascular abdominal aortic aneurysm repair," *Journal of Vascular Surgery*, vol. 55, no. 1, pp. 41–46, 2012.

Adverse Outcome of Early Recurrent Ischemic Stroke Secondary to Atrial Fibrillation after Repeated Systemic Thrombolysis

Luciano A. Sposato,[1] **Valeria Salutto,**[2] **Diego E. Beratti,**[2] **Paula Monti,**[3]
Patricia M. Riccio,[1] **and Claudio Mazia**[2]

[1] *Vascular Research Institute, INECO Foundation, Pacheco de Melo 1860, Ciudad de Buenos Aires (C1126AAB), Buenos Aires, Argentina*
[2] *Department of Neurology, Alfredo Lanari Institute of Medical Investigations, University of Buenos Aires, Buenos Aires, Argentina*
[3] *Department of Medicine, Alfredo Lanari Institute of Medical Investigations, University of Buenos Aires,*
Ciudad de Buenos Aires, Argentina

Correspondence should be addressed to Luciano A. Sposato; lucianosposato@gmail.com

Academic Editors: N. Nighoghossian and J. L. Ruiz-Sandoval

Background. Recurrent ischemic stroke is associated with adverse neurological outcome in patients with atrial fibrillation. There is very scarce information regarding the neurological outcome of atrial fibrillation patients undergoing repeated systemic thrombolysis after early recurrent ischemic stroke. *Clinical Case and Discussion.* We describe a case of a 76-year-old woman with known paroxysmal atrial fibrillation who was admitted because of an acute right middle cerebral artery ischemic stroke and who underwent repeated systemic thrombolysis within 110 hours. The patient underwent systemic thrombolysis after the first ischemic stroke with almost complete neurological recovery. On the fourth day after treatment, an acute left middle cerebral artery ischemic stroke was diagnosed and she was treated with full-dose intravenous recombinant tissue plasminogen activator. A hemorrhagic transformation of the left middle cerebral artery infarction was noted on follow-up cranial computed tomographic scans. The patient did not recover from the second cerebrovascular event and died 25 days after admission. *Conclusion.* To the best of our knowledge, this is the second case reporting the adverse neurological outcome of a patient with diagnosis of atrial fibrillation undergoing repeated systemic thrombolysis after early recurrent ischemic stroke. Our report represents a contribution to the scarce available evidence suggesting that repeated systemic thrombolysis for recurrent ischemic stroke should be avoided.

1. Introduction

There is strong evidence that treatment of acute ischemic stroke with intravenous (IV) recombinant tissue plasminogen activator (rtPA) reduces long-term disability [1]. However, because of the risk of major bleeding, there is a need for careful selection of potentially treatable patients. Eligibility standards are based on inclusion and exclusion criteria used in large randomized clinical trials [2–4]. Among several contraindications, IV rtPA should not be used in patients who had suffered an ischemic stroke within the previous 3 months [1]. The repeated use of IV rtPA in the 3-month window may be associated to a higher risk of cerebral bleeding and to potential anaphylactic reactions [5]. There is scarce information about the repeated use of IV rtPA for early

recurrent ischemic stroke [6–9], and serious concerns have been raised regarding this matter [10].

We report a case of repeated used of IV rtPA within 110 hours in a patient with early recurrent ischemic stroke associated to atrial fibrillation, and we discuss its pathophysiological, clinical, and prognostic implications.

2. Clinical Case and Discussion

A 76-year-old woman was admitted to the Instituto de Investigaciones Médicas "Alfredo Lanari" because of left-sided numbness and slurred speech. On neurologic examination, she was not alert but arousable by minor stimulation. Examination of visual fields revealed a left homonymous hemianopia. A total paralysis of the left lower face was

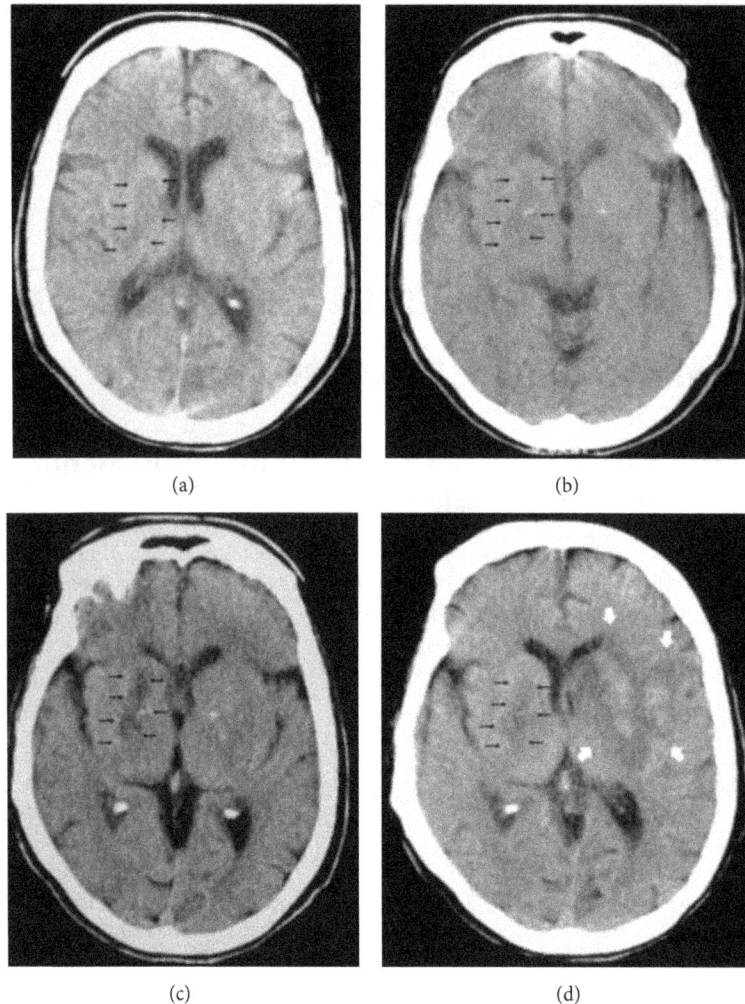

(a)

(b)

(c)

(d)

FIGURE 1: Cranial CT scan performed 100 minutes after first ischemic stroke onset (Panel a) and 24 hours after first IV thrombolysis (Panel b) shows a right lenticular hypodensity compatible with an acute cerebral infarction (black arrows). Cranial CT scan performed 30 minutes after second ischemic stroke onset (Panel c) and 48 hours after second systemic thrombolysis (Panel d) shows a subacute right lenticular infarction (black arrows) and a new predominantly subcortical ischemic lesion in the anterior region of the left middle cerebral artery territory with a PH2 hemorrhage (white arrows).

noted, and no movement could be elicited on the left arm and left leg. A left hemisensory deficit, moderate dysarthria, and profound left hemi-inattention were also evidenced. National Institutes of Health Stroke Scale (NIHSS) score was 18 points. Laboratory results were unremarkable. Head computed tomography (CT) scan performed 100 minutes after symptoms onset showed a subtle hypodensity of the right lenticular nucleus (Figure 1(a)). Electrocardiogram showed sinus rhythm.

The patient had a history hypertension, paroxysmal atrial fibrillation, hyperlipidemia, dilated cardiomyopathy, two acute myocardial infarctions, congestive heart failure, and pulmonary hypertension. She had undergone coronary artery stenting after the second myocardial infarction, and an implantable cardioverter-defibrillator was placed 6 years after. She was taking acetylsalicylic acid (100 mg/day), spironolactone (25 mg/day), furosemide (20 mg/day), carvedilol (6,125 mg BID), and simvastatin (20 mg/day).

IV rtPA (0.9 mg/kg) was started 120 minutes after stroke onset. After 24 hours, there was a significant neurological improvement (NIHSS score of 3). The patient persisted with total lower left facial palsy and mild left leg paresis, and the head CT scan showed the same right lenticular nucleus hypodensity (Figure 1(b)) compatible with an acute cerebral infarction.

Carotid Doppler ultrasound revealed mild bilateral atherosclerotic disease with less than 10% stenoses and transesophageal echocardiography showed left ventricular ejection fraction of 31% and an atherosclerotic debris of the aortic arch. Anticoagulation with low-molecular-weight heparin was initiated 24 hours after IV rtPA.

On the fourth day after treatment, a sudden neurological worsening was noted. The patient was alert but did not respond to simple commands. A conjugate deviation of the eyes that could not be overcome by voluntary or reflexive activity was seen, and visual threat showed a right homonymous hemianopia. Complete inferior bilateral face palsy was evidenced by Foix maneuver. Complete right arm and leg paralysis was noted and the patient was aphasic. NIHSS score was 22 points. The last dose of low-molecular-weight heparin was administered 13 hours before symptoms onset. A new head CT scan showed no significant changes when compared with the one performed 24 hours after first IV rtPA treatment (Figure 1(c)).

A thorough and thoughtful discussion regarding the appropriateness of the second IV thrombolytic treatment was held with the patient's family. Intra-arterial thrombolysis could have been an off-label alternative, but there was no availability at that moment. A second full-dose (0.9 mg/Kg) IV rtPA therapy was started 4 hours after stroke onset. Immediate NIHSS score after treatment was 18. Forty-eight hours later, NIHSS score was 16. The patient persisted with mild-to-moderate right hemiparesis, moderate aphasia, right homonymous hemianopia, and dysphagia. Head CT scan performed 24 and 48 hours (Figure 1(d)) after treatment showed the previous right lenticular infarction and a new predominantly subcortical ischemic lesion in the anterior region of the left middle cerebral artery territory with a PH2 (>30% of the infarcted area with space occupying effect) [11] hemorrhage. A pneumonia was diagnosed on day 20 and the patient died 5 days later. Death was attributed to the latter infectious complication.

We report a case of repeated IV rtPA within less than 5 days in a patient with paroxysmal atrial fibrillation and recurrent acute ischemic stroke. To the best of our knowledge, our case represents the third report on repeated systemic thrombolysis within 5 days between the incident and the recurrent ischemic stroke [6, 7] and the second one reporting on repeated IV rtPA treatment in a patient with early recurrent ischemic stroke associated to atrial fibrillation [7]. The current case raises several relevant issues related to repeated use of IV rtPA that warrant discussion: the potential development of anaphylactic reactions, the risk of hemorrhagic transformation, and the role of atrial fibrillation as a marker of early recurrent ischemic stroke and poor outcome after first and repeated IV thrombolysis.

There are few reports regarding potential anaphylactic reactions triggered by repeated thrombolysis [9]. Animal models have demonstrated the formation of antibodies against rtPA [12, 13]. However, development of these antibodies in humans is unusual [14] and there are only occasional reports of IV rtPA-related anaphylactic reactions in "real-life" clinical practice [15]. Moreover, no anaphylactic reactions have been described among any of the 13 cases of repeated IV thrombolysis for ischemic stroke reported up to date (including ours).

Our patient showed a PH2 hemorrhage on follow-up head CT scans which may have influenced the unfavorable neurological outcome, though this is controversial. Despite the short alpha half-life of rtPA (e.g., 4 to 5 minutes), its repeated use over short periods is contraindicated because of the risk of major bleeding, mainly intracerebral hemorrhage. In our patient, the risk of rtPA-associated hemorrhage was high because of the severity of the second stroke [16], the cardioembolic mechanism of the cerebrovascular event (atrial fibrillation) [17], and her history of congestive heart failure [18]. Damage to cerebrovascular walls due to free radical generation during reperfusion injury [19], the production matrix of metalloproteinases [20], and high concentrations of cellular fibronectin [21] have been implicated in the pathophysiology of rtPA-associated hemorrhage. However, the role of these biomarkers needs to be clarified.

The recovery of our patient was good after the first cerebrovascular event but she remained severely disabled after the second one, possibly because of the combination of recanalization failure and the hemorrhagic transformation. A strong association has been found between atrial fibrillation and early recurrent ischemic stroke after treatment with IV rtPA [22]. This phenomenon may be related to the disintegration of a preexisting intra-atrial thrombus during thrombolysis. As mentioned before, the risk of cerebral bleeding is also higher among atrial fibrillation patients after IV rtPA [17]. However, adverse neurological outcomes in these patients seem to be related more to recurrent embolization than to hemorrhagic transformation [22].

In conclusion, evidence-based medicine is the concept of treating patients according to the best available evidence. However, for many rare diseases and other situations like the very early recurrence of cardioembolic stroke in a patient who has received rtPA, it is often almost impossible to develop any form of randomized controlled trial. As mentioned before, international guidelines recommend avoiding repeated thrombolysis for patients with recurrent ischemic stroke within 3 months of the first event. This recommendation is not founded on randomized clinical trials, but is rather held on for the sake of patients' safety. For medical situations where impending permanent disability is the most probable scenario, "out-of-the-box" treatments could be used after a thorough discussion with patients and their families. We are aware that our medical decision was not supported by current guidelines and that most of the complications of systemic thrombolysis occur when recommendations are not followed. For this reason, based on teaching purposes and hoping to raise awareness about this important issue, we decided to report our case with the aim of further contributing to increase the scarce available evidence suggesting that early repeated systemic thrombolysis for recurrent ischemic stroke should be withheld.

References

[1] G. J. del Zoppo, J. L. Saver, E. C. Jauch, and H. P. Adams, "Expansion of the time window for treatment of acute ischemic stroke with intravenous tissue plasminogen activator: a science advisory from the American heart association/American stroke association," Stroke, vol. 40, no. 8, pp. 2945–2948, 2009.

[2] The National Institute of Neurological Disorders and Stroke rt-PA Stroke Study Group, "Tissue plasminogen activator for acute ischemic stroke," The New England Journal of Medicine, vol. 333, no. 24, pp. 1581–1587, 1995.

[3] W. Hacke, M. Kaste, C. Fieschi et al., "Randomised double-blind placebo-controlled trial of thrombolytic therapy with intravenous alteplase in acute ischaemic stroke (ECASS II)," The Lancet, vol. 352, no. 9136, pp. 1245–1251, 1998.

[4] W. Hacke, M. Kaste, E. Bluhmki et al., "Thrombolysis with alteplase 3 to 4.5 hours after acute ischemic stroke," *The New England Journal of Medicine*, vol. 359, no. 13, pp. 1317–1329, 2008.

[5] I. S. Park, A. H. Cho, S. J. Lee, J. Kim, K. Lee, and Y. Kim, "Life-threatening anaphylactoid reaction in an acute ischemic stroke patient with intravenous rt-PA thrombolysis, followed by successful intra-arterial thrombolysis," *Journal of Clinical Neurology*, vol. 4, no. 1, pp. 29–32, 2008.

[6] R. Topakian, F. Gruber, F. A. Fellner, H. Haring, and F. T. Aichner, "Thrombolysis beyond the guidelines: two treatments in one subject within 90 hours based on a modified magnetic resonance imaging brain clock concept," *Stroke*, vol. 36, no. 11, pp. e162–e164, 2005.

[7] M. A. Simpson and H. M. Dewey, "Should repeat thrombolysis be considered after early ischaemic stroke recurrence?" *International Journal of Stroke*, vol. 4, no. 4, pp. 237–238, 2009.

[8] E. M. Arsava and M. A. Topcuoglu, "De-novo thrombolysis for recurrent stroke in a patient with prior history of thrombolysis," *Blood Coagulation and Fibrinolysis*, vol. 21, no. 6, pp. 605–607, 2010.

[9] R. Sauer, H. B. Huttner, L. Breuer et al., "Repeated thrombolysis for chronologically separated ischemic strokes: a case series," *Stroke*, vol. 41, no. 8, pp. 1829–1832, 2010.

[10] M. Ribo and C. A. Molina, "Repeated tissue plasminogen activator treatment for early stroke recurrence: protocol violation is not an option," *Stroke*, vol. 37, no. 5, pp. 1151–1152, 2006.

[11] B. R. Thanvi, S. Treadwell, and T. Robinson, "Haemorrhagic transformation in acute ischaemic stroke following thrombolysis therapy: classification, pathogenesis and risk factors," *Postgraduate Medical Journal*, vol. 84, no. 993, pp. 361–367, 2008.

[12] C. M. Zwickl, B. L. Hughes, K. S. Piroozi, H. W. Smith, and D. Wierda, "Immunogenicity of tissue plasminogen activators in rhesus monkeys: antibody formation and effects on blood level and enzymatic activity," *Toxicological Sciences*, vol. 30, no. 2, pp. 243–254, 1996.

[13] N. Katsutani, S. Yoshitake, H. Takeuchi, J. C. Kelliher, R. C. Couch, and H. Shionoya, "Immunogenic properties of structurally modified human tissue plasminogen activators in chimpanzees and mice," *Fundamental and Applied Toxicology*, vol. 19, no. 4, pp. 555–562, 1992.

[14] J. Rudolf, M. Grond, W. S. Prince, S. Schmülling, and W. Heiss, "Evidence of anaphylaxy after alteplase infusion," *Stroke*, vol. 30, no. 5, pp. 1142–1143, 1999.

[15] B. R. Reed, A. B. Chen, P. Tanswell et al., "Low incidence of antibodies to recombinant human tissue-type plasminogen activator in treated patients," *Thrombosis and Haemostasis*, vol. 64, no. 2, pp. 276–280, 1990.

[16] D. Tanne, S. E. Kasner, A. M. Demchuk et al., "Markers of increased risk of intracerebral hemorrhage after intravenous recombinant tissue plasminogen activator therapy for acute ischemic stroke in clinical practice: the multicenter rt-PA acute stroke survey," *Circulation*, vol. 105, no. 14, pp. 1679–1685, 2002.

[17] N. Wahlgren, N. Ahmed, N. Eriksson et al., "Multivariable analysis of outcome predictors and adjustment of main outcome results to baseline data profile in randomized controlled trials: safe implementation of thrombolysis in Stroke-MOnitoring STudy (SITS-MOST)," *Stroke*, vol. 39, no. 12, pp. 3316–3322, 2008.

[18] V. Larrue, R. von Kummer, A. Müller, and E. Bluhmki, "Risk factors for severe hemorrhagic transformation in ischemic stroke patients treated with recombinant tissue plasminogen activator: a secondary analysis of the European-Australasian Acute Stroke Study (ECASS II)," *Stroke*, vol. 32, no. 2, pp. 438–441, 2001.

[19] L. Derex and N. Nighoghossian, "Intracerebral haemorrhage after thrombolysis for acute ischaemic stroke: an update," *Journal of Neurology, Neurosurgery and Psychiatry*, vol. 79, no. 10, pp. 1093–1099, 2008.

[20] T. Sumii and E. H. Lo, "Involvement of matrix metalloproteinase in thrombolysis-associated hemorrhagic transformation after embolic focal ischemia in rats," *Stroke*, vol. 33, no. 3, pp. 831–836, 2002.

[21] M. Castellanos, R. Leira, J. Serena et al., "Plasma cellular-fibronectin concentration predicts hemorrhagic transformation after thrombolytic therapy in acute ischemic stroke," *Stroke*, vol. 35, no. 7, pp. 1671–1676, 2004.

[22] M. Awadh, N. MacDougall, C. Santosh, E. Teasdale, T. Baird, and K. W. Muir, "Early recurrent ischemic stroke complicating intravenous thrombolysis for stroke: incidence and association with atrial fibrillation," *Stroke*, vol. 41, no. 9, pp. 1990–1995, 2010.

13

Cerebral Hyperperfusion Syndrome following Protected Carotid Artery Stenting

Rainer Knur

Department of Cardiology and Angiology, Allgemeines Krankenhaus Viersen, Hoserkirchweg 63, 47147 Viersen, Germany

Correspondence should be addressed to Rainer Knur; drrknur@gmx.de

Academic Editors: K. A. Filis and N. Papanas

The cerebral hyperperfusion syndrome is a very rare complication after revascularization of the carotid artery and accompanied by postoperative or postinterventional hypertension in almost all patients. We report a case of a 77-year-old man who developed a complete aphasia and increased right-sided weakness following endovascular treatment of severe occlusive disease of the left internal carotid artery. We discuss the risk and management of cerebral hyperperfusion syndrome after carotid artery stenting.

1. Introduction

Neurological complications following carotid artery stenting (CAS) are usually ischemic in nature, due to embolization or occlusion of the carotid artery. However, in a small subset of patients, cerebral hyperperfusion causes postinterventional neurological dysfunction, characterized by ipsilateral headache, focal seizure activity, focal neurological deficit, and ipsilateral intracerebral edema or hemorrhage. A high clinical suspicion and early diagnosis will allow early initiation of therapy and preventing fatal brain swelling or bleeding in patients with peri- and postinterventional cerebral hyperperfusion syndrome (CHS).

2. Case Report

A 77-year-old man was referred for endovascular treatment after a transient ischemic attack with a right-sided facial and limb weakness. This episode occurred while the patient was undergoing medical treatment consisting of 100 mg acetylsalicylic acid and 75 mg clopidogrel 4 weeks after coronary stenting of the left anterior descending artery. The patient had a history of hyperlipidemia, hypertension, and familiar disposition with coronary heart disease. The neurological examination during the ischemic event revealed a mild right-sided hemiparesis. Brain CT and MRI showed no abnormalities. All hematological and biochemical tests were normal, with a normal platelet count and coagulation screen.

When assessed in our hospital, his blood pressure sometimes jumped up to 180/100 mm Hg. Therefore, the antihypertensive medication consisting of β-blocker, diuretic, and AT1-antagonist was intensified. Another neurological examination was normal. Color Doppler ultrasound showed a severe stenosis of the left internal carotid artery (ICA) with elevation of the peak systolic velocity at 3.9 m/s and an end diastolic velocity of 1.4 m/s (Figure 1). The patient got a loading dose of 500 mg ASS and 300 mg clopidogrel and underwent left carotid stenting the next day via a femoral approach under local anesthesia. The angiography confirmed 95% stenosis of the left ICA (Figure 2(a)). CAS was frictionless performed with distal filter protection, pre- and postdilation, and a self-expandable closed-cell design stent (Figure 2). The peri-interventional blood pressure varied between 140/85 to 160/95 mm Hg. The clinically stable patient was transferred to the intermediate care unit for monitoring.

20 minutes later the patient vomited, described ipsilateral headache, and became very anxious. He then developed a complete aphasia and increased right-sided weakness and became delirious. Blood pressure varied between 160/90 and 200/110 mm Hg. Immediately color Doppler ultrasound of the CCA and ICA revealed a visibly patent vessel. Brain edema and bleeding could be excluded by an urgent cranial CT. Followup within 24 hours with cranial MRI and

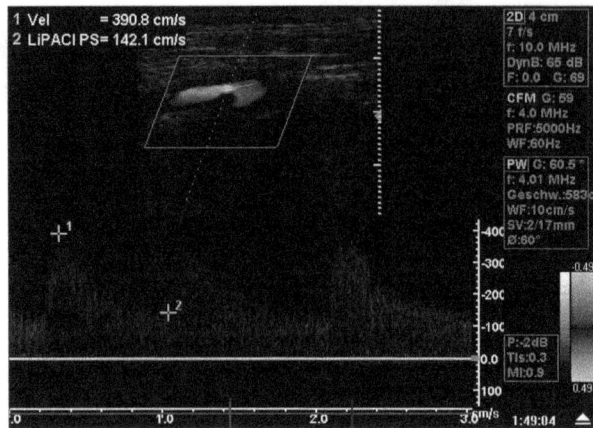

FIGURE 1: Color Doppler ultrasound of the left internal carotid artery (ICA). Severe stenosis of the left internal carotid artery with elevation of the peak systolic velocity at 3.9 m/s and an end diastolic velocity of 1.4 m/s.

TABLE 1: Risk factors for CHS [6–8].

Hypertension
High-grade stenosis with poor collateral flow
Decreased CVR
Increased peak flow velocity
Contralateral carotid occlusion or high-grade stenosis
Recent contralateral CAS or CEA within 3 months
Periprocedural ischemia
Presence of cerebral microangiopathy

CAS: carotid artery stenting, CEA: carotid endarterectomy, CHS: cerebral hypertension syndrome, and CVR: cerebrovascular reactivity.

angiography showed totally normal findings. The patient was transferred to the intensive care to control the hypertension and to monitor the vital parameters. Under intensified treatment of the blood pressure with a β-blocker, diuretic, AT1-, and Ca-antagonist, and temporary intravenous application of nitroglycerin and urapidil the neurological symptoms were totally regressed within few days. The patient was discharged after 10 days from the hospital. Follow-up examinations after 3 and 6 months were normal.

3. Discussion

In 1981, Sundt et al. [1] described a triad of complications that included atypical migrainous phenomena, transient focal seizure activity, and intracerebral hemorrhage after CEA and used the term cerebral hyperperfusion syndrome (CHS). The first report on CHS after CAS was published by Schoser et al. [2]. They described a 59-year-old woman with ipsilateral putaminal hemorrhage that was diagnosed on the 3rd day after CAS of a high-grade stenosis of the left ICA. Outcome in this case was not fatal. The patient recovered with a mild upper limb paresis. McCabe et al. [3] were the first to report the occurrence of fatal ICH soon after CAS. Only a few hours after the procedure, neurological symptoms occurred without any prodromata (severe headache, nausea, and seizures) postulated by Sundt et al. [1] to be an obligate component of CHS. CT of the brain revealed extensive ICH and the patient died 18 days later. Abou-Chebl et al. [4] reported a retrospective single-center study on 450 patients who had been treated with CAS. Three patients (0.67%) developed ICH after the intervention. Further reports on results and complications after CAS have been published [5]. Nearly all reports on CHS after carotid revascularizations in general and CAS in particular have in common patients who had high-grade stenoses in the treated vessel.

CHS following surgical or endovascular treatment of severe carotid occlusive disease is thought to be the result of impaired cerebral autoregulation, hypertension,

ischemia-reperfusion injury, oxygen-derived free radicals, baroreceptor-dysfunction, and intraprocedural ischemia [6]. Chronic cerebral hypoperfusion due to critical stenosis leads to production of vasodilatory substances. Autoregulatory failure results in the cerebral arterioles being maximally dilated over a long period of time, with subsequent loss of their ability to constrict when normal perfusion pressure is restored. The degree of microvascular dysautoregulation is proportional to the duration and severity of ischemia determined by the severity of ipsilateral stenosis and poor collateral flow.

Hypertension plays an important role in the development of CHS. In the absence of cerebral autoregulation, cerebral blood flow is directly dependent on the systemic blood pressure. The restoration of normal blood flow to chronically underperfused brain can result in edema, capillary breakthrough, and perivascular and macroscopic hemorrhages aggravated by peri- and postinterventional hypertension [6, 7]. The risk factors for CHS after CAS are summarized in Table 1.

The classic clinical presentation includes ipsilateral headache, seizures or focal neurological deficit, and ipsilateral intracerebral edema or hemorrhage. The diagnosis can be made readily with color Doppler ultrasound of the carotid artery and especially with transcranial Doppler (TCD) of the middle cerebral artery [9]. An increase in peak blood flow velocity of >100% is predictive of postinterventional hyperperfusion. Diffusion weighted MRI or single photon emission computed tomography (SPECT) could also be performed for diagnosis [10]. Angiography normally shows normal findings.

The prognosis of CHS depends on timely recognition of hyperperfusion and adequate treatment of hypertension before cerebral edema or hemorrhage develops. The prognosis following intracerebral bleeding is very poor, with mortality over 50% and significant morbidity of 80% in the survivors [4, 6]. The prognosis of CHS in patients without cerebral edema or hemorrhage is clearly better especially when they are identified and treated early. The most important aspects in preventing and treating this syndrome are early identification, careful monitoring, and control of blood pressure ideally in a high-dependency unit setting. In our special case, early diagnosis of CHS and immediate intensive medical treatment of blood pressure could prevent devastating cerebral edema or hemorrhage following CAS.

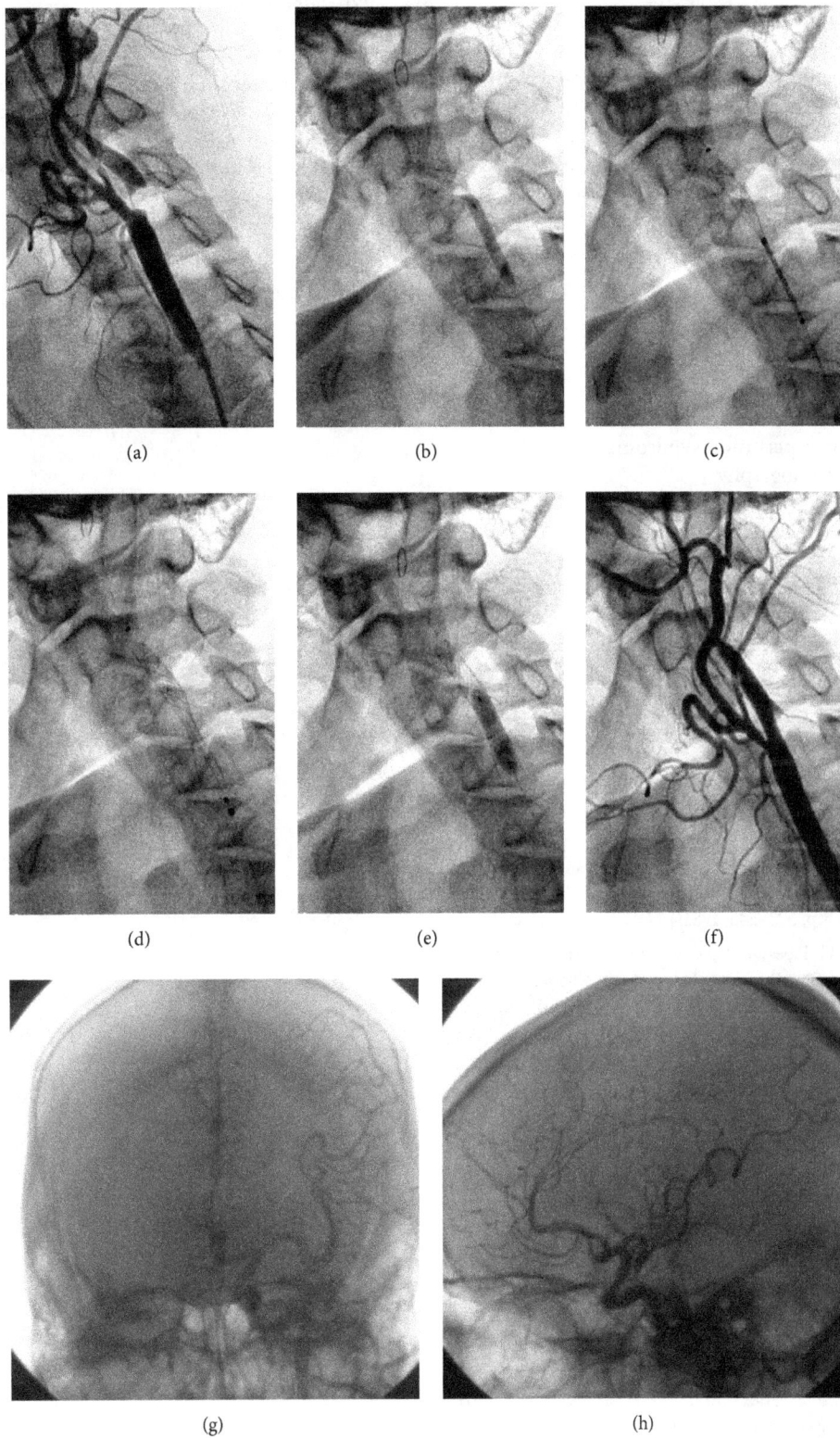

FIGURE 2: Carotid angiogram demonstrating carotid artery stenting (CAS) with distal filter protection in a 77-year-old symptomatic patient. (a) Preprocedural angiogram showing a high-grade stenosis of the left internal carotid artery. (b) After the filter is positioned distal to the lesion the stenosis is predilated with a 3 mm balloon. (c) The self-expanding stent is deployed. (d) Stent after deployment. (e) The stent is postdilated with a 5 mm balloon. (f) The final angiogram shows that the stented site is widely patent. (g), (h) Final angiogram of the intracranial vessels.

4. Conclusion

CHS, which is characterized by ipsilateral headache, hypertension, seizures, and focal neurological deficits, is a rare but devastating complication following carotid artery stenting. Hypertension is the most important risk factor. The diagnosis can be confirmed quickly by TCD, DWI, or SPECT. Especially peri- or postinterventional TCD monitoring should be available to identify patients with hyperperfusion who may benefit from intensive blood pressure management ideally in a specialized intensive care unit.

Abbreviations

CAS: Carotid artery stenting
CCA: Common carotid artery
CEA: Carotid endarterectomy
CHS: Cerebral hyperperfusion syndrome
CT: Computed tomography
CVR: Cerebrovascular reactivity
DWI: Diffusion-weighted imaging
ICA: Internal carotid artery
ICH: Intracerebral haemorrhage
MRI: Magnetic resonance imaging
SPECT: Single photon emission computed tomography
TCD: Transcranial Doppler.

References

[1] T. M. Sundt Jr., F. W. Sharbrough, and D. G. Piepgras, "Correlation of cerebral blood flow and electroencephalographic changes during carotid endarterectomy. With results of surgery and hemodynamics of cerebral ischemia," *Mayo Clinic Proceedings*, vol. 56, no. 9, pp. 533–543, 1981.

[2] B. G. H. Schoser, C. Heesen, B. Eckert, and A. Thie, "Cerebral hyperperfusion injury after percutaneous transluminal angioplasty of extracranial arteries," *Journal of Neurology*, vol. 244, no. 2, pp. 101–104, 1997.

[3] D. J. H. McCabe, M. M. Brown, and A. Clifton, "Fatal cerebral reperfusion hemorrhage after carotid stenting," *Stroke*, vol. 30, no. 11, pp. 2483–2486, 1999.

[4] A. Abou-Chebl, J. S. Yadav, J. P. Reginelli, C. Bajzer, D. Bhatt, and D. W. Krieger, "Intracranial hemorrhage and hyperperfusion syndrome following carotid artery stenting: risk factors, prevention, and treatment," *Journal of the American College of Cardiology*, vol. 43, no. 9, pp. 1596–1601, 2004.

[5] J.-H. Buhk, L. Cepek, and M. Knauth, "Hyperacute intracerebral hemorrhage complicating carotid stenting should be distinguished from hyperperfusion syndrome," *American Journal of Neuroradiology*, vol. 27, no. 7, pp. 1508–1513, 2006.

[6] V. Adhiyaman and S. Alexander, "Cerebral hyperperfusion syndrome following carotid endarterectomy," *QJM*, vol. 100, no. 4, pp. 239–244, 2007.

[7] W. F. Morrish, S. Grahovac, A. Douen et al., "Intracranial hemorrhage after stenting and angioplasty of extracranial carotid stenosis," *American Journal of Neuroradiology*, vol. 21, no. 10, pp. 1911–1916, 2000.

[8] R. Gupta, A. Abou-Chebl, C. T. Bajzer, H. C. Schumacher, and J. S. Yadav, "Rate, predictors, and consequences of hemodynamic depression after carotid artery stenting," *Journal of the American College of Cardiology*, vol. 47, no. 8, pp. 1538–1543, 2006.

[9] M. B. Sánchez-Arjona, G. Sanz-Fernández, E. Franco-Macias, and A. Gil-Peralta, "Cerebral hemodynamic changes after carotid angioplasty and stenting," *American Journal of Neuroradiology*, vol. 28, pp. 640–644, 2007.

[10] Y. Kaku, S. I. Yoshimura, and J. Kokuzawa, "Factors predictive of cerebral hyperperfusion after carotid angioplasty and stent placement," *American Journal of Neuroradiology*, vol. 25, pp. 1403–1408, 2004.

14

Giant Pseudoaneurysm Associated with Arteriovenous Fistula of the Brachial and Femoral Arteries following Gunshot Wounds: Report of Two Cases

Handy Eone Daniel,[1] Ankouane Firmin,[2] Pondy O. Angele,[3] Minka Ngom Esthelle,[1] Bombah Freddy,[1] and Ngo Nonga Bernadette[1]

[1]Department of Surgery, Faculty of Medicine and Biomedical Sciences, University of Yaoundé I, Yaoundé, Cameroon
[2]Department of Medicine, Faculty of Medicine and Biomedical Sciences, University of Yaoundé I, Yaoundé, Cameroon
[3]Department of Pediatrics, Faculty of Medicine and Biomedical Sciences, University of Yaoundé I, Yaoundé, Cameroon

Correspondence should be addressed to Ngo Nonga Bernadette; ngonongab@yahoo.com

Academic Editor: Jaw-Wen Chen

Posttraumatic pseudoaneurysm associated with arteriovenous fistula of the upper or lower limb is exceptional. We are reporting herein the history of two cases in civil life that have been followed and repaired in our service. Both patients were shot more than a year before being referred to our tertiary hospital for an enlarging mass which was a pseudoaneurysm associated with an arteriovenous fistula. The aneurysm was repaired and the fistula closed. Due to the absence of well-trained professionals, vascular injuries and their complications are usually discovered late in Cameroon while these pseudoaneurysms can reach very dramatic sizes. This presentation intends to raise the attention on a careful clinical exam and search of vascular lesion in the case of penetrating wound of the limb associated with profuse bleeding.

1. Introduction

Isolated posttraumatic pseudoaneurysms of the peripheral vessels have been reported in the literature and are more common during war time [1]. Pseudoaneurysms associated with arteriovenous fistula (AVF) are uncommon following penetrating wound trauma of the limbs and have rarely been reported. They have been found more on the upper extremities than the lower extremities [2]. In Africa, few studies on vascular trauma and its complications have been reported [3]. Due to the increasing violence in the fast growing cities in Cameroon, vascular traumas are becoming more common [4]. Yet many of these lesions go unrecognized and are diagnosed at the stages of late complications like pseudoaneurysm and arteriovenous fistula. The combination of both complications can result in a severe treat to the extremity involved [2, 5]. We are reporting two cases of brachial and femoral arteries' pseudoaneurysm associated with arteriovenous fistula to the corresponding venous system, occurring more than a year after gunshot wounds. The following presentation emphasizes the need of careful examination of a patient with penetrating injury near major vessels of the limbs and the development of vascular clinical exam.

Patient 1. This 22-year-old male farmer from a village (150 Km from Yaoundé) was referred to us for a pulsating mass of the left elbow, swollen upper limb, and massively distended veins associated with mild pain. He reported that he was shot with a shotgun 2 years earlier while hunting. He was taken to the hospital just after the injury because he was bleeding profusely. Scattered small wounds were found, a dressing was done, and he was transfused 2 units of blood. There was no other injury elsewhere. He was discharged home with no referral or follow-up appointment. He decided to see a doctor 2 years later because of an enlarging mass of the left elbow. On the physical exam, there was a 6 cm × 8 cm pulsating mass at the left elbow and massively distended

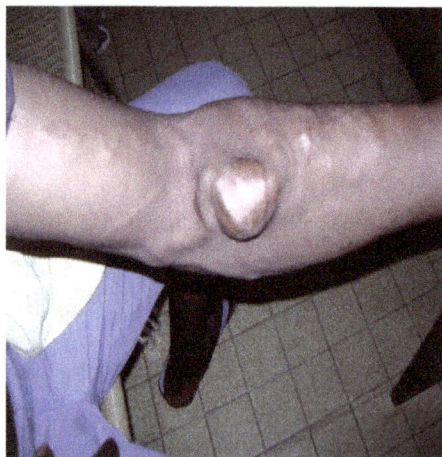

FIGURE 1: Posttraumatic AVF between the brachial artery and the vein comitans with a large pseudoaneurysm and massively distended superficial veins; the distension is from the venous comitans.

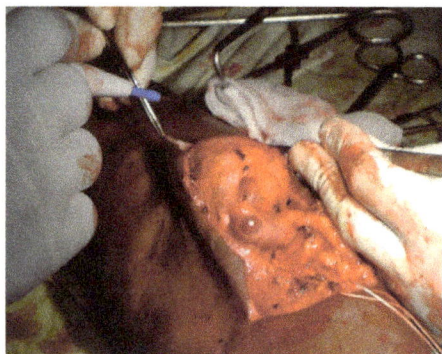

FIGURE 2: Dissection of the pseudoaneurysm. The elastic band is around the brachial artery. The vessels are massively distended. The fistula was between the venous comitans and the brachial artery. So the pseudoaneurysm was just under the skin but having a large communication with the brachial artery.

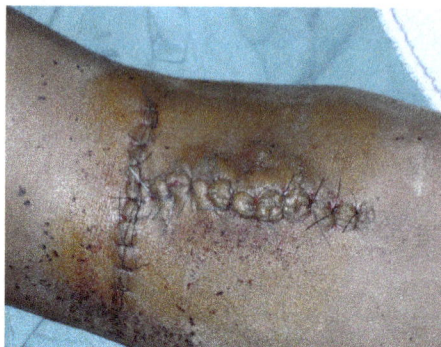

FIGURE 3: Immediate postoperative appearance of the elbow. The distended veins have disappeared.

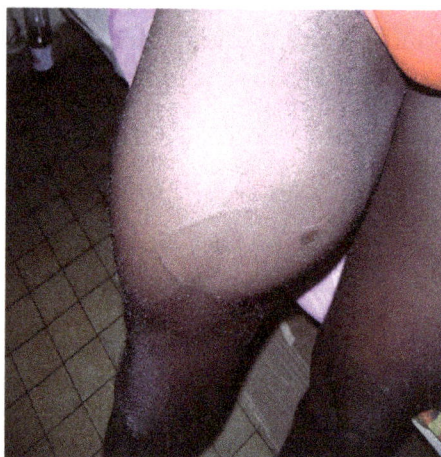

FIGURE 4: Large superficial femoral pseudoaneurysm with AVF fistula with palpable trill and audible machinery murmur.

superficial veins; the radial pulse was present but weak (Figure 1). The left upper limb was mildly swollen and warmer than the right one. There was a strong pulsating and audible thrill at the level of the mass and also a machinery sound audible at the level of the superficial veins. The diagnosis of a posttraumatic pseudoaneurysm of the brachial artery associated with an AVF was made. The young man was very poor and had no money to do any additional work-up test. Because he was a farmer and needed to use his limb, we decided to help him and performed the surgery under local anesthesia. We first controlled the brachial artery just above the elbow and the distal control was obtained just after the pseudoaneurysm (Figure 2); we explored and dissected around the pseudoaneurysm without disrupting it. We found a fistula between the vein comitans (anastomosing the cephalic vein to the brachial vein) and the brachial artery after the elbow. Ligation of the superficial veins was realized, the fistula was divided, and the artery and the veins were repaired using the prolene 6/0. The blood loss was minimal

and no transfusion was necessary. The patient was discharged home the same day and was followed in our clinics. Figure 3 shows the postoperative clinical aspect of the limb.

Patient 2. This young man was a 27-year-old student when he was assaulted and shot on the right thigh. He was taken to a major hospital in Douala. The wounds were found to be small, so no suturing was done and no other exam was requested. The wounds were dressed daily. We have no description of the physical exam at that time. One year later after the incident, he was referred to us complaining of an enlarging mass in the middle of the right thigh associated with intermittent claudication (Figure 4). These symptoms which started after the accident have been increasing gradually and walking for him was more and more difficult. When we saw him for consultation, he was having rest pain, difficulties in walking, and impotence of the right lower limb and he was using crunches to walk. This pain was not responding to codeine based pain medication and was found to be 9/10 in the analogic scale; the pain increased by walking and was located more at the level of the calf. He also complained of paresthesia and mild paralysis. The walking distance has tremendously

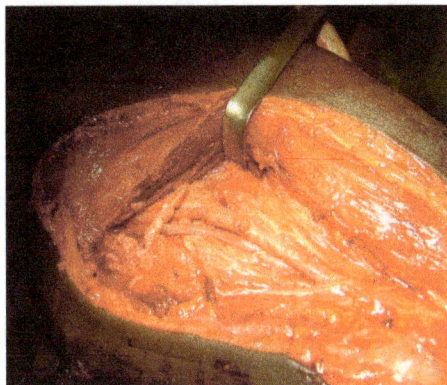

FIGURE 5: Superficial femoral artery and vein after repair using saphenous vein replacement. We have used the inverted larger portion of the vein to repair the artery and the smaller portion to repair the vein.

decreased the last month before consultation and he was feeling pain while being at rest.

On the physical exam, he presented a large mass located on the right thigh measuring 12×9 cm; it was warm, pulsating with an audible and palpable thrill located in the internal surface of the right thigh in the upper third. Besides the thrill, a large machinery murmur was also audible at the level of the Scarpa triangle. We noticed also two small old scars as shown in Figure 4. The foot was cold, and no distal pulse was palpated (popliteal, posterior tibial, or pedal pulse); he had a decreased sensation of the foot and was unable to dorsiflex it. An angioscan showed a large pseudoaneurysm with communication between the femoral vessels. The diagnosis of post traumatic pseudoaneurysm of the superficial femoral artery associated with an AVF between this artery and the corresponding vein complicated by ischemia of the right leg was made. The patient was taken to the operating room on an urgent basis because of impending limb loss due to ischemia. The surgery was done under locoregional anesthesia. We first obtained vascular control at the level of the Scarpa triangle; after a difficult dissection, we were able to find the fistula between the superficial femoral artery and vein. The injured portions of both vessels were resected; the artery and the vein were repaired using saphenous vein grafting (Figure 5). Postoperatively, the patient did not complain of any pain at rest and the foot became warm; there was also a net improvement of the paresthesia, and he was able to dorsiflex the ankle. But no distal pulse was palpated on the right ankle and foot (from the posterior tibial or pedal arteries).

2. Discussion

In Cameroon, some trauma patients are being taken care of by nursing staff (first patient) or general practitioner (second case) who are not trained in vascular injury's clinical presentation. Therefore, with penetrating injuries, patients are usually seen at the time of the trauma; most of them are even transfused blood because of profuse bleeding but the diagnosis is not suspected and the appropriate exams or referrals are not requested. The two cases reported here are illustrative of these facts; the diagnosis was delayed although they have been seen in hospitals at the time of the lesions. Delayed diagnosis is also secondary to the poverty of these patients, very few being able to pay for the exams or the treatment in a tertiary hospital where this diagnosis can be made.

As reported by others, an injury to a peripheral artery should be suspected when one of these clinical signs is present: a penetrating injury next to a major artery, profuse bleeding, expanding hematoma, signs of peripheral ischemia, shock with a need for transfusion, and obvious signs of vascular lesions. All of these signs were found in both patients and it is unlikely that the diagnosis would have been missed if they were seen in a tertiary center as in our hospital [1, 2, 5]. Late complications of peripheral artery's injuries are pseudoaneurysms and AVF. Each complication, though rare, is not uncommon independently [1, 3], but the association of a pseudoaneurysm and AVF has not been reported in Cameroon and is quite rare in the literature. These lesions are easily recognized in a patient with a pulsating mass, associated with distended superficial veins; the extremity is warm, a thrill is palpable, and a machinery murmur is audible. The superficial veins are distended; long standing cases can lead to massive enlargement of both the arteries and the veins involved [6]. In both cases presented here, the extremity was warm and the arteries and veins were massively distended. Although the diagnosis is obvious based on the clinical exam, a duplex ultrasound may be useful. Other exams are MRI angiogram or angioscan. An arteriography may be useful, but it is not available in Cameroon and has been replaced in many cases by MRI angiogram in western countries, because it carries more complications [1, 2, 5]. Complications like rupture and ischemia are life-threatening. To avoid limb loss, rupture, infection, and delayed cardiac failure, the surgery should be realized without delay.

Late complications of vascular injuries due to a shotgun are pseudoaneurysm, arteriovenous fistula, and a combination of both. The aneurysm can reach dramatic proportion with the threat to the life of the patient (Figures 1 and 3). Long standing lesions can also lead to massively distended veins and arteries as in our first case. A high suspicion at the time of the injury is advisable, and a vascular consultation should be sought in any patient with a penetrating injury in the extremity presenting with profuse bleeding and shock even if he does not have signs of ischemia.

References

[1] U. Yetkin and A. Gurbuz, "Post-traumatic pseudo aneurism of the brachial artery and its surgical treatment," Texas Heart Institute Journal, vol. 30, no. 4, pp. 293–297, 2003.

[2] J. Y. Lee, H. Kim, H. Kwon, and S.-N. Jung, "Delayed rupture of a pseudoaneurysm in the brachial artery of a burn reconstruction

patient," *World Journal of Emergency Surgery*, vol. 8, no. 1, article 21, 2013.

[3] H. K. Aduful and W. M. Hodasi, "Peripheral vascular Injuries and their management in Accra," *Ghana Medical Journal*, vol. 41, no. 4, pp. 186–189, 2007.

[4] J. Bahebeck, R. Atangana, E. Mboudou, B. N. Nonga, M. Sosso, and E. Malonga, "Incidence, case-fatality rate and clinical pattern of firearm injuries in two citie's where arm owning is forbidden," *Injury*, vol. 36, no. 6, pp. 714–717, 2005.

[5] V. Loughlin and J. S. Beniwal, "Post-traumatic brachial artery aneurysm and arteriovenous fistulae," *Journal of Cardiovascular Surgery*, vol. 29, no. 5, pp. 570–571, 1988.

[6] C. D. Schunn and T. M. Sullivan, "Brachial arteriomegaly and true aneurysmal degeneration: case report and literature review," *Vascular Medicine*, vol. 7, no. 1, pp. 25–27, 2002.

Right Upper Lobe Partial Anomalous Pulmonary Venous Connection

Christos Tourmousoglou,[1] Christina Kalogeropoulou,[2] Efstratios Koletsis,[1] Nikolaos Charoulis,[1] Christos Prokakis,[1] Panagiotis Alexopoulos,[1] Emmanoil Margaritis,[1] and Dimitrios Dougenis[1]

[1] *Cardiothoracic Department, University Hospital of Patra, 26504 Rio, Patra, Greece*
[2] *Department of Radiology, University Hospital of Patra, 26504 Rio, Patra, Greece*

Correspondence should be addressed to Christos Tourmousoglou; christostourmousoglou@hotmail.com

Academic Editors: N. Espinola-Zavaleta and A. Iyisoy

Partial anomalous pulmonary venous return (PAPVR) is a left-to-right shunt where one or more, but not all, pulmonary veins drain into a systemic vein or the right atrium. We report a case of a 45-year-old male with PAPVR to superior vena cava which was incidentally discovered during a right lower bilobectomy for lung cancer.

1. Introduction

Partial anomalous pulmonary venous connection (PAPVC) is an uncommon congenital anomaly in which one or more pulmonary veins drain into a systemic vein or the right atrium rather than the left atrium. Anomalous right-sided pulmonary veins might drain into the superior vena cava, inferior vena cava, right atrium, azygos vein, portal vein, or hepatic vein. Besides, anomalous left-sided pulmonary veins could drain into the left brachiocephalic vein, coronary sinus, or hemiazygos vein. The PAPVC might occur as an isolated anomaly or might be combined with atrial septal defect (ASD) [1]. The PAPVC to the superior vena cava occurs in about 10–15% of all patients with ASD.

We report a case of a 45-year-old male with PAPVC that was incidentally discovered during a right lower bilobectomy for lung cancer.

2. Case Report

A 45-year-old male had a persistent cough for two months and his chest X-ray showed a nodule in the right lower lobe. A chest computed tomography revealed a mass (5.8 × 6.6 × 6.3 cm) in the right lower lobe that was attached to the right hilum and around the bronchus. Bronchoscopy showed a lesion at the entrance of the right lower lobe that obstructed 30% of the bronchus and pathological examination of a biopsy revealed adenocarcinoma. Spirometry revealed the following values of FVC: 3.17 L (60%) and FEV_1: 2.79 L (77%), while electrocardiography showed normal cardiovascular activity. Clinical examination did not reveal marked abnormalities or evidence of vascular shunt. Surgery was performed through a left posterolateral thoracotomy under one-lung ventilation. An anomalous pulmonary vein was incidentally discovered and the right upper lobe vein drained into the superior vena cava. A right bilobectomy was performed. The right upper lobe with the anomalous variation remained as it was. The patient had an uneventful postoperative course. After the operation, a careful examination and reconstruction of the CT images revealed the anomaly (Figures 1 and 2).

3. Discussion

Partial anomalous pulmonary venous connection is a relatively uncommon congenital anomaly that is found in only 0.5–0.7% of the general population [2, 3]. Asymptomatic PAPVC without an ASD is extremely rare. The greatest number of cases of PAPVC is located in the right lung and

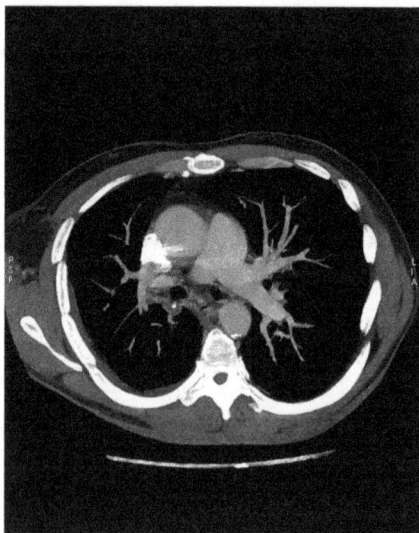

FIGURE 1: Multidetector computed tomography showed a PAPVC from the right upper lobe to the superior vena cava (arrow).

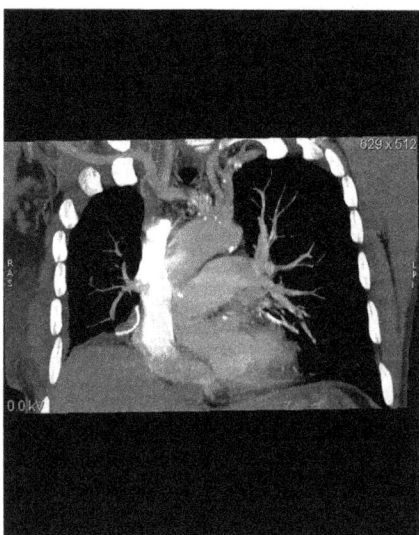

FIGURE 2: Another coronal oblique CT image denoted a PAPVC from the right upper lobe to the superior vena cava (arrow).

the anomalous vein or veins are often connected to the right atrium or the superior vena cava [4].

All PAPVC are left-to-right shunts but more than 50% of the pulmonary flow drain into the right side of the heart and so clinical manifestations such as fatigue, dyspnea, syncope, atrial arrhythmias, right heart failure, and pulmonary hypertension might occur rarely [5, 6]. Generally, PAPVC is symptomatic and it is often associated with other congenital heart defects, especially ASD, reportedly in 80–90% of the cases [7, 8]. No associated risk factors have been identified for its development.

Embryonic development of the pulmonary veins occurs early in development of the cardiovascular system. The main theory is that the initial drainage is via the splanchnic plexus into the cardinal and umbilical vitelline. A craniocaudal

outpouching forms in the sinoatrial region of the heart with extension to lung buds. As caudal regression occurs, the cranial portion develops into the common pulmonary vein, which is incorporated into the left atrial wall. Partial anomalous pulmonary venous return occurs due to failure of connection between the common pulmonary vein and the splanchnic plexus [9, 10].

PAPVC is usually diagnosed by transthoracic echocardiography (TTE), transesophageal echocardiography (TEE), or catheter angiography. The information provided by echocardiography is sometimes not sufficient. Besides, pulmonary angiography by right heart catheterization might not reveal details about the anatomy of small accessory and anomalous vessels [11]. Another examination such as 128-slice multidetector computed tomography (MDCT) scan is helpful in defining ASDs and PAPVR. ECG-gated MDCT offers the possibility of a noninvasive and rapid acquisition with high resolution. All of the anomalous veins and associated cardiovascular defects are observed by MDCT-angiography [12]. The isotropic voxel size and spatial resolution offer the possibility to discover small vessels and shunts with multidimensional reconstructions with the usage of advanced workstations [13]. But it is really a concern about the radiation dose of MDCT especially in young patients [14]. The usage of ECG attenuation techniques limits the exposure during the less informative parts of the cardiac cycle. The success of this technique depends on the usage of premedication, ECG-gating, and special technical protocols. Data processing of multidimensional images might be time consuming but 2D and 3D images are valuable in planning the operation [13].

MRI will also demonstrate the abnormal pulmonary venous connection, but it could better depict an associated ASD. Chest radiography is often normal and secondary signs of a left-to-right shunt such as cardiomegaly, pulmonary vascular prominence, and pulmonary artery hypertension could be seen [8].

If the lung cancer is located in the same lobe as the PAPVC, the patient could have either a lobectomy or an ipsilateral pneumonectomy with an uneventful postoperative course. But if the PAPVC is located in a different lobe, a lobectomy or a contralateral pneumonectomy might result in heart failure [3, 15]. In case that major pulmonary resections are performed for patients with PAPVC, it is critical to correct this anomaly for preventing heart failure.

There are a number of operative procedures for the correction of PAPVR. An anomalous vein on the left side is implanted directly into the left auricular appendage or the left atrium. A number of postoperative complications such as kinking, stenosis of the corrected pulmonary vein, obstruction, and arrhythmias are correlated with these procedures [16, 17]. Surgical repair for PAPVC to SVC consists of complete closure of the septal defect, with redirection of the anomalous pulmonary veins into the left atrium without SVC obstruction, pulmonary venous obstruction, or injury of the sinus node or its blood supply. In case that the veins enter the SVC in an upright position, the surgical treatment is more demanding.

Warden et al. reported a technique for the correction of high PAPVC in which the SVC was divided above the orifices of the anomalous pulmonary veins and the cephalic end of the divided SVC was anastomosed directly to the right atrial appendage. A patch was inserted into the right atrium and diverted the pulmonary blood flow from the orifice of the SVC through the sinus venosus ASD. Then, the caudal end of the divided SVC was closed by sutures. This technique has the advantage of decreased manipulation of the cavoatrial junction while avoiding the creation of conduits inside the SVC [18].

In conclusion, PAPVC is an uncommon congenital anomaly and is incidentally found during an operation for lung cancer. Coronal, sagittal, and 3D volume rendered reformatted CT images could help in the diagnosis of this entity. The best surgical approach for lung resection in patients with PAPVC should be considered carefully for preventing postoperative heart failure.

References

[1] T. C. Demos, H. V. Posniak, K. L. Pierce, M. C. Olson, and M. Muscato, "Venous Anomalies of the Thorax," *American Journal of Roentgenology*, vol. 182, no. 5, pp. 1139–1150, 2004.

[2] H. Boody, "Drainage of the pulmonary veins into the right side of the heart," *Archives of Pathology*, vol. 33, pp. 221–240, 1942.

[3] M. D. Black, F. M. Shamji, W. Goldstein, and H. J. Sachs, "Pulmonary resection and contralateral anomalous venous drainage: a lethal combination," *Annals of Thoracic Surgery*, vol. 53, no. 4, pp. 689–691, 1992.

[4] H. Sakurai, H. Kondo, A. Sekiguchi et al., "Left pneumonectomy for lung cancer after correction of contralateral partial anomalous pulmonary venous return," *Annals of Thoracic Surgery*, vol. 79, no. 5, pp. 1778–1780, 2005.

[5] T. Schertler, S. Wildermuth, N. Teodorovic, D. Mayer, B. Marincek, and T. Boehm, "Visualization of congenital thoracic vascular anomalies using multi-detector row computed tomography and two- and three-dimensional post-processing," *European Journal of Radiology*, vol. 61, no. 1, pp. 97–119, 2007.

[6] J. B. Selby, T. Poghosyan, and M. Wharton, "Asymptomatic partial anomalous pulmonary venous return masquerading as pulmonary vein occlusion following radiofrequency ablation," *The International Journal of Cardiovascular Imaging*, vol. 22, no. 5, pp. 719–722, 2006.

[7] A. Shahriari, M. D. Rodefeld, M. W. Turrentine, and J. W. Brown, "Caval division technique for sinus venosus atrial septal defect with partial anomalous pulmonary venous connection," *Annals of Thoracic Surgery*, vol. 81, no. 1, pp. 224–230, 2006.

[8] M. Gupta, "Partial anomalous pulmonary venous connection," Emedicine, 2010.

[9] J. R. Dillman, S. G. Yarram, and R. J. Hernandez, "Imaging of pulmonary venous developmental anomalies," *American Journal of Roentgenology*, vol. 192, no. 5, pp. 1272–1285, 2009.

[10] C. J. Zylak, W. R. Eyler, D. L. Spizarny, and C. H. Stone, "Developmental lung anomalies in the adult: radiologic-pathologic correlation," *Radiographics*, vol. 22, pp. S25–S43, 2002.

[11] S. Kivistö, H. Hänninen, and M. Holmström, "Partial anomalous pulmonary venous return and atrial septal defect in adult patients detected with 128-slice multidetector computed tomography," *Journal of Cardiothoracic Surgery*, vol. 6, no. 1, article 126, 2011.

[12] H. Kasahara, R. Aeba, Y. Tanami, and R. Yozu, "Multislice computed tomography is useful for evaluating partial anomalous pulmonary venous connection," *Journal of Cardiothoracic Surgery*, vol. 5, no. 1, article 40, 2010.

[13] W. T. Roberts, J. J. Bax, and L. C. Davies, "Cardiac CT and CT coronary angiography: technology and application," *Heart*, vol. 94, no. 6, pp. 781–792, 2008.

[14] P. Cronin, A. M. Kelly, B. H. Gross et al., "Reliability of MDCT in characterizing pulmonary venous drainage, diameter and distance to first bifurcation. An interobserver study," *Academic Radiology*, vol. 14, no. 4, pp. 437–444, 2007.

[15] H. Takei, K. Suzuki, H. Asamura, H. Kondo, and R. Tsuchiya, "Successful pulmonary resection of lung cancer in a patient with partial anomalous pulmonary venous connection: report of a case," *Surgery Today*, vol. 32, no. 10, pp. 899–901, 2002.

[16] C. Van Meter Jr., J. G. LeBlanc, W. S. Culpepper III, and J. L. Ochsner, "Partial anomalous pulmonary venous return," *Circulation*, vol. 82, no. 5, pp. V-195–V-198, 1990.

[17] J. D. Babb, T. J. McGlynn, W. S. Pierce, and P. M. Kirkman, "Isolated partial anomalous venous connection: a congenital defect with late and serious complications," *Annals of Thoracic Surgery*, vol. 31, no. 6, pp. 540–543, 1981.

[18] H. E. Warden, R. A. Gustafson, T. J. Tarnay, and W. A. Neal, "An alternative method for repair of partial anomalous pulmonary venous connection to the superior vena cava," *Annals of Thoracic Surgery*, vol. 38, no. 6, pp. 601–605, 1984.

Pulmonary-Esophageal Variceal Bleeding: A Unique Presentation of Partial Cor Triatriatum Sinistrum

Fortune O. Alabi,[1] Manuel Hernandez,[2] Francis G. Christian,[1] Fred Umeh,[1] and Maximo Lama[1]

[1] *Department of Critical Care Medicine, Florida Hospital Celebration Health, Celebration, FL 34747, USA*
[2] *Department of Radiology, Florida Hospital Orlando, Orlando, FL 32803, USA*

Correspondence should be addressed to Francis G. Christian; francis.g.christian@gmail.com

Academic Editors: H. Matsumoto and H. Nakajima

Cor triatriatum sinistrum is a rare congenital disorder defined as a division of the left atrium by a diaphragmatic membrane resulting in two left atrial chambers. The membranous division of the atrium can be partial or complete and can affect either atrium, with involvement of the right atrium referred to as cor triatriatum dexter. The presence of fenestrations within the membrane allows for communication and forward passage of blood into the true atrium. Absence of fenestrations leads to early symptomatic engorgement of the lungs. We report the case of a young adult male presenting with recurrent hematemesis due to variceal bleeding. On CT imaging the patient was found to have cor triatriatum sinistrum, with a vertical membrane resulting in total obstruction of the pulmonary venous drainage on the right, with normal pulmonary venous drainage on the left. There was extensive pulmonary-systemic arterial collateralization to the right lung suggesting retrograde filling of the right pulmonary artery with effective flow reversal in the right lung.

1. Introduction

Cor triatriatum was first described in 1868 [1]. Since then, reports have described the condition in the pediatric population where presentation is acute and symptomatic. Affected children present with features of congestive heart failure such as decreased cardiac output and pulmonary venous hypertension. With the advent of TTE and TEE, there have been confirmed diagnoses of cor triatriatum presenting in adults with fatigue, dyspnea on exertion, and recurrent infection [2]. When presenting in adulthood, cor triatriatum is mostly isolated; however, the condition has been reported in association with bicuspid aortic valve and atrial septal defects [3].

The unique defect in partial cor triatriatum involving only the right pulmonary veins (with normal flow of left pulmonary veins into left atrium) results in pulmonary venous hypertension and congestion in only the right lung. Subsequent vascular changes of increased mediastinal venous drainage result in development of venous varices. Complete venous obstruction can also result in extensive pulmonary-systemic arterial collateralization providing an effective systemic to pulmonary arterial shunt. In this setting, forward flow to the lung is provided by hypertrophied systemic arteries including phrenic, pleural, aortic, and bronchial artery collaterals, while venous drainage of the lung is successfully provided by retrograde flow within the affected pulmonary artery. To date, there has been no case describing variceal bleeding as a presentation of partial cor triatriatum sinistrum.

2. Case Report

A 26 y/o male was admitted to the critical care service from the emergency department for severe anemia with variceal bleeding. The patient presented with active hematemesis citing a weeklong history of melanotic stool, hematemesis, and lightheadedness. There were no significant past medical or family histories of GI or pulmonary diseases. The patient's social history describes 2 glasses of wine per week

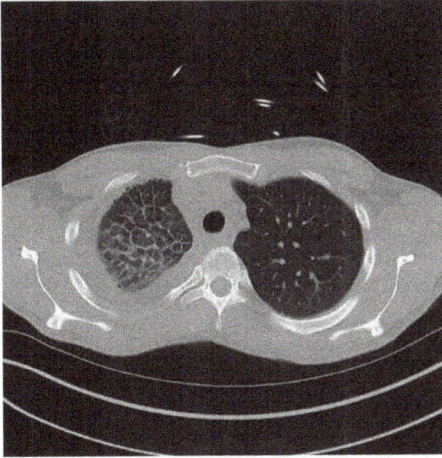

FIGURE 1: Axial plane showing right lung volume loss, secondary lobules, and thickened septa.

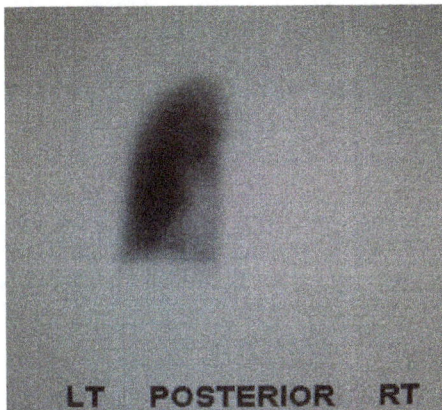

FIGURE 2: Albumin perfusion scan revealing absence of right lung perfusion.

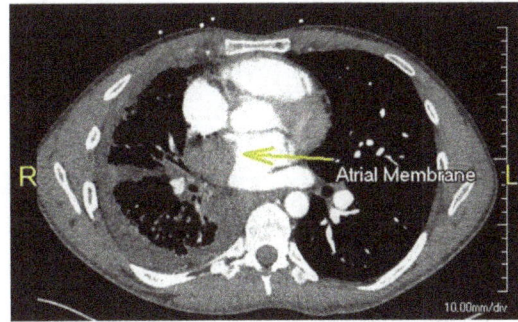

FIGURE 3: Axial plane showing vertical membrane (yellow arrow) in left atria obstructing right pulmonary venous flow.

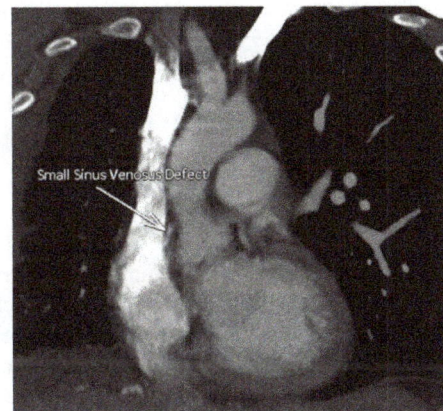

FIGURE 4: Coronal plane showing sinus venosus collateralization between the hypertrophied systemic vessels and the diminutive right pulmonary artery.

for the last 4 years. Physical examination on consultation revealed an alert, young male with mild epigastric tenderness without pulmonary or cardiovascular findings. CT of the abdomen showed supradiaphragmatic "downhill" paraesophageal varices without cirrhosis or splenomegaly and pleural thickening with pleural calcifications. Upper endoscopy revealed numerous 4+ varices from the upper esophagus to the gastroesophageal junction which were banded. High resolution noncontrast CT the following day revealed right lung findings significant for volume loss, septal thickening of the secondary pulmonary lobules, and a "cobble stoning" indicative of pathologic interstitial edema (Figure 1). V/Q scan revealed nearly absent right lung perfusion (Figure 2). Subsequently, a CT of the chest to evaluate for pulmonary vein atresia showed normal left pulmonary veins with near complete functional arterial and venous systemic isolation of the right lung due to chronic right pulmonary vein obstruction. The left atrium was significant for a vertical septation resulting in complete isolation of the right upper and lower pulmonary veins (Figure 3). A small caliber left to right to shunt was noted between the upper portion of

the left atrium and the SVC via a patent sinus venosus (Figure 4). Right lung findings were consistent with chronic pleural congestion, extensive arterial collateralization, and pericardial and peridiaphragmatic lymph node enlargement secondary to vascular congestion. The right lung was supplied by numerous hypertrophied intercostal and peripleural collaterals along the periphery in addition to hypertrophied bronchial artery collaterals. Systemic-pulmonary artery collaterals were also identified as arising directly from the lower thoracic and upper abdominal aorta just superior to the celiac trunk. These collaterals provided retrograde filling of the right pulmonary artery via hypertrophied phrenic artery collaterals forming a series of pulmonary-phrenic arcades and shunts along the diaphragm (Figure 5).

The patient was stabilized and transferred to an outside institution where he underwent surgical resection of the obstructing atrial membrane. After surgery, the patients' hemoptysis, hematemesis, and melena resolved. Repeat upper endoscopy demonstrated no significant residual varices and CT bolus tracking images and echocardiography showed normal anterograde flow in right pulmonary artery.

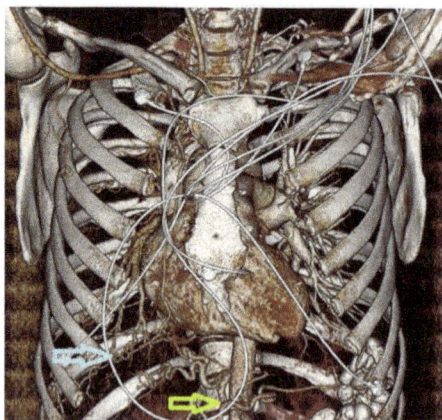

FIGURE 5: Three-dimensional reconstructed image showing origin of anomalous artery (green arrow) supplying diaphragmatic collaterals. Phrenic-pulmonary arcades and marginal pulmonary systemic shunts (blue arrow) are seen draining via the small right pulmonary artery.

3. Discussion

Cor triatriatum sinistrum involves a membranous appendage dividing the left atrium into a proximal (accessory) chamber and distal (true) left atrium. Pulmonary veins returning to the left atria enter the blind ending accessory chamber rather than true left atrium. Without a large orifice of >3 mm or fenestrations in the membrane [4], there will be significantly decreased right lung venous outflow resulting in chronic pulmonary congestion. Subtotal variations of sinistrum may occur as in the presented case, whereby the causative septation affects pulmonary venous drainage from only one lung.

Classification of cor triatriatum into 3 groups was first made by Loeffler [5]. Group 1 has no orifices, in the sinistrum membrane, group 2 has 1 or more small orifices and group 3 has a wide orifice. Groups 1 and 2 present in infants with severe symptomatology and mortality, while group 3, Loeffler postulated, may reach adulthood. This patient likely had no fenestrations in the occluding membrane, having survived till adulthood without significant symptomology due to unilateral involvement and effective left to right shunting. Flow reversal on the right allowed for pulmonary venous return and thus normal lung development.

Unilateral right sided pulmonary vein atresia is the most likely considered differential diagnosis for the case presented. Both conditions have the same physiological incapability of proper forward blood flow from right lung to left atrium. There is physiologic reversal of normal blood flow from the bronchial veins though systemic anastomoses. Normal bronchial venous return occurs through two pathways. First, bronchial veins drain into esophageal veins which flow into the azygous vein and superior vena cava providing return to the right heart. A second pathway is through small bronchopulmonary anastomoses into the pulmonary veins providing deoxygenated return to the left heart, the basis for physiological shunting [6]. Physiologic reversal of flow to the pulmonary veins and increased flow through the esophageal veins results in the formation of "downhill" paraesophageal varices rather than the uphill esophageal varices commonly encountered in portal venous hypertension. Additionally, systemic-pulmonary artery collateralization as seen in this case has also been reported in cases of isolated pulmonary vein atresia [7].

Physiologic similarities between this case of partial cor triatriatum and unilateral right pulmonary vein atresia are manifested in the resemblance of imaging studies. Chest CT demonstrated a small right hemithorax, ground glass pulmonary infiltrates, interlobular septal thickening, and a small caliber right pulmonary artery. V/Q scan revealed nearly absent pulmonary perfusion to right lung with normal ventilation. These findings are almost identical to those reported in previous adult cases of unilateral pulmonary vein atresia [8]. The septated left atrium on CT venous chest and nonatretic pulmonary veins are the only significant differences between imaging studies here and previously reported cases of pulmonary vein atresia.

4. Conclusion

Pulmonary vein atresia is an uncommon but known cause of esophageal varices [9]. When investigating clinical presentations of dyspnea, recurrent infections, and hematemesis, along with concurrent radiological findings significant for pulmonary vein atresia, it would be prudent to consider partial cor triatriatum as a possible differential diagnosis.

References

[1] W. S. Church, "Congenital malformation of heart: abnormal septum in left auricle," *Transactions of the Pathological Society of London*, vol. 19, pp. 188–190, 1868.

[2] Z. Işılak, S. Cay, E. Kardeşoğlu, and M. Uzun, "Fenestrated cor triatriatum sinistrum: a case report," *Türk Kardiyoloji Derneği Arşivi*, vol. 40, no. 4, pp. 347–349, 2012.

[3] R. Hamdan, N. Mirochnik, D. Celermajer, P. Nassar, and L. Iserin, "Cor Triatriatum Sinister diagnosed in adult life with three dimensional transesophageal echocardiography," *BMC Cardiovascular Disorders*, vol. 10, article 54, 2010.

[4] T. B. Karamlou, K. F. Welke, and R. M. Ungerleider, "Congenital heart disease," in *Schwartz's Principles of Surgery*, F. C. Brunicardi, D. K. Andersen, T. R. Billiar et al., Eds., McGraw-Hill, New York, NY, USA, 9th edition, 2010.

[5] E. Loeffler, "Unusual malformation of the left atrium; pulmonary sinus," *Archives of Pathology*, vol. 48, no. 5, pp. 371–376, 1949.

[6] R. A. Rhoades, R. Rhoades, and D. R. Bell, *Medical Physiology, Principles for Clinical Medicine*, Wolters Kluwer Health/Lippincott Williams & Wilkins, Philadelphia, Pa, USA, 4th edition, 2013.

[7] M. Cao, H. Cai, J. Ding, Y. Zhuang, and Z. Wang, "Bronchial varices in congenital unilateral pulmonary vein atresia," *American Journal of Respiratory and Critical Care Medicine*, vol. 187, no. 11, pp. 1267–1268, 2013.

Periodontal Disease and Late-Onset Aortic Prosthetic Vascular Graft Infection

Stephanie Thomas,[1] Jonathan Ghosh,[2] Johnathan Porter,[2] Adele Cockcroft,[2] and Riina Rautemaa-Richardson[1,3]

[1]Department of Microbiology, University Hospital of South Manchester, Wythenshawe Hospital, Southmoor Road, Manchester M23 9LT, UK
[2]Department of Vascular Surgery, University Hospital of South Manchester, Wythenshawe Hospital, Southmoor Road, Manchester M23 9LT, UK
[3]The University of Manchester, Manchester Academic Health Science Centre, Institute of Inflammation and Repair, Oxford Road, Manchester M13 9PT, UK

Correspondence should be addressed to Stephanie Thomas; ssthomas@doctors.org.uk

Academic Editor: Levent Sarikcioglu

Prosthetic vascular graft infection (PVGI) is a rare but significant complication of arterial reconstructive surgery. Although the relative risk is low, the clinical consequences can be catastrophic. Microbiological data on causative bacteria are limited. We present four cases of late-onset PVGI. Using a culture-independent nucleic acid amplification method for analysis of intraoperative samples, the presence of bacteria highly suggestive of an oral source was reported. Examination by an oral health specialist confirmed the presence of chronic periodontal disease. We hypothesize that chronic oral infection may be a previously unreported risk factor for the development of late-onset PVGI.

1. Introduction

Prosthetic vascular graft infection (PVGI) has an incidence of 1–6%, an associated morbidity of 40–70%, limb amputation of up to 70%, and a recognised mortality of 30–50% [1].

Microbiological data on organisms associated with PVGI are rarely published, mainly due to the need for early initiation of broad-spectrum antimicrobial therapy before graft excision and reconstruction. The aim is to disinfect the vascular bed, but this decreases the sensitivity of routine laboratory culture based methods. In addition, PVGIs are associated with polymicrobial biofilm formation around the graft [2]. Bacteria growing within the biofilm disperse sporadically, whereby preoperative blood cultures are unlikely to be positive. Blood cultures are more likely to be positive in patients with an aortodigestive fistula, which provides gut microorganisms with a constant portal of entry into the blood stream.

Epidemiological data on PVGI are similarly poorly defined, but reported risk factors for late-onset infections (>4 months after primary surgery [1]) include postoperative or early wound infection, wound complications at any time, and the presence of a femoral incision [3].

We report four cases where odontogenic bacteria have been implicated in late-onset aortic PVGI, using culture-independent nucleic acid amplification. To our knowledge, this has not been previously reported.

2. Case Reports

We present four cases of late-onset aortic PVGI, diagnosed and treated at our tertiary referral Vascular Surgical Unit between February and May 2013.

Case 1 was a 46-year-old female who presented three years after redo aortobifemoral graft (initial graft insertion, twelve years previously), with bleeding from an opening in the right groin. A CT angiogram aorta carried out on admission reported an infected and occluded aortic bifurcation graft (gas seen along the right limb of the graft) and a probable thrombosed aortoenteric fistula.

Case 2 was a 69-year-old male who presented one year after endovascular aneurysm repair (EVAR), with sudden severe back and abdominal pain and melaena. A CT angiogram aorta reported that a previously noted endoleak had increased significantly with gas seen within the anterior native aortic sac. In addition, the duodenum was reported to be closely applied to the anterior portion of the aneurysm with marked inflammatory stranding around the native aortic aneurysm sac. Appearances were consistent with an aortoenteric fistula.

Case 3 was a 57-year old female who was admitted to our unit three years post axillo-bi-femoral reconstruction following explantation of an infected aortobifemoral graft. She presented with pus discharging from the left groin. A CT angiogram aorta reported a focal collection around the left femoral branch of the graft with an area of infiltration of the adjacent fat likely to represent a focal graft infection.

Case 4 was an 80-year-old male who presented seven years after aortic aneurysm repair with back pain and fever. In view of the prosthetic material in situ, he was admitted to the medical assessment unit and a CT scan was carried out which showed small bowel adherence to the distal aortic graft with gas circling the graft suggestive of an aortoenteric graft fistula.

Cases 1–3 underwent explantation of the infected graft, with debridement of infected tissue and vascular reconstruction. Where debridement was carried out, intraoperative samples were collected and sent for microbiological analysis. In view of multiple comorbidities, case four was unfit for surgical intervention; however, multiple sets of blood cultures were collected on admission.

3. Diagnosis

In addition to routine laboratory culture, the intraoperative samples collected from cases 1–3 were sent for 16S rDNA real-time PCR identification to the Department for Bioanalysis and Horizon Technologies at the Centre for Infections, Colindale, London. In each case, the 16S rDNA analysis detected the presence of a mixture of bacteria highly suggestive of an oral source.

In case 1, analysis of aortic graft fluid, the sequence data displayed a series of overlapping peaks indicative of a mixture of bacteria. Mixed sequence trace file analysis showed that the mixture in the sample was too complex to accurately determine which bacterial species were present. However, it was suggestive of a mixture of oral anaerobic bacteria.

In case 2, aortic thrombus tissue, a 16S rDNA PCR product, was obtained, indicating the presence of a mixture of bacteria in the sample. However, it was not possible to delineate the species. Mixed trace file analysis showed presence of oral anaerobic bacteria including *Fusobacterium* sp., *Prevotella* sp., and *Propionibacterium avidum*.

In case 3, groin pus detected *Pediococcus pentosaceus*. Admission blood cultures collected in case 4 also isolated organisms of oral aetiology, including *Streptococcus oralis*, *Lactobacillus* species, *Klebsiella pneumonia*, and *Enterococcus faecium*.

In view of the microbiology detected, a postoperative clinical oral examination by a specialist in oral medicine

was arranged for cases 2, 3, and 4 who remained in-patients in the unit. Case 2 had evidence of extensive past need for dental care, a number of missing teeth and various dental restorations, and clear clinical signs of past chronic periodontitis. Case 3 was in acute need for dental care with snapped teeth, large carious lesions, and chronic periodontal infection. A number of teeth were missing; partial dentures were in use and moderate denture stomatitis was detected in the underlying mucosa. Case 4 had evidence of extensive past need for dental care including root treatments and crowns and clinical signs of chronic periodontitis. Radiological imaging of the jaws by orthopantomography was carried out in two patients (cases 2 and 3). This was reviewed by a maxillofacial radiologist, confirming the presence of severe periodontal disease in both cases.

4. Discussion

Broad-range 16S ribosomal DNA gene polymerase chain reaction (PCR) is a molecular based technique used for detection and identification of bacterial pathogens in clinical specimens from patients with a high suspicion for infection. Unlike routine culture methods, molecular assays detect bacterial genetic material (DNA). They do not rely on growth of an organism and so results are unaffected by prior antimicrobial use.

It is well known that the oral cavity represents an important reservoir of microorganisms [4]. There have been well-documented associations between periodontal disease and, for example, infective endocarditis, brain, liver and lung abscess, and Lemierre's disease. Low-grade infections can persist asymptomatically and remain dormant for years. In patients with good oral health, only small numbers of mostly facultative bacterial species enter the bloodstream. This occurs following any form of dental manipulation, even daily activities such as eating and tooth brushing [5]. With poor oral hygiene, however, the number of bacteria colonizing the teeth increases, potentially introducing more bacteria into tissues and the bloodstream, leading to an increase in the prevalence and magnitude of bacteraemia [6]. Small numbers of bacteria become quickly cleared by the reticuloendothelial system, but the more intense the bacteraemia, the greater the risk for dissemination and metastatic infections. This is of particular concern for patients with prosthetic material in situ. In line with this, in a recent study, DNA of bacteria typically causing root canal infection was detected in 78.2% of thrombus aspirates of patients with myocardial infarction [7].

In recent years, the role of oral bacteria in endovascular infections has been widely debated. Present United Kingdom National Institute for Health and Care Excellence (NICE) guidance now recommends that the benefits from antibiotic prophylaxis for patients undergoing dental procedures, who are at risk of infective endocarditis, for example, are outweighed by the risks of possible adverse effects to the patient and of antibiotic resistance developing. This guidance is based on one clinical trial of antibiotic prophylaxis in the prevention of infective endocarditis. Patients with prosthetic vascular grafts in situ, who are at subsequent risk of PVGI following dental manipulation, were not included in the cohort [8]. Interestingly, a recent study looking at incidence of infective endocarditis in England from 2000 to 13 shows that prescriptions of antibiotic prophylaxis have fallen substantially and the incidence of infective endocarditis has increased significantly since the introduction of the 2008 NICE guidelines [9].

Successful management of an infected vascular prosthesis remains a significant, occasionally insurmountable challenge. If excision of the infected graft is not possible, patients need broad-spectrum antibiotics for prolonged periods of time, often chosen empirically due to the lack of microbiological data available and often lifelong, with the associated risks of adverse events that include *Clostridium difficile* infection, development of resistance, and treatment failure secondary to poor compliance. For patients undergoing surgery for an infected aortic prosthesis, high operative mortality (reportedly in the range of 10–20% for graft excision [10]) and morbidity, together with the lack of clear national consensus treatment guidelines, are constant reminders that prevention of infection should be the single priority in vascular graft surgery.

Our patients represent a small series and oral health was examined retrospectively. However, the presence of bacteria of an oral source obtained from intraoperative tissue samples and blood, collected from 4 patients with infected aortic grafts and confirmed periodontal disease, suggests revisiting the role of odontogenic bacteria in endovascular infection. Unfortunately, patient 1 died quite soon after the primary sampling and not all investigations were done in his case. Quantitative analysis of bacterial DNA was unavailable and the oral health status was not obtained. In this case, a sample of oral bacteria from either saliva or supra- or subgingival plaque in order to confirm the oral origin of these microorganisms may have been helpful. This may also be a helpful addition to any further studies going forward. In view of the catastrophic consequences of infection, it may be reasonable to recommend a simple presurgical oral assessment for all patients undergoing complex elective aortic graft surgery. In this way, any underlying periodontal disease can be addressed before surgery, the need for good oral hygiene postoperatively can be reinforced, and bacterium of oral origin can be covered when choosing antimicrobial prophylaxis.

In summary, we report four cases where odontogenic bacteria have been associated with late-onset aortic PVGI, using culture-independent nucleic acid amplification. We hypothesize that chronic oral infection may be a risk factor for the development of late-onset PVGI. To our knowledge, this has not been previously reported. We acknowledge that further evaluation of this theory is warranted.

Acknowledgment

The authors would like to thank the Department for Bioanalysis and Horizon Technologies at the Centre for Infections, Colindale, London, UK, for carrying out the molecular analysis.

References

[1] L. Legout, P. V. D'Elia, B. Sarraz-Bournet et al., "Diagnosis and management of prosthetic vascular graft infections," *Médecine et Maladies Infectieuses*, vol. 42, no. 3, pp. 102–109, 2012.

[2] C. E. Edmiston Jr., "Vascular graft acute and late-onset infections," *Infectious Diseases in Clinical Practice*, vol. 3, no. 2, pp. 147–150, 1994.

[3] V. S. Antonios, A. A. Noel, J. M. Steckelberg et al., "Prosthetic vascular graft infection: a risk factor analysis using a case-control study," *Journal of Infection*, vol. 53, no. 1, pp. 49–55, 2006.

[4] T. Pessi, V. Karhunen, P. P. Karjalainen et al., "Bacterial signatures in thrombus aspirates of patients with myocardial infarction," *Circulation*, vol. 127, no. 11, pp. 1219–1228, 2013.

[5] X. Li, K. M. Kolltveit, L. Tronstad, and I. Olsen, "Systemic diseases caused by oral infection," *Clinical Microbiology Reviews*, vol. 13, no. 4, pp. 547–558, 2000.

[6] L. Forner, T. Larsen, M. Kilian, and P. Holmstrup, "Incidence of bacteremia after chewing, tooth brushing and scaling in individuals with periodontal inflammation," *Journal of Clinical Periodontology*, vol. 33, no. 6, pp. 401–407, 2006.

[7] M. J. Pyysalo, L. M. Pyysalo, T. Pessi, P. J. Karhunen, and J. E. Öhman, "The connection between ruptured cerebral aneurysms and odontogenic bacteria," *Journal of Neurology, Neurosurgery and Psychiatry*, vol. 84, no. 11, pp. 1214–1218, 2013.

[8] NICE, *Prophylaxis against Infective Endocarditis. Antimicrobial Prophylaxis against Infective Endocarditis in Adults and Children Undergoing Interventional Procedures*, NICE Clinical Guidelines No. 64, National Institute for Health and Clinical Excellence, London, UK, 2008.

[9] M. Dayer, S. Jones, B. Prendergast, L. Baddour, P. Lockhart, and M. Thornhil, "Incidence of infective endocarditis in England, 2000–13: a secular trend, interrupted time-series analysis," *Journal Scan Summary*, 2014.

[10] P. J. O'Hara, N. R. Hertzer, E. G. Beven, and L. P. Krajewski, "Surgical management of infected abdominal aortic grafts: review of a 25-year experience," *Journal of Vascular Surgery*, vol. 3, no. 5, pp. 725–731, 1986.

Multiple Aneurysms of the Inferior Pancreaticoduodenal Artery: A Rare Complication of Acute Pancreatitis

Chris Klonaris,[1] Emmanouil Psathas,[1] Athanasios Katsargyris,[1] Stella Lioudaki,[1] Achilleas Chatziioannou,[2] and Theodore Karatzas[1]

[1] Second Department of Propaedeutic Surgery, University of Athens Medical School, "Laikon" Hospital, 17 Ag. Thoma Street, 11527 Athens, Greece

[2] Department of Radiology, University of Athens Medical School, "Areteion" University Hospital, 76 Vassilissis Sofias Str., 11528 Athens, Greece

Correspondence should be addressed to Emmanouil Psathas; epsath@gmail.com

Academic Editors: G. Pasterkamp, M. Sindel, and Y.-J. Wu

Inferior pancreaticoduodenal artery (IPDA) aneurysms are uncommon, representing nearly 2% of all visceral aneurysms, and sporadically associated with celiac artery stenosis. Multiple IPDA aneurysms have been rarely reported. We report a case of a 53-year-old female patient with a history of prior pancreatitis, who presented with two IPDA aneurysms combined with median arcuate ligament-syndrome-like stenosis of the celiac trunk. The patient was treated successfully with coil embolization under local anesthesia. The procedure is described and illustrated in detail and the advantages and technical considerations of such an approach are also being discussed.

1. Introduction

Aneurysms of the inferior pancreaticoduodenal artery (IPDAA) represent about 2% of all visceral artery aneurysms and are typically associated with pancreatic or biliary tract disease [1]. Although rare, IPDA aneurysms tend to rupture quite often and unlike other splanchnic artery aneurysms, there is no clear correlation between the size of PDAAs and rupture, which occurs in up to 75% of cases [2]. Thus, incidental diagnosis of asymptomatic IPDAAs warrants prompt evaluation and treatment. Due to their anatomical location in surgically inaccessible regions and the often coexisting pancreatic infection, open surgical repair is challenging even in cases without rupture [3]. Endovascular techniques provide an attractive alternative treatment option with minimal morbidity for patients presenting with IPDAAs. We report on the management of a female patient that was presented to our department with two IPDA aneurysms (26 mm and 20 mm in diameter) two years after an episode of gallstone pancreatitis.

2. Case Report

A 53-years-old female patient was being evaluated by her physician for atypical dyspeptic symptoms over the past eight weeks. Her medical history included gallstone pancreatitis and open cholecystectomy two years previously. At presentation, she was asymptomatic with unremarkable laboratory profile. Duplex ultrasonography of the abdomen revealed two intrapancreatic formations that represented arterial aneurysms. A CTA of the abdominal aorta and splanchnic arteries revealed two saccular aneurysms of the inferior pancreaticoduodenal artery (IPDA), 26 mm and 20 mm in diameter, respectively (Figures 1(a) and 1(b)). These findings were combined with median arcuate ligament-syndrome-like stenosis of the celiac trunk (Figure 1(c)).

Due to the location of the IPDA aneurysms, as well as patient's refusal to primarily undergoing open surgical repair, she was referred to our department for endovascular treatment. Further image processing with 3D volume rendering demonstrated the exact anatomy of the pancreatic arterial arcade and allowed for interventional planning, since both

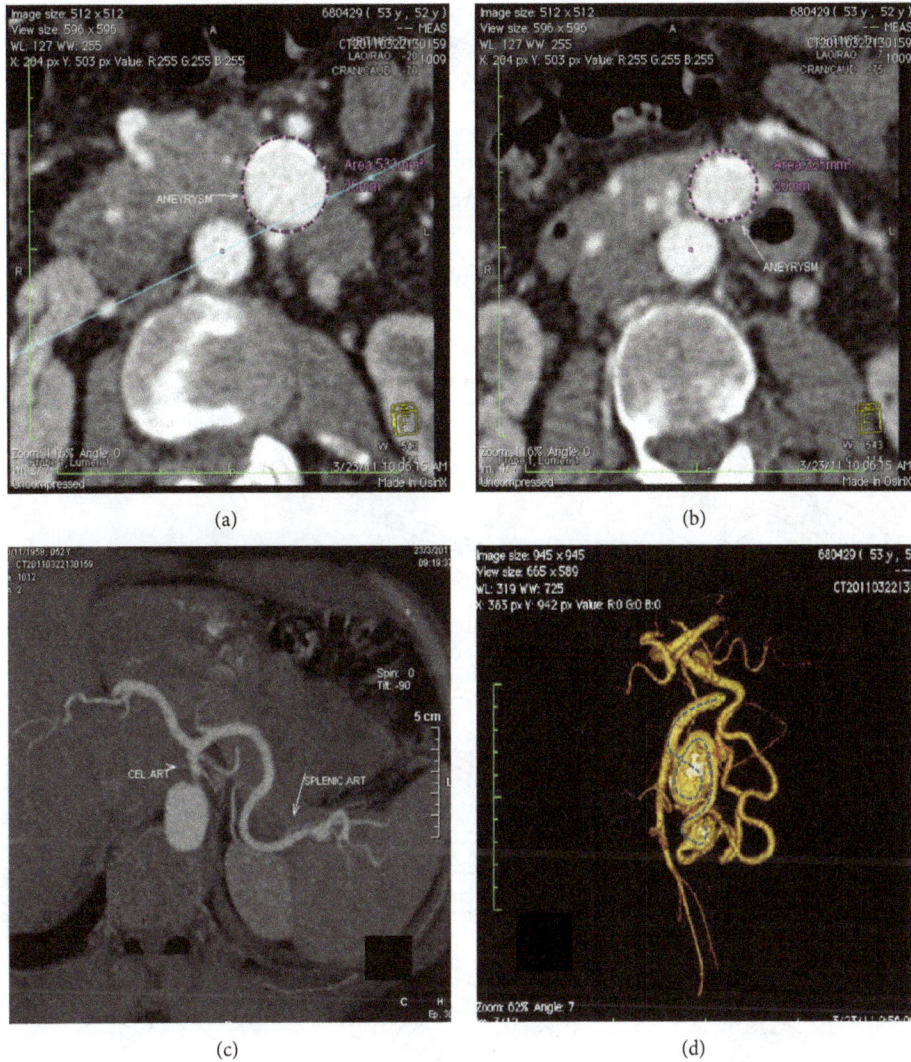

FIGURE 1: (a, b) Intrapancreatic aneurysms of the IPDA on CTA. (c) Median arcuate ligament-syndrome-like stenosis of the celiac trunk origin. (d) 3D volume rendering image processing provides closeup of the superior mesenteric artery, both IPDA aneurysms and their connecting branch.

aneurysms looked morphologically suitable for coil embolization—saccular with narrow neck—and were also connected with a small collateral branch (Figure 1(d)—dashed line). Informed consent was obtained and we proceeded with coil embolization of both aneurysms.

The procedure was performed in the operating room with a C-Arm (Philips, BV 300) under local anesthesia via right brachial access. After intravenous administration of 5.000 IU of heparin, a 6 Fr guiding sheath (Arrow International, Inc., PA, USA) was advanced to the level of the superior mesenteric artery (SMA). The ostium of the SMA was initially catheterized using a 0.035″ hydrophilic stiff Terumo guidewire and a 5F long selective multipurpose catheter using standard coaxial technique (Figure 2(1)). Subsequently, the proximal aneurysm sac was catheterized and the guiding sheath was advanced into it in order to provide additional support for further maneuvers (Figure 2(2) and (3)). Thereafter, we attempted to catheterize

the communicating collateral branch leading to the distal aneurysm. To do so, the wire and the selective multipurpose catheter had to follow a circular route around the sac, since the ostium of the collateral communicating branch was in close proximity and in a steep angle to the aneurysm neck (Figure 2(4)). With the multipurpose catheter placed at the upper proximal part of the communicating branch, the 0.035″ hydrophilic guidewire was exchanged for a BMW 0.014″ wire (Guidant Corporation, Temecula, CA), and the distal IPDA aneurysm was catheterized (Figure 2(5)). A 3F microferret microcatheter (COOK Inc., Bloomington, IN, USA) was then advanced into the distal aneurysm (Figure 2(6)), through which we proceeded to coil embolization with Hilal Embolization Microcoils (COOK Inc., Bloomington, IN, USA) (Figure 2(7)). A total of 30 microcoils were ultimately used. Thereafter, the microcatheter was withdrawn and the multipurpose selective catheter was pulled back into the proximal

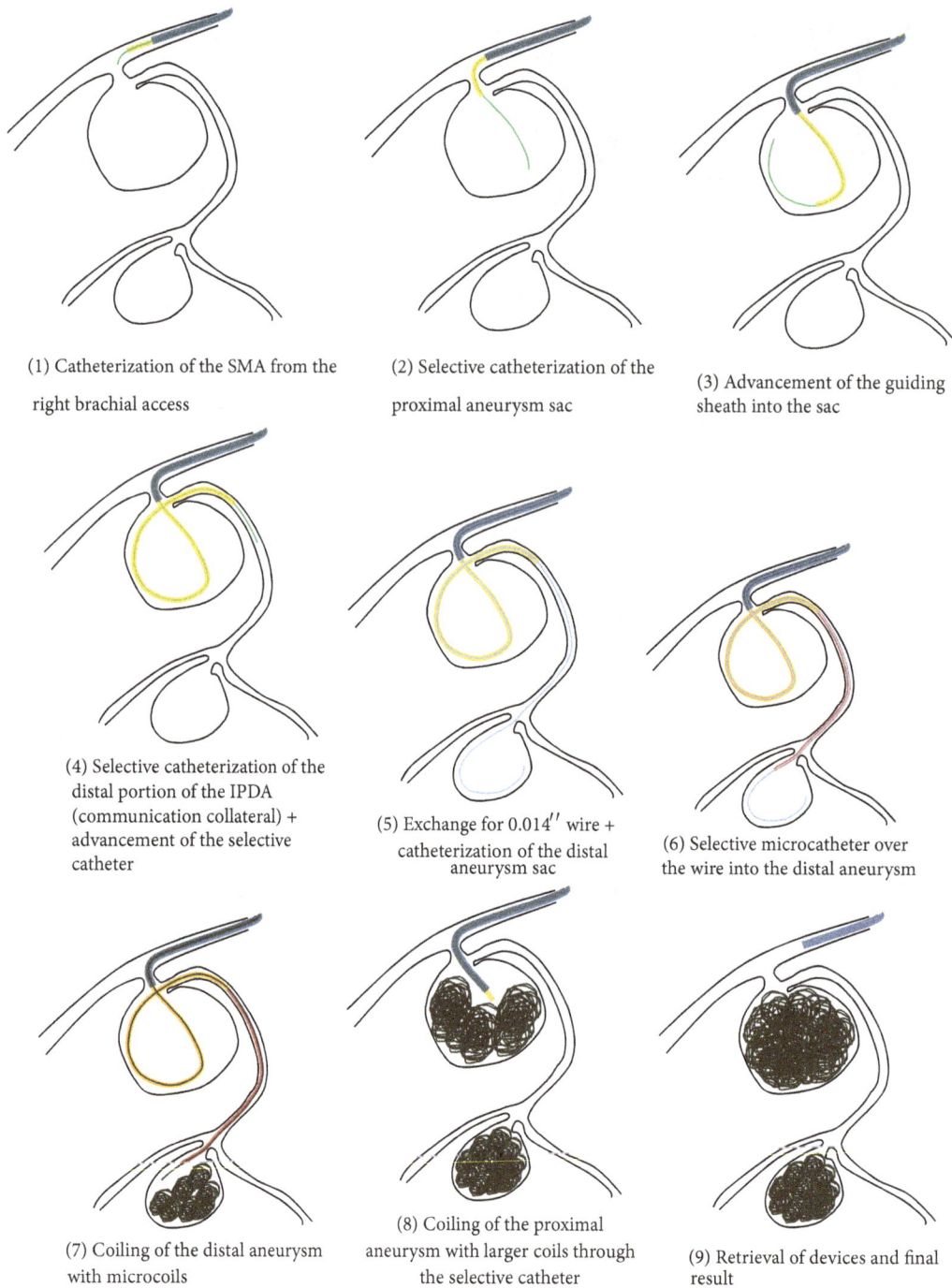

(1) Catheterization of the SMA from the right brachial access

(2) Selective catheterization of the proximal aneurysm sac

(3) Advancement of the guiding sheath into the sac

(4) Selective catheterization of the distal portion of the IPDA (communication collateral) + advancement of the selective catheter

(5) Exchange for 0.014″ wire + catheterization of the distal aneurysm sac

(6) Selective microcatheter over the wire into the distal aneurysm

(7) Coiling of the distal aneurysm with microcoils

(8) Coiling of the proximal aneurysm with larger coils through the selective catheter

(9) Retrieval of devices and final result

FIGURE 2: Diagram demonstrating the steps of the procedure. SMA: superior mesenteric artery, colors—blue: guiding sheath, yellow: selective catheter, green: 0.035″ hydrophilic guidewire, red: microcatheter, Cyan: 0.014″ guidewire, olive gray: coils.

aneurysm sac. The latter was successfully embolized with larger 15 mm MReye Embolization Coils (COOK Inc., Bloomington, IN, USA) (Figure 2(8)). After successful coiling of both aneurysms, the whole system was retrieved and hemostasis was achieved with manual compression (Figure 2(9)). The whole procedure lasted for 94 minutes with total fluoroscopy time of 38 minutes and minimal blood loss (<50 mL). The patient was sent back to the ward and

was discharged the following day. Follow-up imaging with CTA at 1 and 3 months postoperatively revealed patent SMA with preservation of collaterals and successful thrombosis of both IPDA aneurysms without any signs of sac reperfusion or enlargement (Figure 3—blue arrows). The patient remained well 18-month after intervention and is being followed up with duplex ultrasound studies on a 6-month basis.

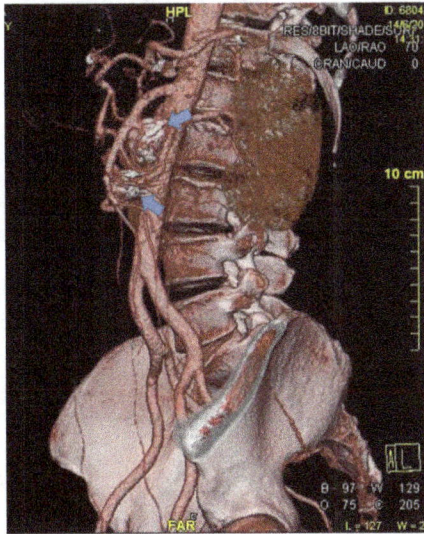

FIGURE 3: Follow-up imaging with volume-rendering lateral CTA views showing patent SMA and branches with thrombosis of both IPDA aneurysms and no sac reperfusion.

3. Discussion

Aneurysms of the pancreaticoduodenal artery (PDA) are rare and most of the time present with rupture, intra-abdominal hemorrhage, or pancreaticus [4]. Mortality in ruptured PDAAs is high, approximating 29% of cases [5], making thus their early detection and prompt treatment mandatory. Asymptomatic PDA aneurysms are diagnosed incidentally during abdominal ultrasound or CT/MRI for other indications. Apart from atherosclerosis PDA aneurysms may be also due to other etiologies including pancreatitis, biliary disease, fibrodysplasia, trauma, and congenital anomalies. The coexistence of a IPDAA with celiac trunk stenosis or occlusion has been well described [6], although the presence of multiple aneurysms—as in our case—is extremely rare [7].

Open surgical repair includes a variety of major operations, ranging from simple ligation with or without revascularization to partial pancreaticoduodenectomy [3]. Mortality rates are high and reported to be up to 19% [8]. On the other hand, endovascular methods including cyanoacrylate glue thrombosis, aneurysm exclusion using a stent graft, and embolization with intravascular coils or detachable balloons [9] provide an attractive alternative with minimal morbidity and mortality compared to open surgery [10].

The use of coils in particular offers many advantages over other endovascular techniques, mostly because of the precision in their deployment and preservation of collateral branches. Nevertheless, selective catheterization of the sac and coiling can be challenging and has also anatomical limitations. In cases of saccular aneurysms, the diameter of the neck and the neck-sac diameter ratio is a crucial point and should not exceed 3 mm and 1.5, respectively, in order to avoid embolization of the coil outside the sac to distal arterial branches [11].

Careful examination of the 3D-CTA images in multiple views can help planning a safe endovascular approach and provides adequate information for the exact anatomic localization of these lesions and especially their correlation to the pancreas that is very important in case of open conversion [12]. With the advent of modern CT and MR angiography, visceral artery aneurysms less than 1 cm in diameter are routinely detected. Multislice computed tomography angiography is also a convenient imaging modality for following up after embolization, although it frequently presents with artifacts in cases of coiling and angiography is occasionally mandatory to exclude aneurysm reperfusion. Duplex ultrasonography performed by a vascular specialist is also an accurate method to follow up these patients and provides hemodynamic information for the whole visceral circulation [13].

Regarding the coexistence of celiac trunk stenosis and PDAAs, Sutton and Lawton [14] have proposed that hemodynamic changes due to celiac artery stenosis could cause aneurysm formation in the PDA. Nevertheless, during our 18-month followup, no new aneurysm or dilatation in the pancreatic arcade was noticed. Stenosis of the celiac trunk in our case was considered to be due to the compression from the median arcuate ligament rather than atherosclerotic, and therefore endovascular intervention either with PTA or stenting of the celiac trunk origin was precluded. Furthermore, due to the asymptomatic nature of the stenosis, we decided to follow up this patient rather than offering open repair.

4. Conclusion

Although inferior pancreaticoduodenal artery aneurysms (IPDAAs) represent a rare entity, they tend to rupture quite often and, unlike other splanchnic artery aneurysms, there is no clear correlation between size and rupture [2]; thus, their detection mandates prompt treatment. Selective embolization of these lesions is a less invasive procedure with minimal mortality and good results [9], although long-term followup is recommended. Multislice computed tomography angiography offers an accurate diagnosis and valuable information for preoperative planning [12].

References

[1] A. Formentini, D. Birk, R. Kunz, K. H. Orend, and H. G. Beger, "Inferior pancreaticoduodenal artery aneurysm as a consequence of traumatic acute pancreatitis: a case report and review of the literature," *International Journal of Pancreatology*, vol. 21, no. 3, pp. 263–267, 1997.

[2] S. Iyomasa, Y. Matsuzaki, K. Hiei, H. Sakaguchi, H. Matsunaga, and Y. Yamaguchi, "Pancreaticoduodenal artery aneurysm: a case report and review of the literature," *Journal of Vascular Surgery*, vol. 22, no. 2, pp. 161–166, 1995.

[3] E. Ducasse, F. Roy, J. Chevalier et al., "Aneurysm of the pancreaticoduodenal arteries with a celiac trunk lesion: current management," *Journal of Vascular Surgery*, vol. 39, no. 4, pp. 906–911, 2004.

[4] S. Santiagu, S. Gananadha, T. J. Harrington, and J. S. Samra, "Direct percutaneous puncture embolization of a peripancreatic pseudoaneurysm presenting with haemosuccus pancreaticus," *Journal of Medical Imaging and Radiation Oncology*, vol. 52, no. 4, pp. 370–373, 2008.

[5] E. Moore, M. R. Matthews, D. J. Minion et al., "Surgical management of peripancreatic arterial aneurysms," *Journal of Vascular Surgery*, vol. 40, no. 2, pp. 247–253, 2004.

[6] P. G. Tarazov, A. M. Ignashov, A. V. Pavlovskij, and A. S. Novikova, "Pancreaticoduodenal artery aneurysm associated with celiac axis stenosis: combined angiographic and surgical treatment," *Digestive Diseases and Sciences*, vol. 46, no. 6, pp. 1232–1235, 2001.

[7] S. V. Sakpal, M. Addis, and R. S. Chamberlain, "Rapid progression of multiple splanchnic artery aneurysms," *Surgery*, vol. 145, no. 5, pp. 573–574, 2009.

[8] D. P. Coll, R. Ierardi, M. D. Kerstein, S. Yost, A. Wilson, and T. Matsumoto, "Aneurysms of the pancreaticoduodenal arteries: a change in management," *Annals of Vascular Surgery*, vol. 12, no. 3, pp. 286–291, 1998.

[9] G. T. Fankhauser, W. M. Stone, S. G. Naidu et al., "The minimally invasive management of visceral artery aneurysms and pseudoaneurysms," *Journal of Vascular Surgery*, vol. 53, no. 4, pp. 966–970, 2011.

[10] S. Murata, H. Tajima, T. Fukunaga et al., "Management of pancreaticoduodenal artery aneurysms: results of superselective transcatheter embolization," *The American Journal of Roentgenology*, vol. 187, no. 3, pp. W290–W298, 2006.

[11] B. Richling, G. Bavinzski, C. Gross, A. Gruber, and M. Killer, "Early clinical outcome of patients with ruptured cerebral aneurysms treated by endovascular (GDC) or microsurgical techniques. A single center experience," *Interventional Neuroradiology*, vol. 30, no. 1, pp. 19–27, 1995.

[12] K. M. Horton, C. Smith, and E. K. Fishman, "MDCT and 3D CT angiography of splanchnic artery aneurysms," *The American Journal of Roentgenology*, vol. 189, no. 3, pp. 641–647, 2007.

[13] L. Y. Zhou, X. Y. Xie, D. Chen, and M. D. Lü, "Contrast-enhanced ultrasound in detection and follow-up of pancreaticoduodenal artery pseudoaneurysm: a case report," *Chinese Medical Journal*, vol. 124, no. 17, pp. 2792–2794, 2011.

[14] D. Sutton and G. Lawton, "Coeliac stenosis or occlusion with aneurysm of the collateral supply," *Clinical Radiology*, vol. 24, no. 1, pp. 49–53, 1973.

Endovascular Repair of a Large Profunda Femoris Artery Pseudoaneurysm

Ahsan Syed Khalid,[1] Omar M. Ghanem,[2] and Seyed Mojtaba Gashti[2]

[1] Saba University School of Medicine, Devens, MA 01434, USA
[2] Medstar Union Memorial Hospital, Baltimore, MD 21218, USA

Correspondence should be addressed to Ahsan Syed Khalid; askhalid24@gmail.com

Academic Editors: R. A. Bishara and T. Fujikawa

Profunda femoris artery aneurysms and pseudoaneurysms are a rare cause of peripheral arterial aneurysms but their risk of rupture is quite high. We have presented a case of a left lower leg pseudoaneurysm. We have shown that endovascular repair with angioplasty and stenting is a suitable treatment method for such a pseudoaneurysm. Due to the limited data on this disease, we suggest multi-institute collaboration to identify and standardize management for the treatment.

1. Introduction

Profunda femoris artery aneurysms (PFAAs) are a rare cause of peripheral arterial aneurysms; however, the risk of rupture associated with such a finding is quite high. PFAAs are mostly asymptomatic and they usually present as an incidental finding. As for symptomatic patients, a swelling in the groin region is the most common presentation [1–3]. True aneurysms of the profunda femoris artery (PFA) are relatively rare (1–2.6%) and are idiopathic in nature without any suggestive cause. On the other hand, pseudoaneurysms of the PFA are more common and are generally secondary to, but are not limited to, orthopedic procedures, fractures, and penetrating or blunt trauma [2, 4]. We present a case of a PFA pseudoaneurysm in a patient with an orthopedic history.

2. Case Report

This is a case of a 38-year-old male who underwent inter-medullary nailing of the left hip for avascular necrosis in September 2012. In March 2013, the patient presented with complaints of increasing edema of his left lower extremity associated with a palpable pulsatile mass in the anterolateral aspect of his thigh. At that point, the patient denied calf claudication on ambulation, nocturnal rest pain, or any other symptoms of the lower extremities. On exam, a palpable pulsatile mass in the anterolateral aspect of his thigh was noticed. He had a palpable thrill over it. Nevertheless, all lower extremity pulses were palpable.

A computed tomography (CT) angiogram (Figure 1) with 3-dimensional reconstructions (Figure 2) was obtained. The imaging revealed a left PFA pseudoaneurysm measuring 5 cm in AP diameter. The neck of the pseudoaneurysm was located 6 cm distal to the femoral bifurcation. In April 2013, the patient underwent exclusion of the left PFA pseudoaneurysm via covered stent placement.

3. Procedure

Right common femoral artery (CFA) access was obtained with a micropuncture needle. A crossover catheter was used to gain access to the left common iliac artery and a 7-French Ansel sheath was introduced over a stiff guidewire and parked in the left CFA. Selective angiography was performed again to precisely delineate the area of the pseudoaneurysm and its neck.

At this time, a 10 × 38 mm iCAST balloon expandable stent was deployed across the aneurysm and dilated using a 12 × 40 mm balloon. Angiography showed exclusion of the pseudoaneurysm; however, there appeared to be an endoleak

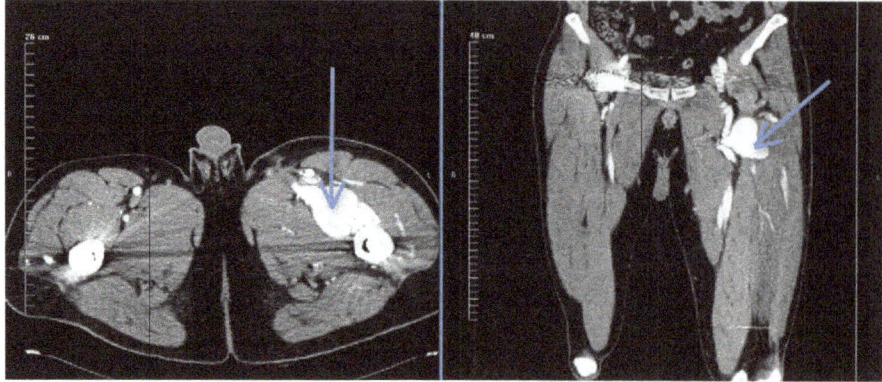

FIGURE 1: CT angiogram showing the left profunda femoris artery pseudoaneurysm.

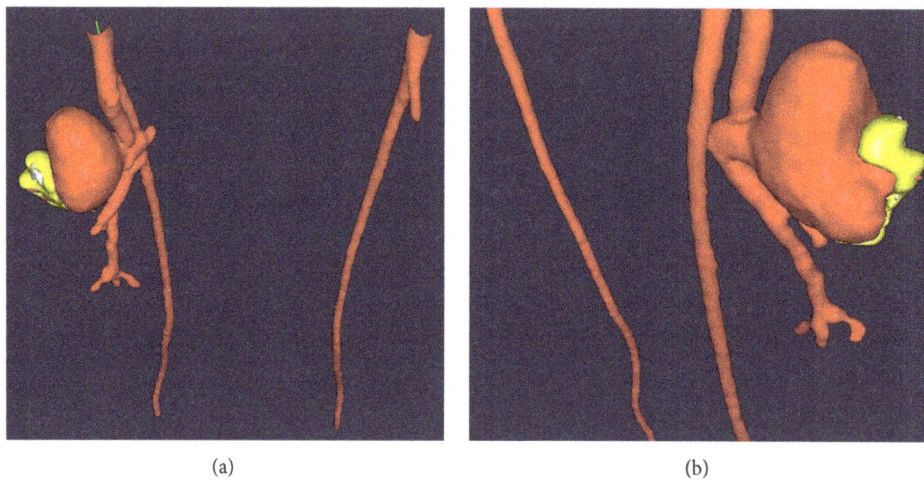

(a)   (b)

FIGURE 2: 3D reconstruction of left profunda femoris artery pseudoaneurysm. (a) Posterior-superior view, (b) left anterolateral view.

from the proximal aspect. Therefore, a second stent was introduced in a similar fashion that overlapped the first one and extended more proximally. A repeat angiogram showed excellent results without any flow into the pseudoaneurysm (Figure 3).

4. Outcome

The patient tolerated the procedure well. One month followup showed significant decrease in the left lower extremity edema. There existed no associated pain or discomfort. Moreover, on his 6-month followup, the patient was clinically asymptomatic and had no bruit or thrills over the profunda femoris site.

5. Discussion

PFAA is an uncommon disease with limited data describing the course and optimal management. After reviewing several publications, solitary PFAAs account for roughly 0.5% of peripheral aneurysms [2, 5]. The risk of rupture in PFAAs is high and it is attributed to the large size of the aneurysm at the

time of diagnosis. The increased size of the PFAA compared to other aneurysms such as a CFA and iliac vessel aneurysms is likely due to its deep location beneath the anterior muscles of the thigh. This makes the diagnosis difficult and thus leads to a delayed presentation [2, 6]. According to Tait et al., this increased size is the reason for the high risk of rupture of 30–45% of PFAAs relative to other peripheral aneurysms [7].

Most patients are asymptomatic and are diagnosed secondary to other diseases. Symptomatic patients most often present with a swelling of the upper thigh. Other symptoms of PFAAs include local compression of surrounding structures such as veins or nerves and thrombosis leading to ischemia and rupture. Moreover, PFAAs can serve as a distal source of emboli [1, 3, 8]. Our patient presented solely with a swelling of the left thigh with an associated palpable thrill. There were no other accompanying symptoms. The average size of PFAAs is difficult to document due to the rarity of the disease but a literature review by Posner et al. reported an average size of 7.4 ± 3 cm and an average age of 73.5 ± 10 years at time of presentation. In our 38-year-old male patient, the pseudoaneurysm measured 5 cm in AP diameter. Posner et al. reviewed 46 cases of PFAAs and found PFAAs to be more common in men (>92%) compared to women.

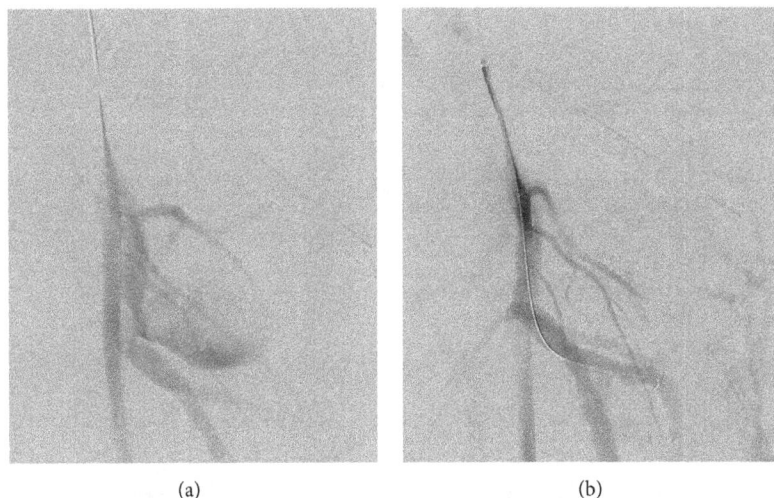

(a)   (b)

FIGURE 3: Angiogram of left lower extremity showing (a) the left profunda femoris pseudoaneurysm and (b) the poststent placement angiogram showing resolution of the pseudoaneurysm.

CT angiography and ultrasound are the appropriate imaging modalities used in the diagnosis of a PFAA [3, 6]. In addition, intraoperative intravenous ultrasound can be used to further characterize the pseudoaneurysm. In our case, we did not utilize intravenous ultrasound since the sizes of the pseudoaneurysm and the neck were characterized by preoperative CT angiography with 3D reconstruction. Previous studies have shown that 65–75% of PFAAs present with an accompanying aneurysm, namely, popliteal (47%), aortic (33%), and iliac (19%); thus, it would be beneficial to investigate for a PFAA in a patient who presents with an aneurysm elsewhere [1, 2]. Treatment options for PFAA should be geared towards removal of the risk of rupture as well as embolization, pain, and any compromised blood flow to the lower extremities. Upon diagnosis, the aneurysm should be repaired at the earliest convenience and reasonable recommendations suggest that repair should be considered immediately at a threshold of 2 cm or greater [1, 9]. However, most aneurysms have been and will be found at a size already greater than that since there is no indication to screen for PFAAs.

Standard treatment of the PFAA has been open surgery with either ligation of the PFA or reconstruction with a vein or a graft. The decision to undergo either one depends on the condition of the SFA. If the SFA is patent, then ligation of the PFA is permissible since there will be blood flow through the femoralpopliteal tract. However, it is suggested that it is best to repair the PFA rather than ligate, as this will maintain optimal flow to the lower extremity. If there is SFA disease or distal vascular disease, which can be associated with PFAA, it is a must to reconstruct the PFA to prevent ischemia to the lower limb, as the PFA is important for collateral circulation [1, 3, 9, 10].

Data on endovascular repair is limited with reports showing successful repair of a PFAA with endovascular coil embolization and others deploying covered stents to exclude the aneurysm [4, 6, 10, 11]. However, an embolization technique may be inappropriate in previous or current SFA occlusive disease [10, 11]. The literature suggests that PFA stenting is a good alternative [11]. Two published cases reported a ruptured PFAA that was successfully repaired with deployment of a stent [4, 10]. In our review of the literature, an endovascular approach was shown to be successful and is a less invasive alternative to open surgery [4, 6]. Although our patient had no history of SFA disease, we decided that endovascular repair with angioplasty and stent placement was the optimal route in management for our patient.

6. Conclusion

We reported a rare case of a pseudoaneurysm of the left PFA. On followup with our patient, he is doing well and there have been no complications with the procedure. We have shown that endovascular repair with angioplasty and stent placement is a reasonably safe and effective and a less invasive option for treatment compared to open surgery. Because of the limited data on endovascular repair of PFAAs, we suggest multi-institute collaboration to identify and standardize the management of this disease.

References

[1] C. Harbuzariu, A. A. Duncan, T. C. Bower, M. Kalra, and P. Gloviczki, "Profunda femoris artery aneurysms: association with aneurysmal disease and limb ischemia," *Journal of Vascular Surgery*, vol. 47, no. 1, pp. 31–35, 2008.

[2] S. R. Posner, J. Wilensky, J. Dimick, and P. K. Henke, "A true aneurysm of the profunda femoris artery: a case report and

review of the english language literature," *Annals of Vascular Surgery*, vol. 18, no. 6, pp. 740–746, 2004.

[3] A. Idetsu, M. Sugimoto, M. Matsushita, and T. Ikezawa, "Solitary profunda femoris artery aneurysm," *Annals of Vascular Surgery*, vol. 25, no. 4, pp. 13–15, 2011.

[4] S. Saha, V. Trompetas, B. Al-Robaie, and H. Anderson, "Endovascular stent graft management of a ruptured profunda femoris artery aneurysm," *European Journal of Vascular and Endovascular Surgery*, vol. 19, no. 4, pp. 38–40, 2010.

[5] J. M. Roseman and D. Wyche, "True aneurysm of the profunda femoris artery. Literature review, differential diagnosis, management," *Journal of Cardiovascular Surgery*, vol. 28, no. 6, pp. 701–705, 1987.

[6] C. Klonaris, J. K. Bellos, A. Katsargyris, E. D. Avgerinos, M. Moschou, and C. Verikokos, "Endovascular repair of two tandem profunda femoris artery aneurysms," *Journal of Vascular and Interventional Radiology*, vol. 20, no. 9, pp. 1253–1254, 2009.

[7] W. F. Tait, R. K. Vohra, H. M. H. Carr, G. J. L. Thomson, and M. G. Walker, "True profunda femoris aneurysms: are they more dangerous than other atherosclerotic aneurysms of the femoropopliteal segment?" *Annals of Vascular Surgery*, vol. 5, no. 1, pp. 92–95, 1991.

[8] C. A. Johnson, J. M. Goff, S. T. Rehrig, and N. C. Hadro, "Asymptomatic profunda femoris artery aneurysm: diagnosis and rationale for management," *European Journal of Vascular and Endovascular Surgery*, vol. 24, no. 1, pp. 91–92, 2002.

[9] G. Gemayel, D. Mugnai, E. Khabiri, J. Sierra, N. Murith, and A. Kalangos, "Isolated bilateral profunda femoris artery aneurysm," *Annals of Vascular Surgery*, vol. 24, no. 6, pp. 11–13, 2010.

[10] A. Ganeshan, M. Hawkins, D. Warakaulle, and M. C. Uthappa, "Endovascular therapy for a profunda femoris artery aneurysm which ruptured following intravenous thrombolysis," *The British Journal of Radiology*, vol. 80, no. 955, pp. 147–149, 2007.

[11] G. Brancaccio, G. M. Celoria, T. Stefanini, R. Lombardi, and E. Falco, "Endovascular repair of a profunda femoris artery aneurysm," *Annals of Vascular Surgery*, vol. 25, no. 7, pp. 11–13, 2011.

20

Successful Implantation of a Coronary Stent Graft in a Peripheral Vessel

Alexander Hess, Britta Vogel, Benedikt Kohler, Oliver J. Müller, Hugo A. Katus, and Grigorios Korosoglou

Department of Cardiology, Angiology and Pneumology, University of Heidelberg, Im Neuenheimer Feld 410, 69120 Heidelberg, Germany

Correspondence should be addressed to Alexander Hess; alexander.hess@med.uni-heidelberg.de

Academic Editor: Nikolaos Papanas

Peripheral artery disease (PAD) is a complex, often underdiagnosed illness with rising prevalence in western world countries. During the past decade there has been a rapid advance especially in the field of endovascular treatment of PAD. Here we present for the first time a case reporting on the placement of coronary stent graft in a peripheral vessel for the management of a peripheral side branch perforation. Interventional angiologists or radiologists may consider such an option for complication management after injury of smaller vessels during peripheral percutaneous interventions. Further specialization and novel options of complication management as described in our case may shift the treatment from surgical to even more endovascular treatment procedures in the future.

1. Introduction

Peripheral artery disease (PAD) is a complex, often under-diagnosed illness with rising prevalence in western world countries [1]. Patients suffering from PAD present with a broad spectrum of symptoms ranging from asymptomatic vascular disease over intermittent claudication to critical limb ischemia (CLI). The overall life expectancy of patients with symptomatic PAD is 80% during 5 years of follow-up [2, 3]. CLI has a significant worse prognosis with an amputation rate of 14–20% and a death rate of 25% within the first year after diagnosis and 50% within five years [4].

Treatment of PAD involves life style modification (e.g., smoking cessation and physical exercise), consequent risk factor control (e.g., statin use), antithrombotic treatment, and endovascular or surgical revascularization. During the past decade there has been a rapid advance especially in the field of endovascular treatment of PAD, contributing to significant reduction of symptoms and improvement of outcomes in such patients. Thus, the number of major amputations decreases, with increasing rates of successful endovascular procedures within the last decade [5]. The recent ERASE study [6], on the other hand, showed that combining endovascular revascularization with supervised exercise training resulted in substantial improvement of clinical symptoms in patients with intermittent claudication. Despite all these technical advances with endovascular treatment option, complications during such procedures may still occur and their appropriate management remains a challenge for clinicians. One of the most feared complications is bleeding, which can lead to large painful hematoma or even to compartment syndrome.

2. Case Presentation

An 88-year-old patient suffering from Fontaine stage IIb peripheral artery disease of his left leg was referred for interventional treatment in our angiology department. Using digital subtraction angiography (DSA) high grade lesions were identified in both his left common iliac and left superficial femoral artery, which were treated by percutaneous trans-luminal angioplasty (PTA) and placement of a bare metal (12 ∗ 40 mm Dynamic, Biotronik, Berlin, Germany) stent and by drug-eluting PTA (6.0 ∗ 120 mm, INPACT Admiral, *Medtronic*, Minneapolis, USA), respectively, using a 0.035″ Terumo Stiff hydrophilic guide wire (Figures 1(a)–1(d)). A minor not flow-limiting dissection was treated with DEB to

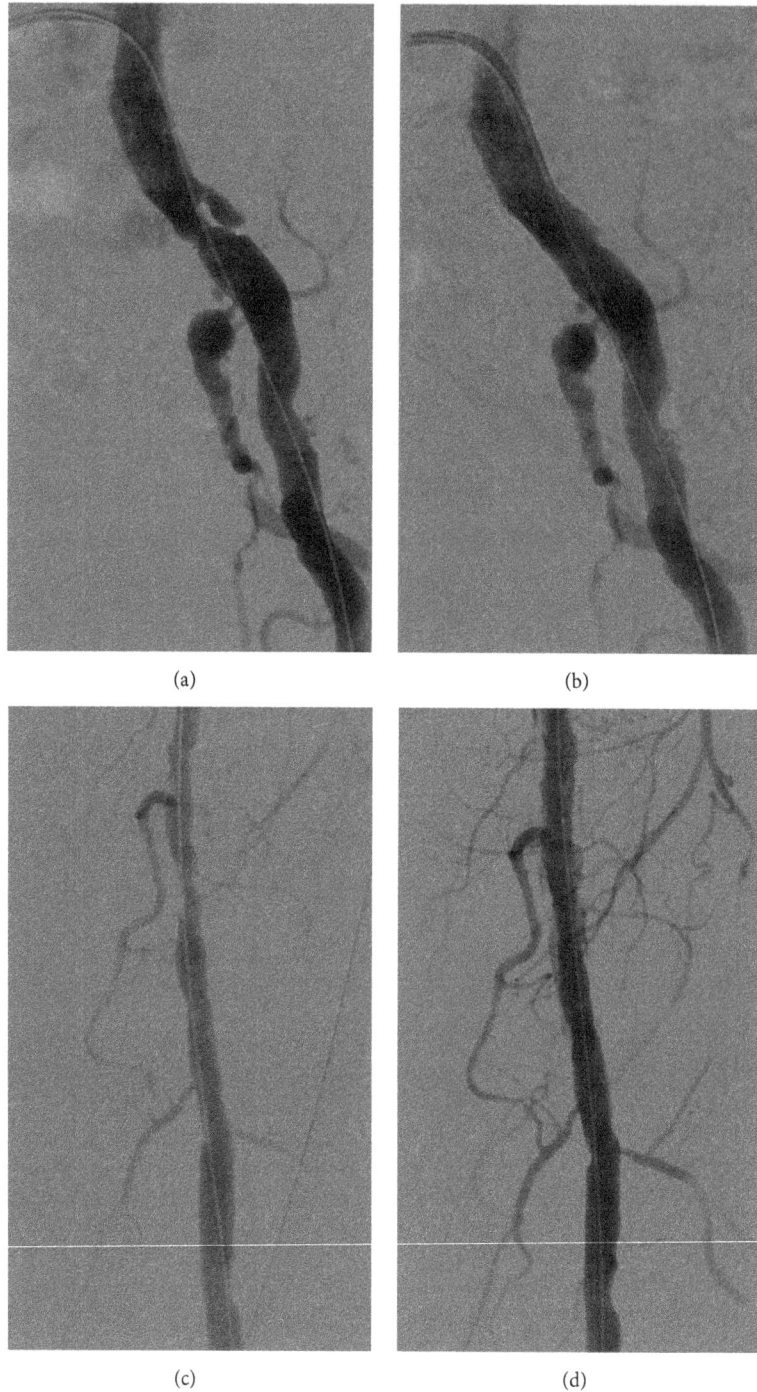

(a)

(b)

(c)

(d)

FIGURE 1: Left common iliac artery before (a) and after (b) percutaneous transluminal angioplasty and placement of one bare metal stent. Left superficial femoral artery before (c) and after (d) percutaneous transluminal angioplasty with a drug eluting balloon.

prevent restenosis. At the end of the procedure a cine angiography of the leg and of the popliteal artery was performed, which revealed that presumably during the intervention a very small side branch of the popliteal artery was accidentally perforated, possibly by the distal end of the 0.035″ guide wire (Figure 2(a), online video 1 in Supplementary Material available online at http://dx.doi.org/10.1155/2015/725168). Visualization of the perforation was performed using DSA

and the small side branch was wired by a 0.014″ coronary guide wire (Figure 2(b), online videos 2 and 3). Repeated hemostasis by balloon occlusion of the popliteal artery (5.0 ∗ 40 mm angioplasty balloon, 3 times over 5 minutes, resp.) and by inflation of a blood pressure cuff proximally to the knee at 20 mmHg over the arterial pressure for another 3 times over 5 minutes, respectively, failed to stop bleeding out of the side branch. Thus, at that time two treatment options appeared

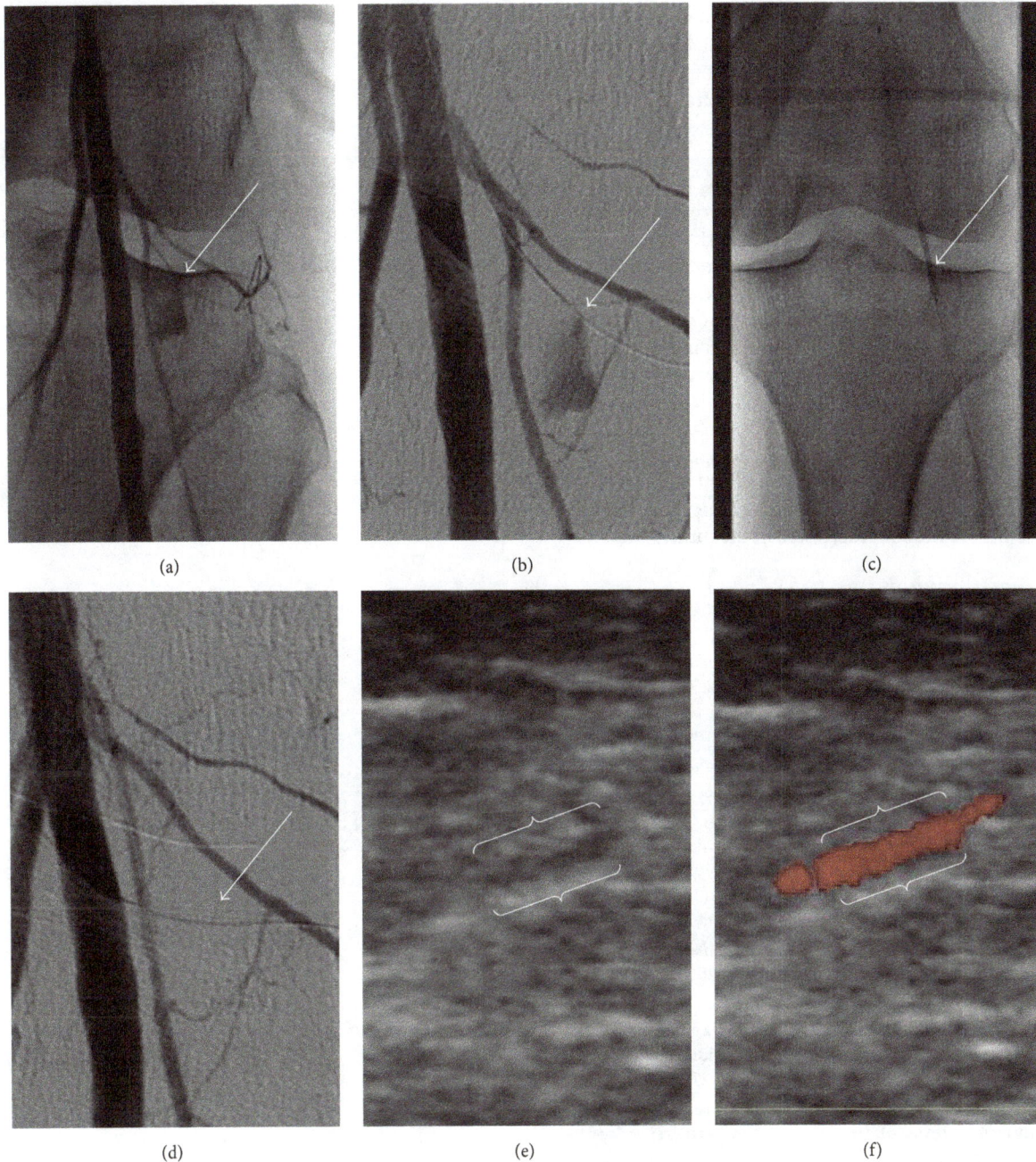

FIGURE 2: Perforation of a small side branch of the popliteal artery presumably by the 0.035″ Terumo guide wire (white arrow in (a)). A 0.014″ wire was subsequently inserted into this side branch (b), and bleeding was stopped after placement of a coronary Direct-Stent stent graft (c and d). Using colour doppler ultrasound the stent graft (white brackets) could be visualized one day after implantation, exhibiting normal blood flow (e and f).

reasonable, including (1) placement of a coated stent graft over the popliteal artery, covering the perforated side branch, or (2) placement of a coated small diameter coronary stent graft in the perforated side branch. In order to avoid long-term stent fracture of a coated stent graft placed in part of the mobile popliteal segment we decided to choose the second treatment option. Firstly, small diameter coronary balloon (Tazuna 1.5 ∗ 10 mm, Terumo Germany GmbH, Eschborn, Germany) was inserted over the wire in the perforated side branch and during balloon inflation with 14 bars bleeding ceased immediately (online video 4). Subsequently, implantation of a Direct-Stent stent graft (2.5 ∗ 19 mm, In Situ Technologies Inc., St. Paul, MN, USA) was performed in the perforated side branch, successfully and permanently stopping bleeding in this segment (Figures 2(c) and 2(d), online video 5). Our patient could be directly mobilized 4 hours after the intervention and did not report any local pain, paraesthesia, or intermittent claudication. Using colour doppler ultrasound the stent graft could be visualized one day after implantation, exhibiting normal blood flow. No signs of haematoma or other bleeding complications could be visualized by ultrasonography (Figures 2(e) and 2(f)).

3. Discussion

To our knowledge this is the first case reporting on the placement of coronary stent graft in a peripheral vessel for the management of a peripheral side branch perforation. Interventional angiologists or radiologists may consider such an option for complication management after injury of smaller vessels during peripheral percutaneous interventions. In the past years significant technical developments have occurred with endovascular therapy, which offer several distinct advantages over open surgical revascularization techniques in selected lesions [7]. Further specialization and novel options of complication management as described in our case may shift the treatment from surgical to even more endovascular treatment procedures in the future.

References

[1] A. Gallino, V. Aboyans, C. Diehm et al., "Non-coronary atherosclerosis," *European Heart Journal*, vol. 35, no. 17, pp. 1112–1119, 2014.

[2] P. M. Rothwell, A. J. Coull, L. E. Silver et al., "Population-based study of event-rate, incidence, case fatality, and mortality for all acute vascular events in all arterial territories (Oxford Vascular Study)," *The Lancet*, vol. 366, no. 9499, pp. 1773–1783, 2005.

[3] L. Norgren, W. R. Hiatt, J. A. Dormandy, M. R. Nehler, K. A. Harris, and F. G. R. Fowkes, "Inter-society consensus for the management of peripheral arterial disease (TASC II)," *Journal of Vascular Surgery*, vol. 45, no. 1, supplement, pp. S5–S67, 2007.

[4] M. Brooks and M. P. Jenkins, "Acute and chronic ischaemia of the limb," *Surgery*, vol. 26, no. 1, pp. 17–20, 2008.

[5] N. Malyar, T. Fürstenberg, J. Wellmann et al., "Recent trends in morbidity and in-hospital outcomes of in-patients with peripheral arterial disease: a nationwide population-based analysis," *European Heart Journal*, vol. 34, no. 34, pp. 2706–2714, 2013.

[6] F. Fakhry and M. G. Hunink, "Randomized comparison of endovascular revascularization plus supervised exercise therapy versus supervised exercise therapy only in patients with peripheral artery disease and intermittent claudication: results of the endovascular revascularization and supervised exercise (ERASE) trial," *Circulation*, vol. 128, pp. 2704–2722, 2013.

[7] C. J. White and W. A. Gray, "Endovascular therapies for peripheral arterial disease: an evidence-based review," *Circulation*, vol. 116, no. 19, pp. 2203–2215, 2007.

21

Onyx Embolization of Ruptured Intracranial Aneurysm Associated with Behçet's Disease

Maher Kurdi,[1] Saleh Baeesa,[2] Mohammed Bin-Mahfoodh,[3] and Khalil Kurdi[4]

[1] Pathology Department, Faculty of Medicine, King Abdulaziz University, Jeddah 21589, Saudi Arabia
[2] Division of Neurological Surgery, Faculty of Medicine, King Abdulaziz University, Jeddah 21589, Saudi Arabia
[3] Neurosciences Department, King Faisal Specialist Hospital and Research Center, Jeddah 21499, Saudi Arabia
[4] Radiology Department, King Faisal Specialist Hospital and Research Center, Jeddah 21499, Saudi Arabia

Correspondence should be addressed to Saleh Baeesa; sbaeesa@kau.edu.sa

Academic Editors: K. A. Filis and Y.-J. Wu

Introduction. Intracranial aneurysms associated with Behçet's disease (BD) are a rare occurrence. They are fragile, thin-walled pseudoaneurysms, which have high tendency to rupture and present a therapeutic challenge. *Case Presentation.* We report a 26-year-old male with BD presented with subarachnoid hemorrhage due to ruptured middle cerebral artery aneurysm. Additionally, two unruptured aneurysms were identified. He underwent endovascular embolization using Onyx with successful obliteration of the ruptured aneurysm. Medical therapy resulted in regression of one and resolution of the other aneurysms. *Conclusion.* We describe the first report of the application of Onyx for obliteration of ruptured cerebral aneurysm in BD as a feasible and safe therapeutic option for patients who are not candidates for other techniques.

1. Introduction

Behçet's disease (BD) is a multisystem inflammatory disorder of unknown etiology characterized by recurrent oral and genital ulcerations, optic manifestations of uveitis, iritis, and retinitis, and dermatological manifestations of erythema nodosum and pseudofolliculitis [1]. The most important morbidity encountered during the disease progression is vascular involvement with overall incidence of 7–29% [2]. Although relatively common in systemic visceral and peripheral vessels, the involvement of intracranial vessels is extremely rare, with overall incidence of 0.3–1.5% [3–5]. Because of the high risk of mortality from ruptured intracranial aneurysms in BD, a high suspicious index and diagnostic imaging surveillance are recommended. Symptomatic intracranial aneurysms are challenging to treat due to their configuration and distal location, and they require either urgent surgical clipping or endovascular treatment.

We describe a patient with BD who experienced a subarachnoid hemorrhage (SAH) secondary to a ruptured right fusiform middle cerebral artery (MCA) aneurysm associated with multiple aneurysms of the anterior and posterior circulations. He was treated by endovascular embolization of the ruptured aneurysm, for the first time in the literature to our knowledge, using liquid embolic agent Onyx (an ethylene vinyl alcohol copolymer) with successful preservation of the parent artery; medical therapy followed for the asymptomatic smaller aneurysm.

2. Case Report

A 26-year-old Saudi Arabian male, with a 9-month diagnosis of BD, presented on October 2010 with sudden onset of headache and generalized tonic clonic seizure. His initial computed tomography (CT) scan of the brain report revealed a significant SAH in the right sylvian fissure. He was then transferred to our institution for definitive management.

General physical examination revealed normal vital signs, with mild neck rigidity. He had a mild sclera injection, and there were with no skin or mucosal lesions. The neurological examination revealed an alert, oriented patient without focal neurological deficit. Routine blood investigations, including complete blood count, electrolytes, and renal and coagulation profiles, were within normal values. A subsequent brain CT

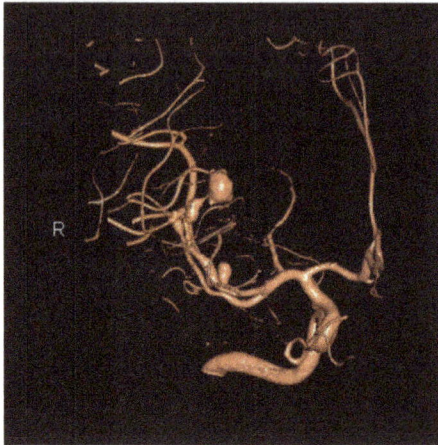

FIGURE 1: Oblique CTA scans demonstrating an ectatic fusiform dilatation of the involved MCA distal branch with aneurysm, in addition to saccular smaller aneurysm at the origin of MCA bifurcation.

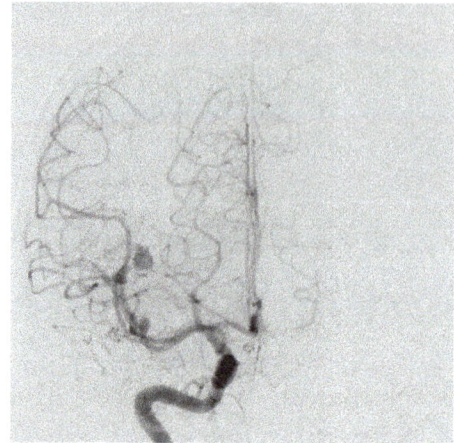

FIGURE 2: Lateral CTA scans demonstrating an ectatic fusiform dilatation of the involved MCA distal branch with aneurysm. In addition, a saccular smaller aneurysm at the origin of MCA bifurcation and another fusiform smaller aneurysm at the first segment of PCA were demonstrated.

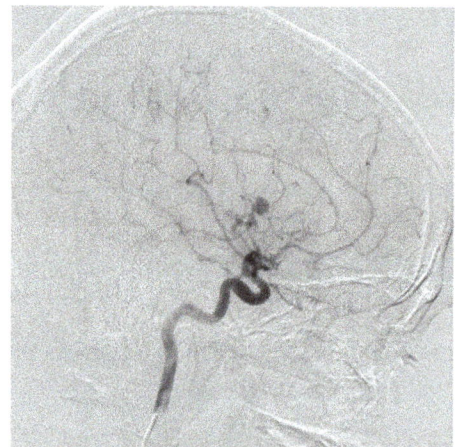

FIGURE 3: Anterior-posterior view of cerebral angiographic (DSA) image demonstrating an 8 mm right M3-MCA fusiform aneurysm and a 4 mm M2-MCA saccular aneurysm.

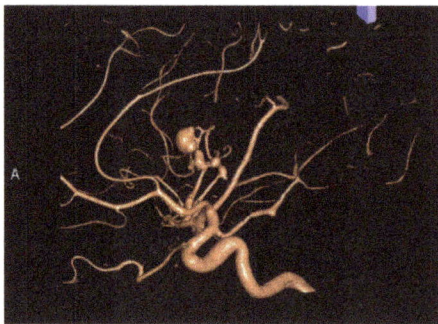

FIGURE 4: Lateral view of cerebral angiographic (DSA) image demonstrating an 8 mm right M3-MCA fusiform aneurysm with disease ectatic parent artery.

scan, on the 5th SAH day, was negative for SAH but 3D-CT angiogram revealed one large distal fusiform and another 2 smaller aneurysms: one at the right MCA and another at the right PCA (Figures 1 and 2). A conventional four-vessel cerebral angiogram (DSA) revealed an ectatic fusiform dilatation of insular M3-segment of the right MCA with 4 mm proximal (M2-segment) aneurysm and 8 mm distal (M3-segment) fusiform aneurysms (Figures 3 and 4). The left carotid and posterior circulations were normal, apart from a 3 mm proximal PCA aneurysm.

The patient was deemed ineligible for conventional therapy due to the small size of the parent artery which makes its preservation and protection not possible and carries a higher risk of rerupture and bleeding. The procedure was discussed with the patient and his family and an informed consent was obtained. Endovascular embolization using Onyx within the ruptured aneurysm was considered as a viable treatment option.

Under general anesthesia, a cerebral angiogram was performed through a right femoral artery puncture. A size 6

French guiding catheter (Guider Soft-tip, Boston Scientific) was placed in the right internal carotid artery. A Marathon microcatheter (1.5F/1.7F eV3 Neurovascular) was advanced over a silver speed 10 microwire and placed in the ruptured aneurysm against the wall. Onyx 18 was injected slowly into the aneurysm with slow lamination of the precipitated amount within the aneurysm (Figure 5). Control of Onyx 18, to avoid any penetration of the normal distal artery, was assured to allow retrograde filling of the distal normal artery via collaterals. Complete occlusion of the ruptured aneurysm was successful and filling with Onyx 18 achieved. This also resulted in cessation of flow within the fusiform dilated parent artery and the associated proximal aneurysm. Immediate retrograde filling of normal branch distal to the aneurysm was observed on the late arterial phase. A postprocedural cerebral angiogram confirmed the complete obliteration of the diseased segment in the right MCA, including the ruptured fusiform aneurysm, and the smaller aneurysm was left for medical therapy.

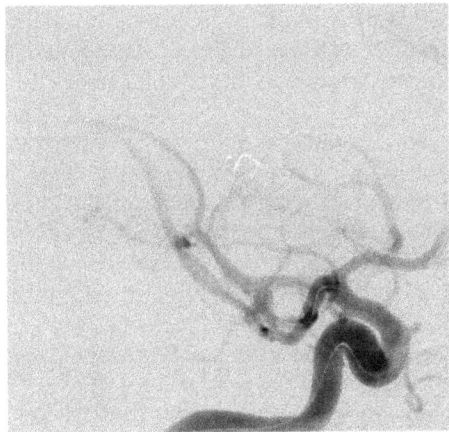

FIGURE 5: Intraprocedure cerebral angiogram demonstrating microcatheter tip placement within the fusiform aneurysm and Onyx embolization completion.

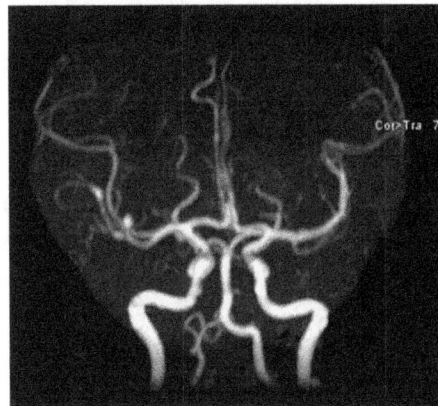

FIGURE 7: 24-hour post-Onyx embolization MRA scan in AP view demonstrating resolution of the embolized MCA aneurysm.

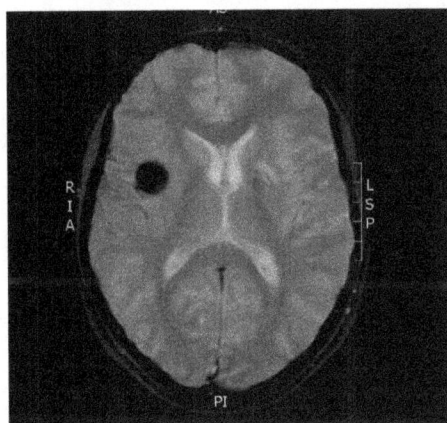

FIGURE 6: MRI-GE image scan 24 hours after Onyx embolization showing an area of low intensity at the site of embolic material within the aneurysm without ischemic complication.

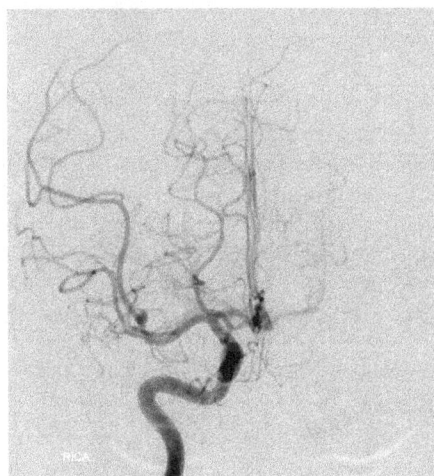

FIGURE 8: Cerebral angiographic (DSA) image in AP view of right ICA at 6-month follow-up, demonstrating complete obliteration of the embolized aneurysm with retrograde filling of the normal artery distal to the aneurysm. The smaller aneurysm has shown significant reduction in size.

Postprocedure period was uneventful; the patient was extubated and had no neurological deficits. There was no evidence of postendovascular complications on follow-up magnetic resonance imaging (MRI) and MR angiogram (MRA) scans in the next day. An area of low intensity at the site of embolic material has been revealed with resolution of the ruptured MCA aneurysm (Figure 6). Furthermore, there was no evidence of any ischemic insult (Figure 7). The patient was started on a 6-month course of prednisolone (1 mg/kg/day), azathioprine (150 mg/day), and colchicine (1 mg/day) for treatment of the remaining small aneurysm.

At 6 months of follow-up, DSA showed persistent occlusion of the right MCA fusiform aneurysm with 40% decrease in the size of the proximal MCA aneurysm, and resolution of proximal PCA aneurysm (Figures 8 and 9).

3. Discussion

The pathophysiology of vascular involvement in BD is believed to be an inflammatory related process where lymphocytic infiltrations of the vasa vasora occur leading to vasculitis and thickening of the vascular wall with subsequent thrombosis and occlusion. Less commonly, thinning of the tunica media and rupture of the internal and external membranes leading to weakness of the vessel wall and subsequent ectasia and aneurysm formation [1, 2, 5].

The overall incidence of vascular involvement in BD is 7–29% and much more frequently in men [1, 2]. Venous involvement in the form of venous thrombosis is more common (up to 85%) than arterial involvement, although both can coexist; arterial involvement, usually aortic and pulmonary vessels, occurs in 7% of patients with BD and consists of occlusion, aneurysm, or peudoaneurysm [2, 5]. Intracranial arterial aneurysm, usually of a peripheral location, is extremely rare in patients with BD. Three studies, two Moroccans and one Saudi Arabian, reported one case in each series with an incidence of 0.3–1.5% [3–5].

We reviewed the literature through PubMed search engine searching for intracranial aneurysms/SAH in BD, similar to our case. The search revealed description of reported

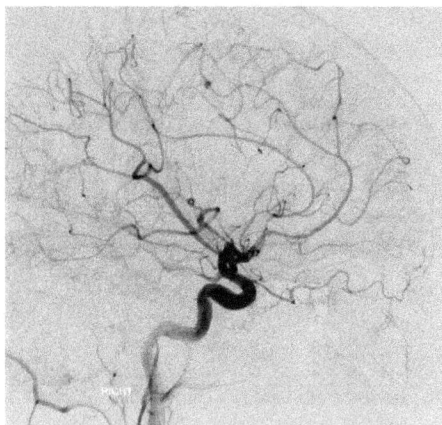

FIGURE 9: Cerebral angiographic (DSA) image in lateral view of right ICA at 6-month follow-up, demonstrating complete obliteration of the embolized aneurysm with retrograde filling of the normal artery distal to the aneurysm.

cases for intracranial aneurysms in 22 patients with BD, in addition to our case, which were summarized in Table 1 [6–27]. Few reports mentioning the occurrence of aneurysms without patient data were not added to the table. Eighteen patient (78%) were males with mean age of 40 years (range, 12–65 years). The majority (87%) presented with ruptured aneurysm causing SAH, one with MCA thrombosis leading to hemispheric infarction, one with vertebral dissecting aneurysm causing lateral medullary syndrome, and one was an incidental finding. The ethnic distribution revealed that the majorities are from far eastern (Japan) and Mediterranean (Turkey) regions. Thirty-five aneurysms were identified on angiograms in these cases, 25 (71%) in the anterior circulation and 13 of them involving MCA as the commonest artery involved. Multiple aneurysms occurred in 7 patients (30%), which predominately involved the anterior circulation, particularly MCA. Our case suffered from SAH and presented with 2 saccular and fusiform aneurysms located in the MCA, which is extremely rare and the only case reported.

Treatment of the reported cases of ruptured cerebral aneurysms in BD varied from only medical treatment to microsurgical clipping or endovascular treatment (Table 1). Microsurgical treatment was performed in 10 patients; 8 had clipping of the aneurysms and 2 had excision, with postexcision grafting performed in one. Endovascular treatment was performed in 8 patients. Coiling technique was utilized in 5 patients; one patient had VA stent, and another one had NBCA embolization, and Onyx embolization was used in our patient. Endovascular treatment has recently been the first choice of therapy despite the concern that insertion of the catheter may induce formation of pseudoaneurysm at the puncture site, or thrombosis of the vessels. Two patients with ruptured aneurysm were treated only medically with immunosuppressive drugs (corticosteroids plus azathioprine or cyclophosphamide and colchicine). One patient received no therapy after spontaneous thrombosis of the VA aneurysm, and 2 died before they receive any treatment.

There was no consistency about the indication for adjuvant immunosuppressive therapy after securing the

aneurysm. Five patients did not receive medical therapy after clipping or coiling of the aneurysm or after spontaneous resolution of the aneurysm [6, 15, 21, 22, 26]. Three patients, 2 with endovascular coiling and one with excision, did not receive adjuvant medical therapy [7, 9, 16]. Some authors emphasized the importance of receiving immunosuppressive drugs for few months, after clipping or coiling of the aneurysm, to prevent new aneurysm formation [11, 13, 14, 18–20, 23, 24]. Nevertheless, the use of immunosuppressive therapy for treatment of unruptured aneurysms may not be successful [10], which emphasizes the regular surveillance with noninvasive methods, such as MRI and MRA or CTA with high sensitivity instead of invasive procedure (DSA) [22].

Outcome could not be extracted in detail from all the reports but there was a mortality of 6 patients (26%). One patient gradually worsened and died due to the progression of the disease, and 3 patients died of severe subarachnoid bleeding and intracranial clot; the remaining patients were reported to be alive after treatment. Prognosis of ruptured intracranial aneurysms in patients with BD is unclear but is likely to be influenced by both the severity of the hemorrhage and the course of the disease [25]. On 2-year follow-up of our patient, he remained in a good condition and there were persistent occlusion of the Onyx embolized aneurysm and resolution of the smaller aneurysm after medical therapy.

The choice of treatment modality in our case was based on the presence of a small sized and diseased parent artery where preservation and protection were not possible; therefore, we did not consider surgical clipping. Endovascular treatment using coils would be technically difficult for the distal locating aneurysm, not protecting the parent artery, and carry a higher risk of rupture. Therefore, we decided to use Onyx 18 as a reasonable alternative therapeutic modality.

Onyx is a liquid embolic material, a polymer mixture of EVOH (ethylene vinyl alcohol copolymer) and DMSO (diethyl sulfoxide, opacified in micronized tantalum powder) which has a different concentration; Onyx 18 contains 6% copolymer and 94% DMSO. When onyx comes in contact with blood or water, the EVOH precipitates because of the rapid diffusion of DMSO solvent. Therefore, Onyx would precipitate and solidify into a spongy material capable of achieving permanent vascular occlusion. In contrast to other embolic materials (e.g., NBCA), Onyx has nonadhesive quality and longer working time, which minimize gluing to microcatheters or fracture and migration of embolized materials. It also can be injected several times without removing the catheter. Onyx embolization is used initially in the treatment of aneurysms associated with an AVM in the form of an intranidal ruptured aneurysm or postnidal ruptured venous varix. Its unique features for treating distally located and vasculitic thin-walled ruptured aneurysms have been demonstrated first by Utoh and colleagues (1995) using Onyx 18 to embolize a ruptured infectious PCA aneurysm [27]. With the recent advances in endovascular technology, flow diverters (pipeline embolization device) and high concentration Onyx (Onyx HD 500) have been used for treatment of large intracranial aneurysms with equally effective results [28]. Recently, cerebral aneurysm multicenter European Onyx trial, the first multicenter prospective study

TABLE 1: Summary of reported cases in the literature of ruptured intracranial aneurysms associated with Behçet's disease.

	Authors (Year)	Age (yrs.)/sex	Presentation	Ethnicity	Location	Intervention	Additional
1	Katoh et al. (1985)	29/M	SAH	Japanese	MCA	Clipping	NS
2	Buge et al. (1987)	43/M	Cerebral infarction	Moroccan	ACA, ICA, MCA. PComA	No	Medical therapy
3	Kerr et al. (1989)	12/M	SAH	Caucasian	AComA, PComA, AChor	Clipping	Medical therapy
4	Tsuji et al. (1990)	62/F	SAH	Japanese	Bilateral MCA, ICA	Clipping	NS
5	Bahar et al. (1993)	40/M	SAH	Chinese	VA	Stent	Medical therapy
6	Khodja et al. (1991)	43/M	NS	Tunisia	AComA	No	Medical therapy
7	Dietl et al. (1994)	47/F	SAH/ICH	Turkish	Bilateral ICA	Coiling	Medical therapy
8	Ildan et al. (1996)	28/M	SAH	Turkish	AComA	Clipping	Medical therapy
9	Itoh et al. (1996)	65/M	Medullary infarction	Japanese	VA	No	No
10	El Abbadi et al. (1999)	44/M	SAH	Moroccan	Bilateral MCA	Clipping	NS
11	Nakasu et al. (2001)	57/M	SAH	Japanese	Bilateral MCA	Clipping	Medical therapy
12	Rosensting et al. (2001)	36/M	SAH	Armenian	SCA	Coiling	Medical therapy
13	Kizilkilic et al. (2003)	38/M	SAH	Turkish	SCA	Coiling	Medical therapy
14		55/M	SAH	Turkish	VA	NBCA embolization	
15	Koçak et al. (2004)	37/M	SAH	Turkish	MCA	Clipping	Medical therapy
16	Zsigmond et al. (2005)	38/M	SAH	Mediterranean	AComA	Clipping	No
17	Chi and Deruytter (2005)	30/F	SAH	Japanese	SCA	Excision	No
18	Agrawal et al. (2007)	36/F	SAH	Indian	ICA	Coiling	Medical therapy
19	Kaku et al. (2007)	19/F	SAH	Japanese	Bilateral MCA	Excision and grafting	Medical therapy
20	Aktas et al. (2008)	38/M	SAH	Turkish	BA	No	No, patient died
21	Ozveren et al. (2009)	38/M	Unruptured	Japanese	ICA	Coiling	No
22	Senel et al. (2010)	45/M	SAH	Turkish	PCA	No, spontaneous thrombosis	No
23	Present Case (2010)	26/M	SAH	Saudi Arabian	Multiple MCA	Onyx embolization	Medical therapy

NS: not specified, MCA: middle cerebral artery, ICA: internal carotid artery, PComA: posterior communicating artery, PCA: posterior cerebral artery, AChorA: anterior choroidal artery, AComA: anterior communicating artery, VA: vertebral artery, BA: basilar artery, SCA: superior cerebellar artery, NBCA: N-butyl cyanoacrylate, SAH: subarachnoid hemorrhage, ICH: intracerebral hemorrhage.

using Onyx embolization for cerebral aneurysms, demonstrated decreased risk for recanalization and complications of smaller aneurysms compared with coil embolization [29].

4. Conclusion

A high index of suspicion should be raised for the incidence of cerebral aneurysms in patients with BD. Medical treatment including corticosteroid and immunosuppressive therapies should be the initial part of the management of asymptomatic aneurysms with regular imaging surveillance. However, if they rupture, endovascular treatment using Onyx should be considered as a curative therapy among other treatment modalities.

Abbreviations

NS: Not specified
MCA: Middle cerebral artery
ICA: Internal carotid artery
PComA: Posterior communicating artery
PCA: Posterior cerebral artery
AChorA: Anterior choroidal artery
AComA: Anterior communicating artery
VA: Vertebral artery
BA: Basilar artery
SCA: Superior cerebellar artery
NBCA: N-Butyl cyanoacrylate
SAH: Subarachnoid hemorrhage
ICH: Intracerebral hemorrhage.

References

[1] R. C. Wong, C. N. Ellis, and L. A. Diaz, "Behçet's disease," *International Journal of Dermatology*, vol. 23, no. 1, pp. 25–32, 1984.

[2] J. H. Park, M. C. Han, and M. A. Bettman, "Arterial manifestation of Behçet's disease," *American Journal of Roentgenology*, vol. 143, pp. 821–825, 1984.

[3] A. N. Al-Dalaan, S. R. Al Balaa, K. El Ramahi et al., "Behçet's disease in Saudi Arabia," *Journal of Rheumatology*, vol. 21, no. 4, pp. 658–661, 1994.

[4] L. Essaadouni, H. Jaafari, C. H. Abouzaid, and N. Kissani, "Neurological involvement in Behçet's disease: evaluation of 67 patients," *Revue Neurologique*, vol. 166, no. 8-9, pp. 727–733, 2010.

[5] S. Benamour, B. Zeroual, R. Bennis, A. Amraoui, and S. Bettal, "Behçet's disease. 316 Cases," *Presse Medicale*, vol. 19, no. 32, pp. 1485–1489, 1990.

[6] K. Senel, O. Pasa, T. Baykal et al., "Behcet's disease associated with subarachnoid hemorrhage due to intracranial aneurysm," *Acta Reumatologica Portuguesa*, vol. 35, no. 3, pp. 391–392, 2010.

[7] K. Katoh, K. Matsunaga, and Y. Ishigatsubo, "Pathologically defined neuro-, vasculo-, entero-Behçet's disease," *Journal of Rheumatology*, vol. 12, no. 6, pp. 1186–1190, 1985.

[8] A. Buge, D. Vincent, G. Rancurel, H. Dechy, M. Dorra, and B. C. Betourne Cl., "Behçet's disease with multiple intracranial arterial aneurysms," *Revue Neurologique*, vol. 143, no. 12, pp. 832–835, 1987.

[9] J. S. Kerr, E. S. Roach, S. H. Sinal, and J. M. McWhorter, "Intracranial arterial aneurysms complicating Behçet's disease," *Journal of child neurology*, vol. 4, no. 2, pp. 147–149, 1989.

[10] S. Tsuji, Y. Suzuki, Y. Tomii, Y. Matsuoka, H. Kishimoto, and S. Irimajiri, "Behçet's disease associated with multiple cerebral aneurysms and downhill esophageal varices caused by superior vena cava obstruction: a case report," *Ryumachi*, vol. 30, no. 5, pp. 375–381, 1990.

[11] S. Bahar, O. Coban, I. H. Gurvit, G. Akman-Demir, and A. Gokyigit, "Spontaneous dissection of the extracranial vertebral artery with spinal subarachnoid haemorrhage in a patient with Behçet's disease," *Neuroradiology*, vol. 35, no. 5, pp. 352–354, 1993.

[12] R. H. Khodja, S. Declemy, M. Batt, B. Daune, G. Avril, and P. Le Bas, "Behcet disease with multiple arterial lesions and intracerebral angiodysplasia," *Journal des Maladies Vasculaires*, vol. 16, no. 4, pp. 383–386, 1991.

[13] F. Ildan, A. I. Göçer, H. Bağdatoğlu, M. Tuna, and A. Karadayi, "Intracranial arterial aneurysm complicating Behçet's disease," *Neurosurgical Review*, vol. 19, no. 1, pp. 53–56, 1996.

[14] S. Dietl, M. Schuhmacher, H. Menninger, and J. T. Lie, "Subarachnoid hemorrhage associated with bilateral internal carotid artery aneurysms as a manifestation of Behçet's disease," *Journal of Rheumatology*, vol. 21, no. 4, pp. 775–776, 1994.

[15] K. Itoh, F. Umehara, Y. Utatsu, Y. Maruyama, and M. Osame, "Medullary infarction due to vertebral dissecting aneurysm in a patient with Behçet's disease," *Clinical Neurology*, vol. 36, no. 8, pp. 986–989, 1996.

[16] N. El Abbadi, B. El Mostarchid, A. Ababou, A. Mosadik, A. Semlali, and F. Bellakhdar, "Behçet's disease with multiple intracranial arterial aneurysms: a case report," *Journal des Maladies Vasculaires*, vol. 24, no. 3, pp. 225–228, 1999.

[17] S. Nakasu, M. Kaneko, and M. Matsuda, "Cerebral aneurysms associated with Behçet's disease: a case report," *Journal of Neurology Neurosurgery and Psychiatry*, vol. 70, no. 5, pp. 682–684, 2001.

[18] S. Rosensting, E. Dupuy, O. Alves, B. George, and G. Tobelem, "Maladie de Behcet revelee par un anevrisme intracranien," *La Revue de Médecine Interne*, vol. 22, no. 2, pp. 177–182, 2001.

[19] A. Koçak, S. Cayli, O. Ates, and K. Saraç, "Middle cerebral artery aneurysm associated with Behçet's disease," *Neurologia Medico-Chirurgica*, vol. 44, pp. 368–371, 2004.

[20] O. Kizilkilic, S. Albayram, I. Adaletli, H. Ak, C. Islak, and N. Kocer, "Endovascular treatment of Behçet's disease-associated intracranial aneurysms: report of two cases and review of the literature," *Neuroradiology*, vol. 45, no. 5, pp. 328–334, 2003.

[21] P. Zsigmond, L. Bobinski, and S. Boström, "Behçet's disease, associated with subarachnoid heamorrhage due to intracranial aneurysm," *Acta Neurochirurgica*, vol. 147, no. 5, pp. 569–571, 2005.

[22] L. H. Chi and M. J. Deruytter, "Manifestations of Neuro-Behçet's disease: report of two cases and review of the literature," *Clinical Neurology and Neurosurgery*, vol. 107, no. 4, pp. 310–314, 2005.

[23] S. Agrawal, R. Jagadeesh, A. Aggarwal, R. V. Phadke, and R. Misra, "Aneurysm of the internal carotid artery in a female patient of Behçet's disease: a rare presentation," *Clinical Rheumatology*, vol. 26, no. 6, pp. 994–995, 2007.

[24] Y. Kaku, J.-I. Hamada, J.-I. Kuroda, Y. Kai, M. Morioka, and J.-I. Kuratsu, "Multiple peripheral middle cerebral artery aneurysms

associated with Behçet's disease," *Acta Neurochirurgica*, vol. 149, no. 8, pp. 823–827, 2007.

[25] E. Aktas, M. Kaplan, and M. F. . Ozveren, "Basilar artery aneurysm associated with Behcet's disease: a case report," *Turkish Neurosurgery*, vol. 18, pp. 35–38, 2008.

[26] M. F. Ozveren, Y. Matsumoto, R. Kondo, and A. Takahashi, "Coil embolization of an unruptured intracranial aneurysm associated with Behçet's diseas—case report," *Neurologia Medico-Chirurgica*, vol. 49, no. 10, pp. 471–473, 2009.

[27] J. Utoh, Y. Miyauchi, H. Goto, H. Obayashi, and T. Hirata, "Endovascular approach for an intracranial mycotic aneurysm associated with infective endocarditis," *Journal of Thoracic and Cardiovascular Surgery*, vol. 110, no. 2, pp. 557–559, 1995.

[28] N. Chalouhi, J. F. McMahon, L. A. Moukarzel et al., "Flow diversion versus traditional aneurysm embolization strategies: analysis of fluoroscopy and procedure times," *Journal of neurointerventional surgery*, 2013.

[29] S. Simon, K. Archer, and R. Mericle, "Multicenter registry of liquid embolic treatment of cerebral aneurysms," *World Neurosurgery*, 2013.

22

Medial Clavicular Osteophyte: A Novel Cause of Paget-Schroetter Syndrome

Keagan Werner-Gibbings and Steven Dubenec

Department of Vascular Surgery, Royal Prince Alfred Hospital, Sydney, NSW 2006, Australia

Correspondence should be addressed to Keagan Werner-Gibbings; kwer2596@uni.sydney.edu.au

Academic Editor: Atila Iyisoy

Paget-Schroetter syndrome is a form of upper limb deep venous thrombosis usually seen in younger patients in association with repetitive activities of the affected limb. When occurring in more elderly patients or in those where it is difficult to appreciate a causative mechanism, other aetiologies should be considered. We present a case in which degenerative osteoarthritis of the sternoclavicular joint with osteophyte development impinged on the subclavian vein, leading to extensive upper limb thrombosis. The difficulties in identifying and managing this unusual cause of Paget-Schroetter are presented and discussed.

1. Introduction

Paget-Schroetter Syndrome is a deep venous thrombosis (DVT) of the subclavian-axillary vein complex usually seen in association with repetitive upper limb activity [1]. Anatomical variations that act to narrow the thoracic outlet such as cervical ribs and hypertrophied musculature are known to predispose towards the development of this condition. Less common causative mechanisms such as posterior dislocation of the clavicular heads and Langer's axillary arch have also been reported. We report a unique case of the investigation and management of Paget-Schroetter Syndrome caused by a large clavicular head osteophyte.

2. Case Report

A 69-year-old former competitive rower and active sportsman presented to the emergency department with a 10-day history of pain and increasing swelling to his left arm. His background history included hypertension and paroxysmal atrial fibrillation. Physical examination revealed a neurovascularly intact left arm with extensive swelling distal to the axilla. No other abnormality was detected on physical examination. The patient was left-handed. Venous duplex ultrasound demonstrated occlusive thrombus in the left upper limb venous system involving the proximal subclavian, axillary and basilic veins, and the brachial veins to the level of midhumerus. Laboratory testing showed no evidence of a coagulation disorder.

Contrast venography confirmed thrombus extending from the brachial vein to the left brachiocephalic vein (Figure 1). Mechanical thrombectomy (Angiojet, MEDRAD Inc.) was employed to decrease thrombotic burden in the affected vessels. Subsequently an infusion catheter was placed in the left brachiocephalic vein. A urokinase infusion was initiated through with daily venography demonstrating resolution of thrombus distal to the first rib following 48 hours of treatment. Angioplasty of the subclavian-axillary system with a 12 mm balloon demonstrated impingement at the level of the first rib. CT angiography of the thoracic outlet showed poor filling of the left upper limb venous system with focal narrowing of the left subclavian artery as it passed over the first rib, suspecting the presence of a fibromuscular band of the first rib causing subclavian vein compression.

Following thrombolysis, the patient underwent a left-sided transaxillary first rib resection to decompress the thoracic outlet with the aim of subsequently placing a stent across the affected portion of subclavian vein. During stent placement, performed 10 days after his first rib resection, the patient's left-sided central veins had again thrombosed, necessitating further mechanical thrombectomy to restore patency. A venous stent was then placed at the level of

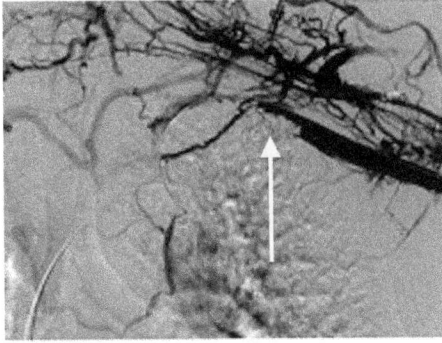

FIGURE 1: Venogram of Left subclavian vein demonstrating thrombus extending into the left brachiocephalic vein.

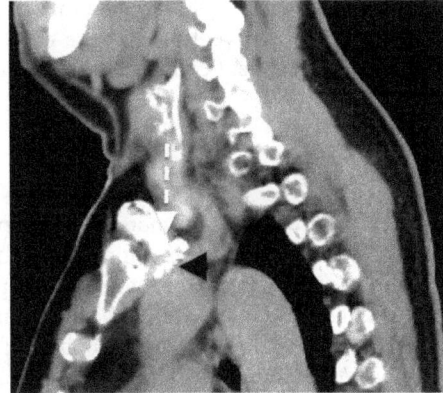

FIGURE 3: Sagittal view of left subclavian stent impingement.

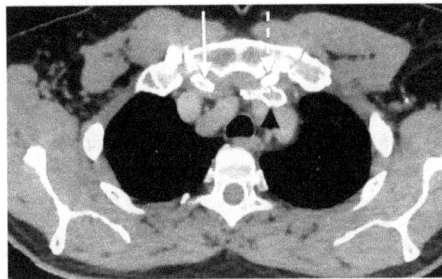

FIGURE 2: Axial view of large osteophytic projection arising from the posterior surface of the left clavicular head impinging the left subclavian stent.

venous stenosis with poststenting venography, demonstrating a widely patent vessel. The patient was discharged on oral anticoagulation therapy.

The patient was symptom-free at his 3-month follow-up; however, a CT at that time demonstrated compression of the subclavian vein stent with significant architectural distortion. The causative mechanism of this impingement was a large osteophytic projection arising from the posterior surface of the left clavicular head (Figures 2 and 3). Dedicated imaging of the sternoclavicular joints bilaterally exposed further signs of severe arthrosis and posterosuperior joint subluxation, indicating advanced osteoarthritic degenerative disease of the joint. The significance of the compression exerted by this large projection was not appreciated on the initial imaging and was likely the initiating factor of the primary thrombotic event.

A specialist shoulder surgeon was consulted on the possibility of surgical resection of the osteophytic prominence to relieve the obstruction. The expert orthopaedic opinion was that resection of the entire medial segment of clavicle was the only available course of treatment. This procedure would necessarily result in a significant functional deficit for the patient where previously none existed. The decision was therefore made to treat medically with anticoagulation and ongoing review. The patient remains symptom-free 6 months after the initial event.

3. Discussion

Effort thrombosis or Paget-Schroetter Syndrome is a form of upper limb DVT that occurs when strenuous activity of the upper limb results in subclavian vein endothelial microtrauma and activation of the coagulation cascade [2]. Anatomical variations that act to narrow the thoracic outlet such as cervical ribs, fibromuscular bands, and hypertrophied musculature are well known to exacerbate the development of Paget-Schroetter syndrome [3]. Less frequent causative mechanisms such as posterior dislocations of the clavicular head [4], pseudoarthrosis of the clavicle [5], and Langer's axillary arch [6] have previously been reported as precipitating upper limb DVT. This is the first reported case of a sternoclavicular osteophyte secondary to osteoarthritis causing subclavian vein obstruction and upper limb deep venous thrombosis.

Degenerative osteoarthritis of the sternoclavicular joint is a relatively common condition, especially in the elderly population [7], with osteophytic projections being a frequent part of the pathological process [8]. It is seen more commonly in active people and extensive rowing experience of the patient presented in this case was likely a contributing factor to the development of his degenerative joint changes.

This anatomical variant presents diagnostic and therapeutic challenges. The presence and impact of the osteophytic projection could not be fully appreciated on initial presentation as extensive thrombus in the vasculature rendered visualisation of the course and calibre of the subclavian vein difficult on CT imaging. The significance of the osteophytic projection and the severe compression it imparted on the subclavian vein could only be appreciated after surgical intervention and placement of the radiolucent stent.

The management of this condition, once identified, is challenging. The accepted treatment for sternoclavicular arthrosis causing significant pain or functional impairment is surgical resection of the medial clavicular head, as less invasive treatment is unlikely to be effective [9, 10]. In an appropriate management plan in patients with symptomatic sternoclavicular arthrosis refractory to conservative management, this procedure imparts significant functional impairment and a substantial impact on quality of life [9]. In view of the patient's active lifestyle, clavicular head resection was not an appropriate intervention and the decision was made to continue the treatment conservatively with ongoing anticoagulation.

4. Conclusion

Paget-Schroetter syndrome is common in younger active patient groups. When occurring in more elderly patients other aetiologies such as abnormal anatomical compression of the subclavian vein should be considered. As seen in this case, degenerative osteoarthritis with osteophytic development can significantly compress posterior structures and may not be appreciated until the full course of the subclavian vein is possible to be visualized.

Disclosure

There has been no duplicate or alternate submission of this work or any part thereof. All the authors of this paper have reviewed the document in its entirety and are in agreement with the structure and content.

References

[1] K. A. Illig and A. J. Doyle, "A comprehensive review of Paget-Schroetter syndrome," *Journal of Vascular Surgery*, vol. 51, no. 6, pp. 1538–1547, 2010.

[2] V. Vijaysadan, A. M. Zimmerman, and R. E. Pajaro, "Paget-Schroetter syndrome in the young and active," *The Journal of the American Board of Family Practice*, vol. 18, no. 4, pp. 314–319, 2005.

[3] G. L. Oktar and E. G. Ergul, "Paget-Schroetter syndrome," *Hong Kong Medical Journal*, vol. 13, no. 3, pp. 243–245, 2007.

[4] E. Turan, C. Suat, P. Gökhan, and D. Enver, "Bilateral retrosternal dislocation and hypertrophy of medial clavicular heads with compression to brachiocephalic vein," *The Internet Journal of Thoracic and Cardiovascular Surgery*, vol. 6, no. 1, 2003.

[5] K. Hahn, R. Shah, Y. Shalev, D. H. Schmidt, and T. Bajwa, "Congenital clavicular pseudoarthrosis associated with vascular thoracic outlet syndrome: case presentation and review of the literature," *Catheterization and Cardiovascular Diagnosis*, vol. 35, no. 4, pp. 321–327, 1995.

[6] C. Magee, C. Jones, S. McIntosh, and D. W. Harkin, "Upper limb deep vein thrombosis due to Langer's axillary arch," *Journal of Vascular Surgery*, vol. 55, no. 1, pp. 234–236, 2012.

[7] S. Kopp, G. E. Carlsson, T. Hansson, and T. Öberg, "Degenerative disease in the temporomandibular, metatarsophalangeal and sternoclavicular joints: an autopsy study," *Acta Odontologica Scandinavica*, vol. 34, no. 1, pp. 23–32, 1976.

[8] R. A. Yood and D. L. Goldenberg, "Sternoclavicular joint arthritis," *Arthritis & Rheumatism*, vol. 23, no. 2, pp. 232–239, 1980.

[9] C. A. Rockwood Jr., G. I. Groh, M. A. Wirth, and F. A. Grassi, "Resection arthroplasty of the sternoclavicular joint," *The Journal of Bone & Joint Surgery—American Volume*, vol. 79, no. 3, pp. 387–393, 1997.

[10] A. Pingsmann, T. Patsalis, and I. Michiels, "Resection arthroplasty of the sternoclavicular joint for the treatment of primary degenerative sternoclavicular arthritis," *Journal of Bone and Joint Surgery—British Volume*, vol. 84, no. 4, pp. 513–517, 2002.

23

A Giant Pseudoaneurysm of the Forearm as Unusual Complication of Bacterial Endocarditis

Michele Arcopinto, Teresa Russo, Antonio Ruvolo, Antonio Cittadini, Luigi Saccà, and Raffaele Napoli

Department of Translational Medical Sciences, School of Medicine, Federico II University, 5 Via Sergio Pansini, 80131 Napoli, Italy

Correspondence should be addressed to Michele Arcopinto; micarcopinto@hotmail.it

Academic Editors: N. Espinola-Zavaleta, A. Iyisoy, R. Zbinden, and A. Zirlik

A 59-year-old man with fever was diagnosed with endocarditis due to *Streptococcus bovis*. Two weeks after antibiotic therapy was started, he presented with red and painful swelling of the forearm without any sign of systemic inflammation. A giant hematoma connected to the radial artery was detected with ultrasound. Surgical intervention with the removal of multiple, sterile clots from the hematoma was performed, and the multiple lacerations of the artery detected were corrected. This is the first case reporting rupture of the radial artery as a complication of infective endocarditis.

1. Background

Endocarditis is a potentially life-threatening inflammation of the inner layer of the heart, mainly involving epithelium of the mitral valve. In addition to local damage and secondary hemodynamic impairment, endocarditis could cause a wide array of systemic and/or organ-specific complications with several mechanisms [1]. In the current paper, we describe the sudden development of a giant pseudoaneurysm of the forearm due to rupture of the radial artery in a patient with bacterial endocarditis diagnosed two weeks earlier and the surgical repair of the artery wall.

2. Case Description

A 59-year-old man with no history of major diseases was admitted to the hospital for the presence of fever during the previous 8 weeks, asthenia, myoarthralgia, and abdominal pain. Before being hospitalized, the patient was prescribed an offhand antibiotic therapy (amoxicillin 2 g/die for five days) without any improvement of his symptoms. On arrival, the physical examination performed showed no clear sign of disease, except for a mild systolic murmur detectable at the cardiac apex. Body temperature was between 37.5 and 38.7°C during the day, heart rate was 90 bpm, respiration

rate 20/min, and blood pressure 130/80 mmHg. Blood check showed mild neutrophilic leukocytosis, high C-reactive protein and fibrinogen. Chest radiogram and urinalysis were normal. During the following days, three consecutive venous blood samples were taken one day apart from each other for culture. In these blood cultures *Streptococcus bovis*, was constantly present. Transthoracic echocardiography showed vegetations on the anterior leaflet of the distal third of the mitral valve, associated with moderate regurgitation. According to modified Duke criteria [2], diagnosis of bacterial endocarditis was established and treatment with ceftriaxone (2 g IV, daily), based on actual bacterial susceptibility, was started and continued for the following 4 weeks. Right from the first week of treatment, the blood cultures were negative, fever disappeared, and the clinical conditions improved. The patient was then discharged. Two weeks after diagnosis, the patient returned to the hospital with a giant, red, and painful swelling on the anterior side of the left forearm (about 10 × 12 cm). This swelling appeared suddenly and was associated with rise in body temperature for a few days. No signs of ischemia in the left hand were present. Laboratory data showed an increase of inflammatory markers (C-reactive protein and erythrocyte sedimentation rate), whereas two consecutive blood cultures were negative for germs. A major trauma as a possible explanation of the forearm swelling

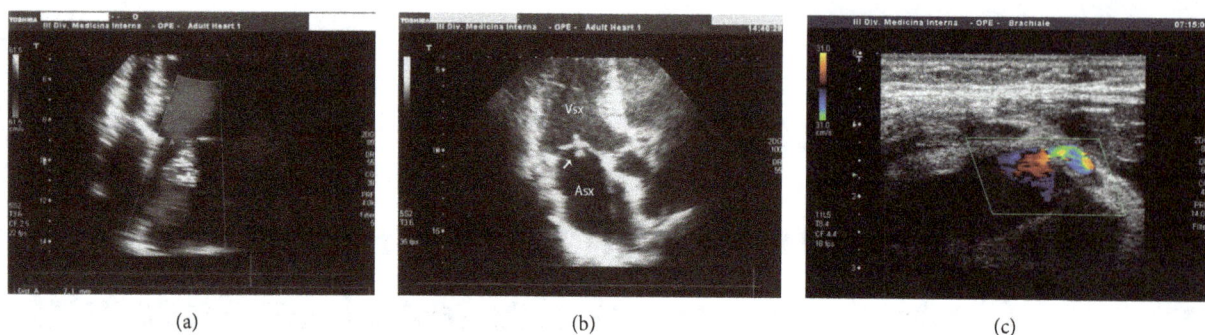

FIGURE 1: (a) Color Doppler imaging showing mild-to-moderate mitral regurgitation; (b) three-chamber apical view showing vegetation on distal third of mitral anterior leaflet; (c) echography of anterior aspect of right forearm showing color Doppler imaging of radial artery refueling perivascular blood collection.

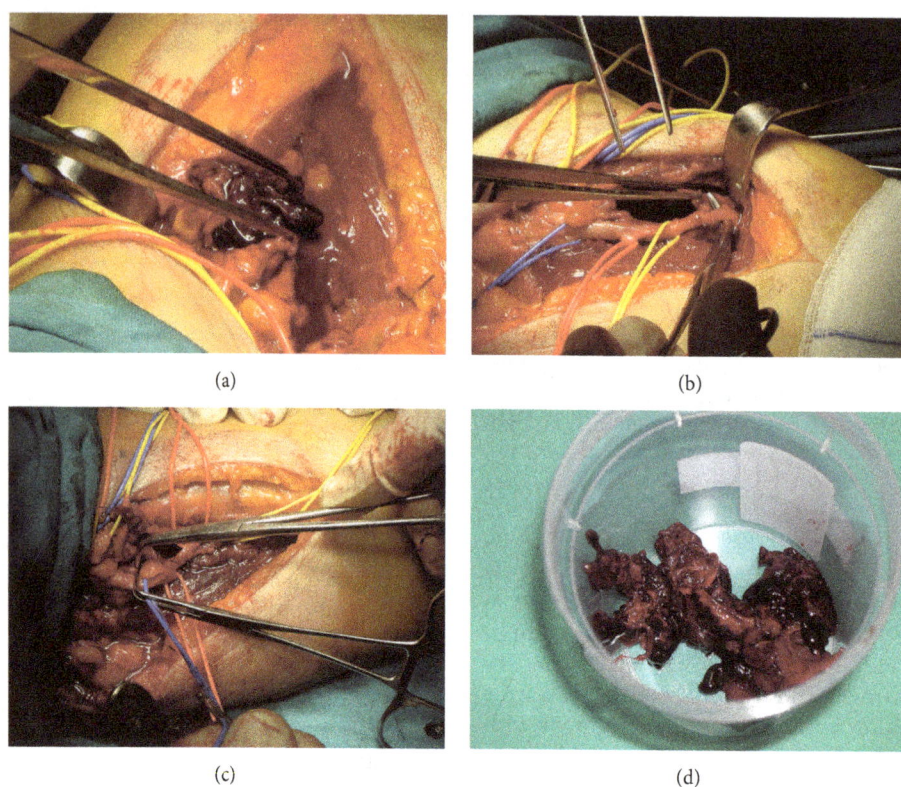

FIGURE 2: Consecutive phases of vascular intervention. (a) Clot detection immediately below muscular fascia; (b) isolation of vessels and recognition of multiple and point lacerations on the anterior and medial sides of radial artery; (c) radial arterial repair with application of 6-0 prolene sutures; (d) thrombus removed from periarterial collection.

was easily ruled out with careful patient's interview. An echography of the forearm was performed and an ~8 cm, low-echogenic, blood collection connected with the radial artery was clearly visible (Figure 1). On the basis of the results of the antibiotic testing on the *Streptococcus bovis* isolated in the original blood culture, medical therapy was upgraded with Gentamicin, 1 mg/kg every 8 hours. To stop the refueling of the pseudoaneurysm by the artery, since the surgical support was not immediately available, two consecutive 20-minute compressions of the forearm were applied, but the results were unsatisfactory. Therefore, the patient underwent

surgery for diagnostic and therapeutic purposes. During the surgery, after the incision of the brachial fascia, a big clot was evident. Several lacerations on different sides of radial artery were also visible, providing possible explanation for the blood extravasation. No vegetations or other major abnormalities of the arterial wall were found. The vessel integrity was then reconstructed with excision of the damaged segments and primary end-to-end anastomosis of the mobilized extremities with application of 6-0 prolene sutures was performed (Figure 2). Microbiological examination of the tissues removed showed complete sterility. After two additional weeks of antibiotic treatment, medical therapy was discontinued and a strict follow-up was planned. Thereafter, the patient has been checked several times till a year later and no recurrence of systemic or local signs or symptoms has been detected. Radial arterial patency and hand hemodynamics have been assessed through serial ultrasound examinations of ulnar and radial arteries. As *S. bovis* is known to be associated to colonic neoformations, we carried out also a screening colonoscopy, and four adenomatosis masses were removed from the gut.

3. Discussion

Complications of endocarditis are quite frequent and severe despite the progress made in antibiotic therapy and cardiac surgery [3]. Vascular complications are generally due to septic embolization from valve vegetations with subsequent thrombosis or hemorrhage in target organs. The most often observed complication in left-sided native valve endocarditis is cerebral ischemia due to septic embolization. Hemorrhagic strokes are less frequent and account for 12–30% of neurologic complications [4]. Intracranial hemorrhage in the setting of infective endocarditis recognizes different pathophysiologic mechanisms: transformation of primary ischemic lesions, formation and rupture of mycotic aneurysms, and rupture of intraparenchymal vessels due to necrotizing arteritis [5]. Although vascular complication of infective endocarditis might involve virtually every district in the body, far fewer cases of extracerebral arterial complications have been reported. In a multicenter prospective study including 384 cases of definite infective endocarditis, 7.3% of patients developed embolic complications after initiation of antibiotic therapy, with total embolic events (before and after antibiotic therapy) occurring in 34.1% of them [3]. Among 28 cases of complication during therapy, common sites of embolization were central nervous system (14 cases), spleen (9 cases), and peripheral artery (5 cases). Excluding vascular disease presenting as the first symptom of subclinical endocarditis, 71.4% of complications occurred in the first 15 days of adequate antibiotic treatment (median time of 7 days).

We describe the case of a patient with the rupture of radial artery secondary to subacute bacterial endocarditis sustained by *S. bovis*. As the clinical presentation of vascular involvement was atypical (no clinical findings of ischemia downstream the vascular bed), possible differential etiology including preexisting vasculitis or autoimmune diseases was considered, but no history or signs were found.

Local predisposing factors, such as previous trauma, prior surgical interventions, or professional, chronic, and mechanical solicitation, were also ruled out. Timing of onset was well in agreement with previous reports of vascular complications occurring under antibiotic therapy (14 days), but some novel aspects were present in this case. First of all, the rupture of the radial artery has not yet been reported as complication of infective endocarditis. Secondly, sterility of the clot removed during the surgical procedure makes the interpretation of arterial injury further challenging. Classic mechanisms postulated for cerebral hemorrhagic lesions, mainly mediated by aneurysm formation and rupture, do not apply in our case. Although, the patient had a low cardiovascular risk profile, and radial artery is a district poorly affected by atherosclerotic alterations, we cannot rule out preexisting, subclinical plaques of the artery tract before overlying events. A prior lesion may have served as predisposing condition for metastatic bacterial colonization and then for parietal infection/inflammation with subsequent vulnerability to physiologic mechanical stress. As we found sterile field at the moment of surgical artery repair, inflammation might self-perpetuate even in the absence of antigenic stimulation. Two conditions make this multistep hypothesis reliable: (1) *S. Bovis* is considered among germs with the highest risk for embolization [3, 6]; (2) time between endocarditis diagnosis and arterial rupture is consistent with subclinical embolization in the first days after antibiotic therapy initiation (period at the highest risk for embolism [7]) and may be considered sufficient for the subsequent damage of the arterial wall induced by inflammation. However, since the patient was on proper, effective, antibiotic therapy and the vascular tissues removed by the surgeon were sterile, damage to the vascular wall must have been triggered before the therapy become effective to eliminate bacteria. To our knowledge, this report describes, for the first time, a case of endocarditis complicated by the rupture of radial artery. Vascular damage, although probably initiated by microbial infection, can become insensitive even to effective antibiotic therapy and lead to dangerous complications, particularly when involving vital organs.

References

[1] G. Habib, B. Hoen, P. Tornos et al., "Guidelines on the prevention, diagnosis, and treatment of infective endocarditis (new version 2009): the task force on the prevention, diagnosis, and treatment of infective endocarditis of the European society of cardiology (ESC)," *European Heart Journal*, vol. 30, no. 19, pp. 2369–2413, 2009.

[2] J. S. Li, D. J. Sexton, N. Mick et al., "Proposed modifications to the Duke criteria for the diagnosis of infective endocarditis," *Clinical Infectious Diseases*, vol. 30, no. 4, pp. 633–638, 2000.

[3] F. Thuny, G. Disalvo, O. Belliard et al., "Risk of embolism and death in infective endocarditis: prognostic value of echocardiography—a prospective multicenter study," *Circulation*, vol. 112, no. 1, pp. 69–75, 2005.

[4] I. Corral, P. Martín-Dávila, J. Fortún et al., "Trends in neurological complications of endocarditis," *Journal of Neurology*, vol. 254, no. 9, pp. 1253–1259, 2007.

[5] J. Masuda, C. Yutani, R. Waki, J. Ogata, Y. Kuriyama, and T. Yamaguchi, "Histopathological analysis of the mechanisms of intracranial hemorrhage complicating infective endocarditis," *Stroke*, vol. 23, no. 6, pp. 843–850, 1992.

[6] V. Pergola, G. Di Salvo, G. Habib et al., "Comparison of clinical and echocardiographic characteristics of *Streptococcus bovis* endocarditis with that caused by other pathogens," *The American Journal of Cardiology*, vol. 88, no. 8, pp. 871–875, 2001.

[7] I. Vilacosta, C. Graupner, J. San Román et al., "Risk of embolization after institution of antibiotic therapy for infective endocarditis," *Journal of the American College of Cardiology*, vol. 39, no. 9, pp. 1489–1495, 2002.

24

Upper Limb Ischemic Gangrene as a Complication of Hemodialysis Access

Shamir O. Cawich, Emil Mohammed, Marlon Mencia, and Vijay Naraynsingh

Department of Clinical Surgical Sciences, University of the West Indies, St. Augustine Campus, St. Augustine, Trinidad and Tobago

Correspondence should be addressed to Shamir O. Cawich; socawich@hotmail.com

Academic Editor: Halvor Naess

Upper limb ischemia is a well-recognized complication of dialysis access creation but progression to gangrene is uncommon. We report a case of upper limb ischemic gangrene and discuss the lessons learned during the management of this case. Clinicians must be vigilant for this complication and they should be reminded that it requires *urgent* management to prevent tissue loss.

1. Introduction

Hemodialysis is the commonest form of renal replacement therapy for patients with chronic kidney disease in the Caribbean [1, 2]. With an increasing number of persons being diagnosed with chronic kidney disease and more hemodialysis accesses being created, we have noticed a concomitant rise in access-related complications [3, 4].

We report the case of a patient with a steal syndrome that was neglected until there was gangrene requiring amputation. Our message is to remind clinicians who encounter patients with hemodialysis accesses that a steal syndrome is a complication that requires emergent intervention to avert the threat of limb loss.

2. Presentation of a Case

A 58-year-old woman with diabetes mellitus and stage V chronic kidney disease received maintenance hemodialysis through a brachioaxillary PTFE graft in the left upper limb. The graft was in use for three years prior to presentation.

Approximately one week prior to presentation, graft thrombosis developed. She sought attention at a facility in North America where her original graft was implanted. Reportedly, significant thrombus load was evacuated and a self-expanding metallic stent was placed across a stenosed area near the arterial anastomosis. The procedure was reported to be uneventful, although technical details and

stent size were not reported. She was discharged within 24 hours and returned to her country of residence in the Caribbean.

Within 36 hours, she presented to the emergency room complaining of persistent pain in the ipsilateral upper limb, affecting mostly the fingers and hand. The pain was associated with numbness in the fingers and exacerbated by hand movements. She was evaluated by the emergency room physician and discharged with an increased analgesic prescription. She returned to the emergency room on two further occasions with similar complaints. At her last presentation, the emergency physician detected a thrill in the graft but the radial and ulnar pulses were weak. Therefore, a duplex Doppler ultrasound was ordered and suggested the presence of a steal syndrome (Figure 1). She was referred to the surgical team on call.

Upon assessment by the surgeons, she was noted to be in severe pain. Dry gangrene was already present at the ipsilateral limb extending up to the distal third of the forearm (Figure 2). There was a strong thrill and bruit at the graft but the pulses at the wrist were absent. As there was no vascular surgeon at the facility in which she was admitted, she was airlifted to our service for definitive management.

She was taken immediately to the operating room where an incision was made over the arterial anastomosis in the left antecubital fossa. The anastomotic site was identified in preparation for access ligation (Figure 3). We attempted ligation by leaving a 1 cm cuff of PTFE graft distal to the

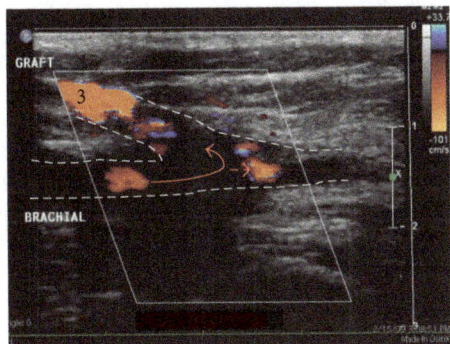

FIGURE 1: Duplex Doppler ultrasound of the left antecubital fossa demonstrating a significant steal syndrome. Blood enters the proximal brachial artery (1) and >70% is shunted through the PTFE graft (3) with <30% flow through the native distal artery (2).

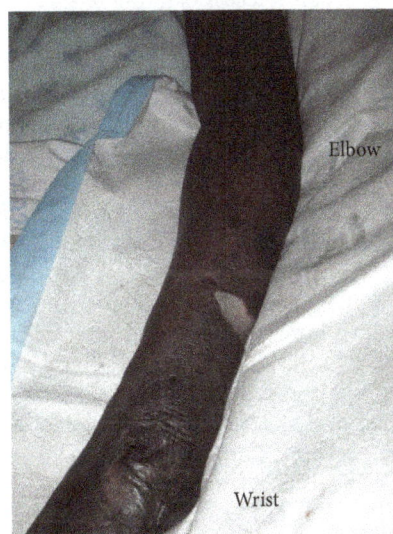

FIGURE 2: Clinical photograph of the left upper limb of a patient with dry gangrene to the midforearm level. Note the presence of blebs in the midforearm and distal forearm.

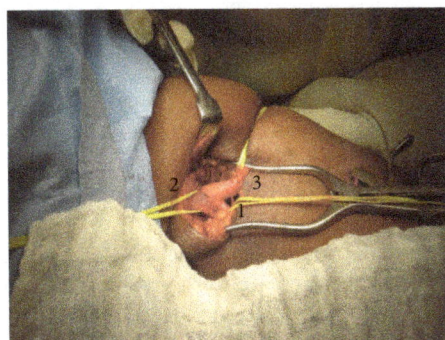

FIGURE 3: Operative photograph of the dissection in the antecubital fossa demonstrating the proximal (1) and distal (2) brachial artery. The anastomosis (3) is seen clearly and the PTFE graft is seen coursing proximally to the axillary vein.

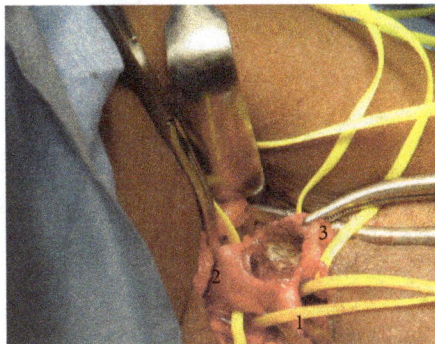

FIGURE 4: Operative photograph showing the proximal (1) and distal (2) native brachial artery. The anastomosis has been opened and reveals the metallic stent traversing the anastomosis and coursing up the graft (3). This required excision of the anastomosis and repair with a PTFE cuff.

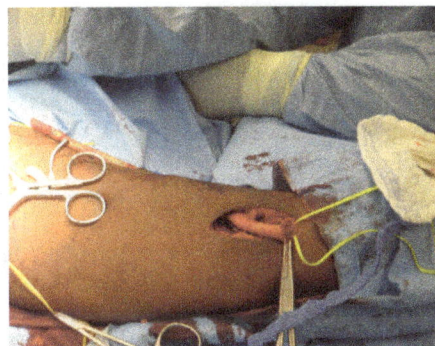

FIGURE 5: The anastomosis has been excised completely and the remnant defect repaired. The graft is being excised from the upper limb.

anastomotic site but this was not feasible due to the presence of the metallic stent (Figure 4). The anastomosis was taken down, PTFE and metallic stent were excised completely, and the native vessel was repaired with a patch (Figure 5). The forearm was turgid and gangrenous. Therefore, we proceeded with a midforearm amputation at the same sitting (Figure 6). A temporary catheter was also introduced into the right internal jugular vein for continued hemodialysis.

Postoperatively, she had a prolonged recovery but the wounds healed uneventfully with no further wound-related complications.

3. Discussion

Storey et al. [5] was the first to report a "steal syndrome" after upper limb hemodialysis access creation in 1969. It is now a well-recognized complication of hemodialysis accesses, but the progression to upper limb gangrene is uncommon. On review of the literature, we only encountered 11 reports of upper limb gangrene related to hemodialysis accesses [6–15]. Once gangrene develops, an amputation is inevitable and brings associated morbidity and increased mortality. Therefore, upper limb ischemia should be considered a serious

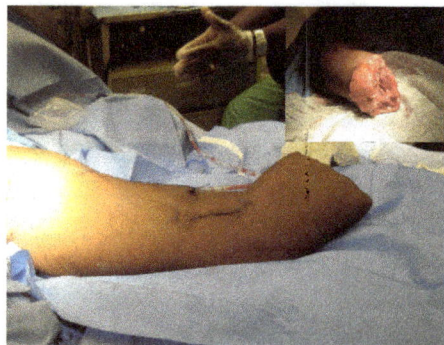

FIGURE 6: Viable tissue was only present at the proximal third of the forearm (inset). An amputation at the proximal third of the forearm was required.

complication and treated with urgency to avert the threat of limb loss.

The literature contains many reports of steal syndromes after access creation. Davidson et al. [16] proposed a standardized clinical definition characterized by persistent severe ischemic symptoms (pain or weakness) distal to the access with a temporal relationship to access creation or manipulation. Using this definition, the incidence of steal syndrome varies from 1.6% [17] to 6.2% [16].

Many have explored the factors that may predict a risk of developing the steal syndrome. The presence of diabetes mellitus seems to be a strong predictor [5–7, 16, 18], with incidence of steal syndrome ranging from 5.5% [19] to 6.2% [16] in persons with diabetes. Other risk factors include increased age [7, 16, 20], female gender [17], smoking [17, 21], presence of peripheral arterial occlusive disease [7], use of PTFE grafts [17], and proximal access sites [17]. Several of these factors were present in our patient.

There is a wide variation of symptomatology in these patients, with the clinical manifestations allowing disease categorization into four stages [22]. In stage I there are pallor, cyanosis, and decreased temperature of the fingers and palm and in stage II there is pain only during hemodialysis; stage III indicates pain at rest and stage IV indicates the presence of ischemic ulcers, apical necrosis, and/or gangrene. Our patient presented initially with stage III disease but delayed intervention allowed rapid progression to stage IV. This reinforces the need for vigilant surveillance in patients who have had access creation and/or manipulation.

Although this is usually a clinical diagnosis made on history and examination, duplex Doppler ultrasound may provide confirmation when the classic signs are present: reduced pulse volume distal to the access, flow inversion at the anastomosis site, monophasic distal flow, arterial pressures <50 mmHg, and wrist-brachial index <0.4 [23]. Although the Doppler in this case was clearly suggestive of a steal syndrome, there was a disappointing lack of urgency in treatment, highlighting the need to remind clinicians of this diagnosis and the appropriate therapeutic regimes.

In stages I and II disease, medical management is an option using combinations of aspirin, clopidogrel, calcium antagonists, Pentoxifylline, naftidrofuryl, peripheral vasodilators, and anticoagulation [23]. Close surveillance is still mandatory because the disease will progress in up to 33% of patients despite medical management [23, 24].

In this case, however, immediate operative intervention would have been more appropriate. Operative intervention has two aims: the priority is to increase flow through the forearm arteries and a secondary goal is to maintain sufficient flow through the access to maintain dialysis. Several operative options would have been available.

3.1. Access Ligation. Access ligation can rapidly correct limb ischemia [22, 25, 26] and provides the greatest chance of limb salvage but sacrifices the access. This is usually reserved for patients who have impending tissue loss in stage III or stage IV disease. Access ligation was eventually performed in this case in an attempt to limit the rapid progression of ischemic necrosis but was too late to preserve the limb.

3.2. Access Restriction. Access banding refers to a procedure that limits flow through the access by reducing the diameter of the conduit just distal to the anastomosis. The resultant increased resistance redirects flow into the forearm vessels. This, however, has been greeted with inconsistent results because it is difficult to standardize the restriction created [27]. Some have advocated a modified banding technique known as the MILLER (Minimally Invasive Limited Ligation Endoluminal Revision) procedure to create a standardized restriction [28, 29]. This involves the use of a balloon catheter that is inflated just distal to the anastomosis until there is 60–80% reduction in luminal diameter at the access limb [30]. The balloon is left inflated and the access limb is dissected to allow a polypropylene suture to be passed 360° around the access and tied over the balloon, thereby restricting access inflow. Miller et al. [30] studied a cohort of 183 patients with steal syndromes and reported 89% technical success after the initial MILLER banding and 96% success with repeated bandings. This resulted in 75% primary patency at 6 months and 89% secondary patency at 24 months. Zangan and van Ha [28] described a similar technique using an external ligature over a constrained stent within the graft lumen to reduce the inflow diameter to 4 mm.

3.3. Access Revision. Distal Revascularization and Interval Ligation (DRIL) was initially described by Schanzer et al. in 1988 [31] on three patients with steal syndromes. The DRIL procedure aims to preserve the access but increase distal flow in the limb. This is achieved with an arterial bypass from the brachial artery at least 7 cm proximal to the access jumped into the artery just distal to the access anastomosis. The native artery is then ligated just distal to the access. By creating a low resistance conduit proximal to the access anastomosis with a concomitant relative increase in the resistance in the access limb due to ligation, there is a change in hemodynamics with preferential flow down the lower resistance bypass limb.

Schanzer et al. [14] reported 96% access patency and 100% symptom relief after 2 years in 23 patients post-DRIL procedures. The largest series to date was reported by Huber et al. [32] who performed 64 DRIL procedures. They reported 78% symptom relief, 77% primary patency, and 81% secondary patency at one year. Others have reported up to 90% ischemic ulcer healing rates after DRIL procedures [27].

An alternative to interrupting the native brachial artery is to perform a Revision Using Distal Inflow (RUDI) procedure as described by Minion et al. [33] in 2005. Here, the access is ligated just distal to the anastomosis and a new anastomosis is created using a smaller artery more distal in the limb. The RUDI procedure leaves intact flow in at least one forearm vessel, thereby increasing flow to the hand while maintaining access patency [33].

The final surgical option is Proximalization of Arterial Inflow (PAI) [24]. Here the existing access is taken down and a new one is created using a proximal artery, commonly the axillary artery [20]. There are two theories explaining how PAI works [20]. Firstly, there is increased pressure at the split point between the arm and the access (because the access takes blood from a higher-flow vessel), thereby leaving an increased amount of flow to descend in the normal vasculature. Secondly, with a higher access takeoff there will be a greater propensity for collaterals to form, taking advantage of the scapular anastomoses.

There are several operative options available to restore arterial flow to the limb threatened by a steal syndrome, but the majority of experience exists between the DRIL and MILLER procedures, which have comparable intermediate term results. There is ongoing debate about the indications and it is still unsettled which of these should be the first line procedure.

4. Conclusion

Although upper limb ischemia is a well-recognized complication of dialysis access creation, there are few reports of gangrene as a result of ischemia. Clinicians must be vigilant for this complication and they should be reminded that it requires emergent management to prevent tissue loss.

In the long term, dialysis patients should be monitored closely to identify potential graft complications that may require intervention. This must be facilitated by free communication between nephrologists, interventional radiologists, and vascular surgeons in the management of these cases.

References

[1] S. O. Cawich, N. Iheonunekwu, F. Hendriks, and G. Hoeksema, "Renal replacement therapy for stage 5 chronic kidney disease in the Cayman Islands," *International Urology and Nephrology*, vol. 42, no. 2, pp. 461–464, 2010.

[2] A. K. Soyibo and E. N. Barton, "Report from the Caribbean renal registry, 2006," *West Indian Medical Journal*, vol. 56, no. 4, pp. 355–362, 2007.

[3] S. O. Cawich, H. Brown, A. Martin, M. S. Newnham, R. Venugopal, and E. Williams, "Arteriovenous fistulas as vascular access for hemodialysis: the preliminary experience at the University Hospital of the West Indies, Jamaica," *International Journal of Angiology*, vol. 18, no. 1, pp. 29–32, 2009.

[4] S. O. Cawich, N. Iheonunekwu, F. Hendriks, L. V. H. de Jonge, M. A. C. Frankson, and G. Hoeksema, "Access surgery for hemodialysis in the Cayman Islands: preliminary results of a vascular access service," *International Journal of Angiology*, vol. 18, no. 2, pp. 71–74, 2009.

[5] B. G. Storey, C. R. P. George, J. H. Stewart, D. J. Tiller, J. May, and A. G. R. Sheil, "Embolic and ischemic complications after anastomosis of radial artery to cephalic vein," *Surgery*, vol. 66, no. 2, pp. 325–327, 1969.

[6] O. Cebesoy and E. T. Baltaci, "Acute gangrene that developed in the fingers of the hand with arteriovenous fistule in a chronic hemodialysis patient," *Journal of the National Medical Association*, vol. 98, no. 10, pp. 1707–1709, 2006.

[7] R. A. Yeager, G. L. Moneta, J. M. Edwards et al., "Relationship of hemodialysis access to finger gangrene in patients with end-stage renal disease," *Journal of Vascular Surgery*, vol. 36, no. 2, pp. 245–249, 2002.

[8] G. B. Piccoli, M. Quaglia, P. Quaglino et al., "Acute digital gangrene in a long-term dialysis patient—a diagnostic challenge," *Medical Science Monitor*, vol. 8, no. 11, pp. CS83–CS89, 2002.

[9] G. Bathini, M. Yadla, S. Burri et al., "Bilateral upper limb digital gangrene in a patient on maintenance hemodialysis," *Renal Failure*, vol. 36, no. 8, pp. 1348–1350, 2014.

[10] C.-H. Hsieh, H.-H. Tsai, J.-W. Yin, T.-S. Lin, and S.-F. Jeng, "Salvage of the hand with a free flap in a hemodialysis patient with finger gangrene and ipsilateral arteriovenous fistula: a case report," *Annals of Vascular Surgery*, vol. 18, no. 3, pp. 365–368, 2004.

[11] B. B. Chang, S. P. Roddy, R. C. Darling III et al., "Upper extremity bypass grafting for limb salvage in end-stage renal failure," *Journal of Vascular Surgery*, vol. 38, no. 6, pp. 1313–1315, 2003.

[12] M. Haimov, H. Schanzer, and M. Skladani, "Pathogenesis and management of upper-extremity ischemia following angioaccess surgery," *Blood Purification*, vol. 14, no. 5, pp. 350–354, 1996.

[13] A. H. Tzamaloukas, G. H. Murata, A. M. Harford et al., "Hand gangrene in diabetic patients on chronic dialysis," *ASAIO Transactions*, vol. 37, no. 4, pp. 638–643, 1991.

[14] H. Schanzer, M. Skladany, M. Haimov et al., "Treatment of angioaccess-induced ischemia by revascularization," *Journal of Vascular Surgery*, vol. 16, no. 6, pp. 861–866, 1992.

[15] R. A. Mactier, W. K. Stewart, D. M. Parham, and J. A. Tainsh, "Acral gangrene attributed to calcific azotaemic arteriopathy and the steal effect of an arteriovenous fistula," *Nephron*, vol. 54, no. 4, pp. 347–350, 1990.

[16] D. Davidson, G. Louridas, R. Guzman et al., "Steal syndrome complicating upper extremity hemoaccess procedures: incidence and risk factors," *Canadian Journal of Surgery*, vol. 46, no. 6, pp. 408–412, 2003.

[17] M. K. Lazarides, D. N. Staramos, G. Kopadis, C. Maltezos, V. D. Tzilalis, and G. S. Georgiadis, "Onset of arterial 'steal' following proximal angioaccess: immediate and delayed types," *Nephrology Dialysis Transplantation*, vol. 18, no. 11, pp. 2387–2390, 2003.

[18] S. J. Eliades and J. Eliades, "Hemodynamic changes during dialysis in the arms and digits of patients with polytetrafluoroethylene arteriovenous grafts," *Journal of Vascular Technology*, vol. 22, no. 3, pp. 143–151, 1998.

[19] C. D. Goff, D. T. Sato, P. H. S. Bloch et al., "Steal syndrome complicating hemodialysis access procedures: can it be predicted?" *Annals of Vascular Surgery*, vol. 14, no. 2, pp. 138–144, 2000.

[20] J. Zanow, U. Kruger, and H. Scholz, "Proximalization of the arterial inflow: a new technique to treat access-related ischemia," *Journal of Vascular Surgery*, vol. 43, no. 6, pp. 1216–1221, 2006.

[21] C. Combe, J. M. Albert, J. L. Bragg-Gresham et al., "The burden of amputation among hemodialysis patients in the Dialysis Outcomes and Practice Patterns Study (DOPPS)," *The American Journal of Kidney Diseases*, vol. 54, no. 4, pp. 680–692, 2009.

[22] V. Mickley, "Steal syndrome-strategies to preserve vascular access and extremity," *Nephrology Dialysis Transplantation*, vol. 23, no. 1, pp. 19–24, 2008.

[23] P. N. Suding and S. E. Wilson, "Strategies for management of ischemic steal syndrome," *Seminars in Vascular Surgery*, vol. 20, no. 3, pp. 184–188, 2007.

[24] M. R. Scheltinga, F. van Hoek, and C. M. A. Bruyninckx, "Surgical banding for refractory hemodialysis access-induced distal ischemia (HAIDI)," *Journal of Vascular Access*, vol. 10, no. 1, pp. 43–49, 2009.

[25] J. Malik, V. Tuka, Z. Kasalova et al., "Understanding the dialysis access steal syndrome. A review of ethiology, diagnosis, prevention and treatment strategies," *Journal of Vascular Access*, vol. 9, no. 3, pp. 155–166, 2008.

[26] H. Schanzer and D. Eisenberg, "Management of steal syndrome resulting from dialysis access," *Seminars in Vascular Surgery*, vol. 17, no. 1, pp. 45–49, 2004.

[27] G. S. Tynan-Cuisinier and S. S. Berman, "Strategies for predicting and treating access induced ischemic steal syndrome," *European Journal of Vascular and Endovascular Surgery*, vol. 32, no. 3, pp. 309–315, 2006.

[28] S. M. Zangan and T. G. van Ha, "Percutaneous placement of a constrained stent for the treatment of dialysis associated arteriovenous graft steal syndrome," *Journal of Vascular Access*, vol. 8, no. 4, pp. 228–230, 2007.

[29] N. Goel, G. A. Miller, M. C. Jotwani, J. Licht, I. Schur, and W. P. Arnold, "Minimally invasive limited ligation endoluminal-assisted revision (MILLER) for treatment of dialysis access-associated steal syndrome," *Kidney International*, vol. 70, no. 4, pp. 765–770, 2006.

[30] G. A. Miller, N. Goel, A. Friedman et al., "The MILLER banding procedure is an effective method for treating dialysis-associated steal syndrome," *Kidney International*, vol. 77, no. 4, pp. 359–366, 2010.

[31] H. Schanzer, M. Schwartz, E. Harrington, and M. Haimov, "Treatment of ischemia due to 'steal' by arteriovenous fistula with distal artery ligation and revascularization," *Journal of Vascular Surgery*, vol. 7, no. 6, pp. 770–773, 1988.

[32] T. S. Huber, M. P. Brown, J. M. Seeger, and W. A. Lee, "Midterm outcome after the distal revascularization and interval ligation (DRIL) procedure," *Journal of Vascular Surgery*, vol. 48, no. 8, pp. 926–932, 2008.

[33] D. J. Minion, E. Moore, and E. Endean, "Revision using distal inflow: a novel approach to dialysis-associated steal syndrome," *Annals of Vascular Surgery*, vol. 19, no. 5, pp. 625–628, 2005.

25

Unique Nutcracker Phenomenon Involving the Right Renal Artery and Portal Venous System

Maximilian Stephens,[1,2] **Sarah Kate Ryan,**[1] **and Roger Livsey**[1,2]

[1] *University of Queensland School of Medicine, Herston Road, Herston, Brisbane, QLD 4006, Australia*
[2] *Department of Medical Imaging, Mater Misericordiae Hospital, Raymond Terrace, South Brisbane, QLD 4101, Australia*

Correspondence should be addressed to Maximilian Stephens; maximilian.stephens@uqconnect.edu.au

Academic Editor: Nilda Espinola-Zavaleta

The nutcracker phenomenon is usually caused by compression of the left renal vein by the superior mesenteric artery anteriorly and the aorta posteriorly, although variations of this anatomy have previously been reported. We observed a nutcracker phenomenon in a 42-year-old female who underwent portal venous phase computed tomography of the body for oncologic workup. She had no documented proteinuria or hematuria. Multiplanar reconstructions demonstrated an enhancing left renal vein draining into the left ovarian vein without draining into the inferior vena cava due to external compression immediately before the renocaval junction. The left renal vein was compressed between the right renal artery and the portal vein. This type of nutcracker has not been previously reported in the literature and represents a new variation.

1. Introduction

The nutcracker phenomenon (NCP) and the nutcracker syndrome (NCS) have been recognized more frequently in the literature over the last few years. These reports describe external compression of the left renal vein (LRV), typically between the superior mesenteric artery (SMA) and the aorta, as was first described clinically by El-Sadr and Mina in 1950 [1]. This compression of the LRV restricts venous outflow and causes reciprocal dilatation of the hilar portion of the LRV and often the tributary left gonadal vein. NCP differs from NCS in that NCS is "symptomatic" or detectable with urinalysis, although no strict criteria exist as to the necessary extent of symptoms to define NCS [2]. NCS may manifest as macro- or microscopic hematuria, flank pain, proteinuria, varicocele, or orthostatic intolerance [2, 3]. Although compression of the LRV between the SMA and aorta is the most common scenario, variations to this have been reported:

(i) aorta and spinal column or "posterior" nutcracker phenomenon [4];

(ii) arching left gonadal artery and psoas major muscle [5];

(iii) SMA and right renal artery [6, 7];

(iv) circumferential fibrous tissue [2, 8];

(v) retroperitoneal neoplasms/lymphadenopathy [2].

Here we describe external compression of the LRV by the right renal artery (RRA) and the portal vein (PV), which resulted in a nutcracker phenomenon with collateral outflow through the left ovarian vein.

2. Case Report

A 42-year-old Asian female presented with a 6-month history of left neck pain. This was on a background of left mastectomy for invasive ductal carcinoma 12 months prior, with post-operative chemoradiation. She also had chronic e-antigen negative hepatitis B but had unremarkable liver enzymes and hepatitis B DNA levels whilst on tenofovir. Examination was unremarkable except for postradiotherapy changes to the left chest wall. Portal venous phase computed tomography (CT) of the neck, chest, abdomen, and pelvis was performed (Philips Brilliance-64 MDCT, Philips Healthcare, Cleveland, OH, USA) to rule out metastatic disease. All studies were normal except for an observed nutcracker phenomenon (Figures 1 and 2).

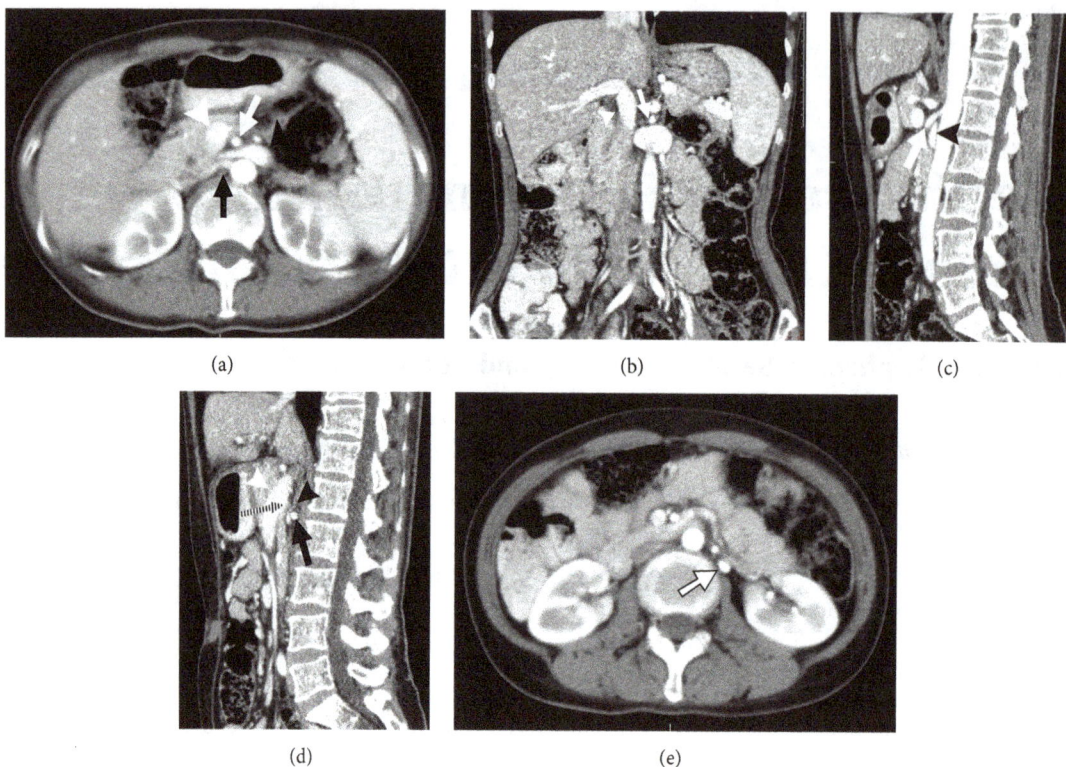

FIGURE 1: Multiplanar reconstruction of a nutcracker phenomenon. (a) Axial view: the left renal vein is compressed between the portal vein anteriorly and the right renal artery posteriorly. The left renal vein is patent after it traverses behind the superior mesenteric artery although minor compression occurs at this point. (b) Coronal view: the left renal vein ceases abruptly before the renocaval junction. (c) Sagittal view: the left renal vein is patent as it traverses behind the superior mesenteric artery. (d) Sagittal view: the left renal vein is compressed between the right renal artery and the portal vein. Adjacent retroperitoneal fat is present but not the offending structure. (e) Axial view: the left ovarian vein is dilated and enhancing, whilst the right ovarian vein is not appreciated. White arrowhead: portal vein; white arrow: superior mesenteric artery; black arrowhead: left renal vein; black arrow: right renal artery; white arrow with black border: left ovarian vein; black and white striped arrow: posterior bend of portal vein compressing left renal vein.

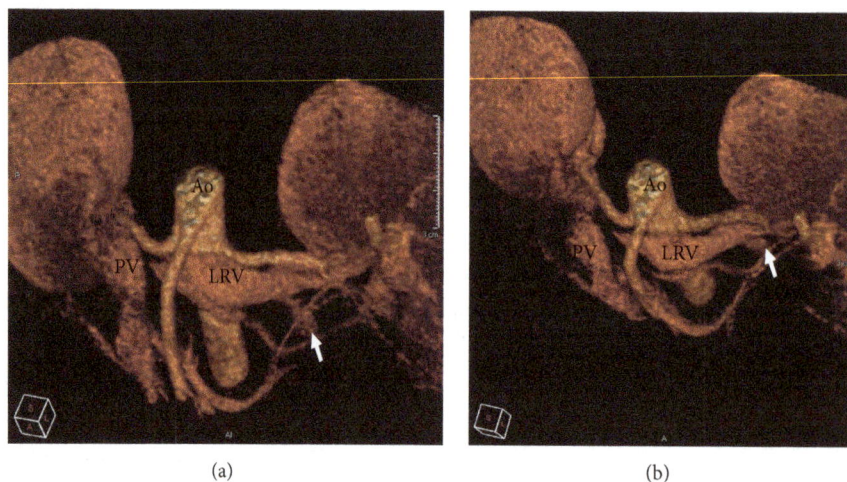

FIGURE 2: (a) and (b) 3D reconstructions of a nutcracker phenomenon. The left renal vein is compressed as it approaches the right renal artery and portal vein. Ao: aorta; PV: portal vein; LRV: left renal vein; LOV: left ovarian vein.

The LRV appeared to be dilated, measuring 10.8 mm anteroposterior (AP) × 19.2 mm craniocaudal (CC) at its most dilated point, then tapering to complete occlusion, measuring 1.5 mm AP × 7.7 mm CC before the obstruction. This yielded a decrease in functional diameter by 86% and a cross-sectional proportion of 18 : 1. These measurements far exceed the suggested nutcracker phenomenon criteria of >50% and >4 : 1, respectively [2, 3]. The LRV appeared to be externally compressed anteriorly by the PV and posteriorly by the RRA immediately after its takeoff from the aorta. Compression of the LRV occurred proximally to the renocaval junction. Contrast filled the entire LRV; however, no contrast was seen in the inferior vena cava (IVC) (Figure 1). Of note, the right renal vein was patent with contrast seen to reach the right renocaval ostium; however, this occurred in a minute amount, inferior to the LRV, leaving the IVC predominantly unenhanced. Contrast was also seen to enhance the left ovarian vein (LOV) from the LRV to the level of the left ovary whilst the right ovarian vein did not enhance. The LOV appeared dilated, measuring 6.7 mm AP × 5.9 mm transverse at its most dilated point, although its caliber did not change significantly throughout its course. Blood analysis performed 3 weeks prior showed a creatinine of 58 μmol/L (reference range 64–108 μmol/L); however, no urinalysis was performed.

3. Discussion

The exact prevalence of NCS or NCP is unknown, although one series found evidence of asymptomatic "renal venous distension" in 72% of abdominal CTs [10]. There appears to be a slight predilection for females in their second to fourth decades of life [2, 8]. Although there is no concrete delineation between NCS and NCP, it is generally accepted that NCS is simply NCP with classical symptoms or evidence of renal damage.

Our patient matched the classic demographic, yet was asymptomatic, and had a normal blood creatinine, favoring NCP over NCS. A urinalysis would have added considerably to the clinical picture to rule out proteinuria and hematuria. Although there was no evidence of decompensation by the left kidney, there were radiological findings that indicated significant venous shunting had been occurring through the left ovarian vein. The lack of contrast filling of the IVC, despite a contrast-laden LRV, in conjunction with a dilated and enhancing full length LOV suggests that venous blood from the LRV was shunted by collateral outflow through the LOV due to obstruction of the LRV. Blood entering the LOV was probably shunted through the connecting uterine veins and possibly the ipsilateral ovarian vein as shown in Figure 3 [9]. Indeed, on more inferior axial slices, the left uterine veins appeared mildly congested and showed enhancement; however, this may be due to normal anterograde venous flow. The source of LRV obstruction was due to external compression by the PV and RRA and was seen on CT multiplanar reconstructions. Further imaging such as MRI or angiography would have added considerably to the results; however, they were not performed as there was no clinical justification.

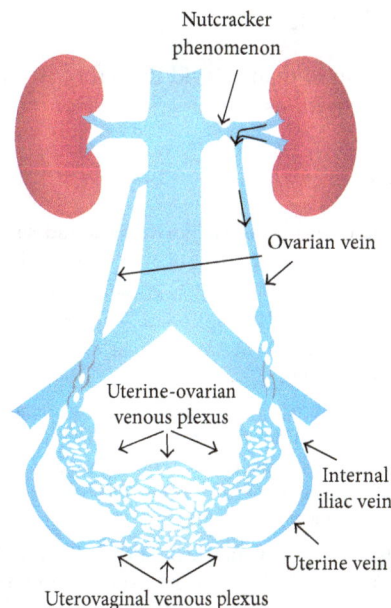

FIGURE 3: Anatomic illustration demonstrating the key venous anastomoses that facilitate shunting of renal blood when a nutcracker scenario arises. Image adapted with permission from Umeoka et al., Radiographics, 2004, 24 : 197, RSNA [9].

NCP involving the RRA has been reported twice previously, although neither involved the PV. The authors of the first case observed a ventral takeoff of the RRA [6] whilst the authors of the second case noted a precipitously inferior course of the RRA being the driving factor [7]. We identified neither of the above observations in our case and suggest that a "tight" posterior course of the PV is the main cause to the left renal vein compression seen in our patient.

Whilst NCP is untreated due to its benign nature, a wide variety of operative and nonoperative treatments have been employed to treat NCS. If patients are younger than 18 years, conservative management with a 2-year-old observational period is considered best practice as up to 75% of symptomatic patients in this demographic will have complete resolution of their symptoms [2]. There is weak evidence to support angiotensin converting enzyme inhibitors and aspirin as part of nonoperative therapy, although larger studies are needed to confirm efficacy [2, 3]. Common operative approaches include LRV transposition ± Dacron wedge insertion, LRV bypass, medial nephropexy, and more recently extra-/intraluminal LRV stenting [2, 6]. Larger operations such as renal autotransplant, SMA transposition, and nephrectomy tend to be less efficacious although no large trials exist [2].

A more complete understanding of the possible pathologic anatomy that may underlie NCP/NCS is imperative to aid treating teams in diagnosis and management. NCP/NCS due to compression from the PV and the RRA has not been previously reported, making our case an important addition to the understanding of these conditions.

Acknowledgment

The authors wish to thank David Ryan for assisting with the images and illustrations.

References

[1] A. R. El-Sadr and E. Mina, "Anatomical and surgical aspects in the operative management of varicocele," *The Urologic and Cutaneous Review*, vol. 54, no. 5, pp. 257–262, 1950.

[2] A. K. Kurklinsky and T. W. Rooke, "Nutcracker phenomenon and nutcracker syndrome," *Mayo Clinic Proceedings*, vol. 85, no. 6, pp. 552–559, 2010.

[3] T. Scholbach, "From the nutcracker-phenomenon of the left renal vein to the midline congestion syndrome as a cause of migraine, headache, back and abdominal pain and functional disorders of pelvic organs," *Medical Hypotheses*, vol. 68, no. 6, pp. 1318–1327, 2007.

[4] B. Ali-El-Dein, Y. Osman, A. B. Shehab El-Din, T. El-Diasty, O. Mansour, and M. A. Ghoneim, "Anterior and posterior nutcracker syndrome: a report on 11 cases," *Transplantation Proceedings*, vol. 35, no. 2, pp. 851–853, 2003.

[5] M. C. Rusu, "Human bilateral doubled renal and testicular arteries with a left testicular arterial arch around the left renal vein.," *Romanian Journal of Morphology and Embryology*, vol. 47, no. 2, pp. 197–200, 2006.

[6] A. Basile, D. Tsetis, G. Calcara et al., "Nutcracker syndrome due to left renal vein compression by an aberrant right renal artery," *The American Journal of Kidney Diseases*, vol. 50, no. 2, pp. 326–329, 2007.

[7] M. Polguj, M. Topol, and A. Majos, "An unusual case of left venous renal entrapment syndrome: a new type of nutcracker phenomenon?" *Surgical and Radiologic Anatomy*, vol. 35, no. 3, pp. 263–267, 2013.

[8] L. Wang, L. Yi, L. Yang et al., "Diagnosis and surgical treatment of nutcracker syndrome: a single-center experience," *Urology*, vol. 73, no. 4, pp. 871–876, 2009.

[9] S. Umeoka, T. Koyama, K. Togashi, H. Kobayashi, and K. Akuta, "Vascular dilatation in the pelvis: identification with CT and MR imaging," *Radiographics*, vol. 24, no. 1, pp. 193–208, 2004.

[10] A. J. Buschi, R. B. Harrison, A. Norman et al., "Distended left renal vein: CT/sonographic normal variant," *American Journal of Roentgenology*, vol. 135, no. 2, pp. 339–342, 1980.

26

Treatment with Aortic Stent Graft Placement for Stanford B-Type Aortic Dissection in a Patient with an Aberrant Right Subclavian Artery

Yohei Kawatani, Yujiro Hayashi, Yujiro Ito, Hirotsugu Kurobe, Yoshitsugu Nakamura, Yuji Suda, and Takaki Hori

Department of Cardiovascular Surgery, Chiba-Nishi General Hospital, 107-1 Kanegasaku, Matsudo-Shi, Chiba-ken 2702251, Japan

Correspondence should be addressed to Takaki Hori; hori@tokushima-cvs.info

Academic Editor: Paolo Vanelli

A 71-year-old man visited our hospital with the chief complaint of back pain and was diagnosed with acute aortic dissection (Debakey type III, Stanford type B). He was found to have a variant branching pattern in which the right subclavian artery was the fourth branch of the aorta. We performed conservative management for uncomplicated Stanford type B aortic dissection, and the patient was discharged. An ulcer-like projection (ULP) was discovered during outpatient follow-up. Complicated type B aortic dissection was suspected, and we performed thoracic endovascular aortic repair (TEVAR). The aim of operative treatment was ULP closure; thus we placed two stent grafts in the descending aorta from the distal portion of the right subclavian artery. The patient was released without complications on postoperative day 5. Deliberate sizing and examination of placement location were necessary when placing the stent graft, but operative techniques allowed the procedure to be safely completed.

1. Introduction

Acute aortic dissection, in which the tunica intima and tunica media are separated due to a tear in the tunica intima, is characterized by abdominal or chest pain and high mortality [1]. Conservative management is recommended in patients with Stanford type B dissections, where dissection of the ascending aorta is not present. Operative treatment is recommended for complicated cases in which findings such as reperfusion injury, continuing chest pain, or a progression of dissection are present and the risk of rupture is high [2].

There are many subtypes of aortic arch branching patterns. Here, we describe a patient who had an aberrant right subclavian artery (ARSCA) and developed acute aortic dissection. Placement of stent grafts in the aorta after emergence of an ulcer-like projection (ULP) during the subacute phase was an effective treatment. Concomitant ARSCA and acute dissection are rare. Patients with this condition who receive a stent graft are even more rare.

2. Case Presentation

A 71-year-old hypertensive man presented to hospital with a 1-day history of chest pain and dyspnea. Enhanced computed tomography (CT) revealed type B aortic dissection. He was transferred to our hospital for further investigation and care. His medical history included medically managed hypertension, untreated diabetes mellitus, and a 50-year smoking habit (Brinkman index: 1500).

On presentation, blood pressure was controlled below 120 mmHg with nicardipine. The patient complained of back pain. Abdominal and peripheral pulse examinations revealed no abnormality. Enhanced CT showed dissection and coagulation in the false lumen from distal to left subclavian artery at the renal artery level. Contrast-enhanced CT and echocardiographic findings did not reveal any congenital heart defects such as right-sided aortic arch or cardiac malformation. Two arterial anomalies were observed. The right subclavian artery arose from the aortic arch posterolateral to the origin of the left subclavian artery. The right vertebral artery arose

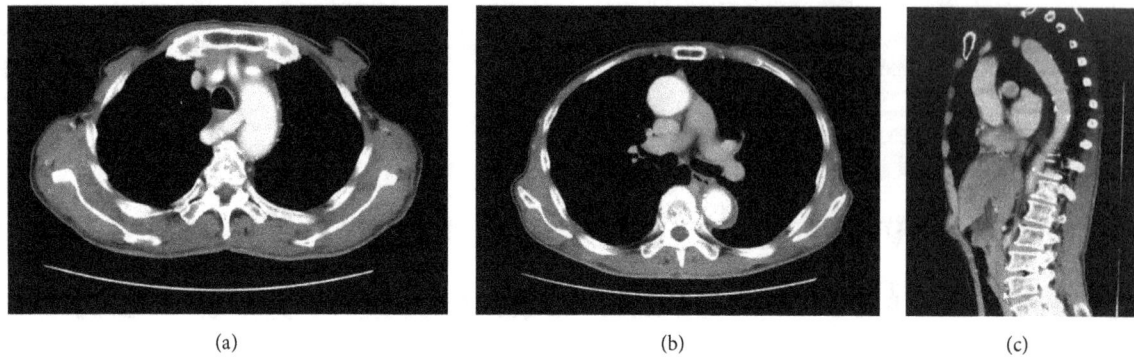

(a)   (b)   (c)

FIGURE 1: Contrast-enhanced CT images at time of onset. (a, b) Horizontal cross section. The origin of the right subclavian artery is identified as the fourth branch of the aortic arch and runs posteriorly to the right of the esophagus. No dissection of the right subclavian artery was present. Thrombosis of the false lumen from the origin to periphery of the right subclavian artery was observed. (c) Sagittal section. False lumen was observed. Total false lumen thrombosis was observed, and no signs of ULP were noted.

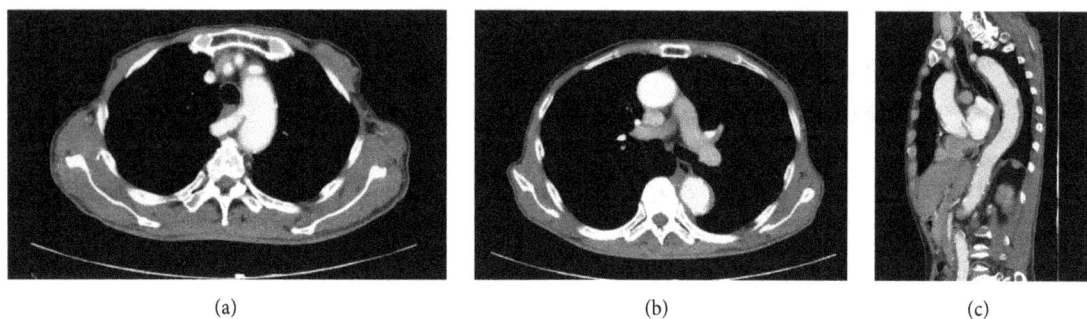

(a)   (b)   (c)

FIGURE 2: Contrast-enhanced CT findings after onset. (a) Horizontal cross section. False lumen thrombosis was observed. No changes in the origin of the right subclavian artery were noted. (b) Horizontal cross section. (c) Coronal cross section. The emergence of ULP in the descending aorta was observed.

from the right common carotid artery (Figure 1). All aortic branches including the aberrant right subclavian artery arose from the true lumen.

Upon admission, antihypertensive and analgesic treatment with bed rest were initiated. The symptoms were gradually ameliorated; therefore we performed rehabilitation in accordance with the type B acute aortic dissection rehabilitation protocol utilized by our hospital. Contrast-enhanced CT was performed on hospitalization days 2, 4, 7, and 12 to assess the aortic condition. No changes such as dilation or emergence of ULP were noted. After the rehabilitation protocol was completed, the patient was discharged. Hypotensive drugs were prescribed to control blood pressure, and the patient was scheduled for outpatient follow-up aortic imaging.

On day 11 after discharge (day 25 after onset), the patient visited our hospital for outpatient follow-up. Contrast-enhanced CT findings revealed a ULP (Figure 2). We determined that the patient had complicated type B dissection, and an urgent operation was required. After the necessary presurgical checkups, we performed endovascular repair under general anesthesia, with tracheal intubation for mechanical ventilation. The right brachial artery was accessed, and a pigtail catheter was positioned in the ascending aorta for contrast enhancement. The left common femoral artery was exposed and used as the access route for stent graft placement.

Contrast-enhanced CT imaging of the thoracic aorta was used to visualize the ULP in the descending aorta. We confirmed the origin of the right subclavian artery that had arisen as the fourth aortic branch. The diameter of the proximal landing zone was 30 mm and the diameter around the ULP was 27 mm. The treatment length was 150 mm, which was between the position of just distal to ARSCA and 50 mm distal to the ULP. A guide wire (Amplatz Super Stiff wire) was inserted from the left common femoral artery to the ascending aorta and used as a guide for the stent grafts (Relay plus 26 ∗ 26 ∗ 10, Bolton) that were placed to cover the ULP. Care was taken to place the bare stent in a sufficiently peripheral site to prevent the tip from contacting the aortic arch. Furthermore, the stent was positioned 2 cm medially to the medial part of the ULP.

For Proximal part, we selected a stent graft that was considered appropriate for long-term treatment, at the aortic diameter (Valiant 32 ∗ 32 ∗ 10, Medtronic). We placed the second stent graft in the descending aorta from the region distal to the origin of the ARSCA. Angiography using a pigtail catheter confirmed that the ULP had disappeared on contrast-enhanced imaging and that no occlusion existed in the fourth branch of the aortic arch (Figure 3).

No postoperative complications, including cerebral infarcts, paraplegia, or right upper limb claudication, were observed. On hospital day 5, the patient was discharged

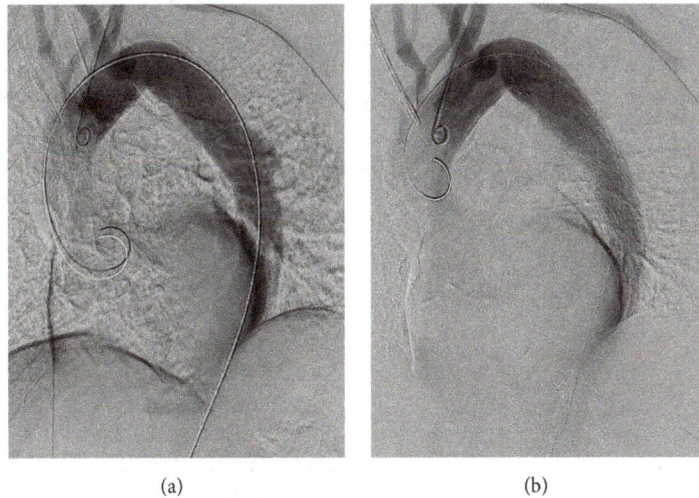

(a)   (b)

FIGURE 3: Image of angiographic findings taken during operative treatment. (a) Angiographic findings before treatment. The origin of the right subclavian artery was confirmed, and ULP was observed on contrast-enhanced CT. (b) Angiographic contrast-enhanced CT findings after placement of the stent grafts. The stent grafts were inserted so that the tips did not come into contact with the curve of the arch. The disappearance of the ULP was confirmed by contrast-enhanced CT.

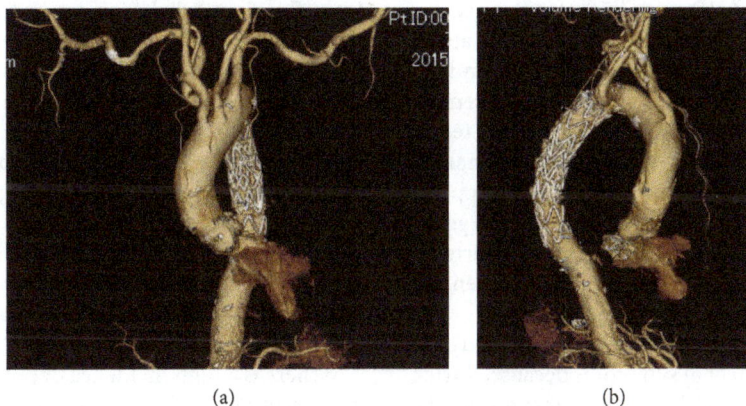

(a)   (b)

FIGURE 4: Three-dimensional CT findings at postoperative day 12. (a) Anterior view. (b) Right lateral view. The disappearance of ULP was confirmed by contrast-enhanced CT, and no endoleaks were observed. The stent grafts were placed distal to the origin of the right subclavian artery so the tips of the bare stents did not come into contact with the aortic wall.

in ambulatory condition. At postoperative day 12, contrast-enhanced CT findings revealed that the ULP had disappeared, and no other abnormal findings such as occlusion or stenosis of the arch branch were observed (Figure 4).

3. Discussion

The majority of cases of ARSCA are asymptomatic. ARSCA is the most common congenital aortic arch anomaly, found in 0.5–1.8% of humans [3]. ARSCA is due to the persistence of the embryonic right dorsal aorta with involution of the arch segment between the right common carotid artery and right subclavian artery [4]. In the present patient, the right subclavian artery was the fourth branch of the aortic arch, and after branching from the most distal region of the artery arch, it ran posteriorly to the right of the esophagus. The right vertebral artery did not originate from the right subclavian artery, but rather from the right common carotid artery,

which was the first branch. There are many variations of the aortic arch branches, which are classified according to the system proposed by Williams et al. (Figure 5) [5]. The present patient was similar to type G or type GC. However, in type G, the right vertebral artery branches from the subclavian artery, whereas, in the present patient, the right vertebral artery originated from the common carotid artery. In type GC, the right vertebral artery branches from the right subclavian artery, similar to the present case, but type GC differs in the fact that the left vertebral artery branches normally from the subclavian artery. While type G is the most common of all the variations, it seems that there are few cases that completely match the type seen in the present patient. The frequency of this morphology has not been elucidated. ARSCA can be involved in aortic dissection, either as the site of the primary intimal tear or as a dissected aortic branch [6, 7].

Conservative treatment is recommended for uncomplicated type B dissection [2]. Since our patient was hospitalized

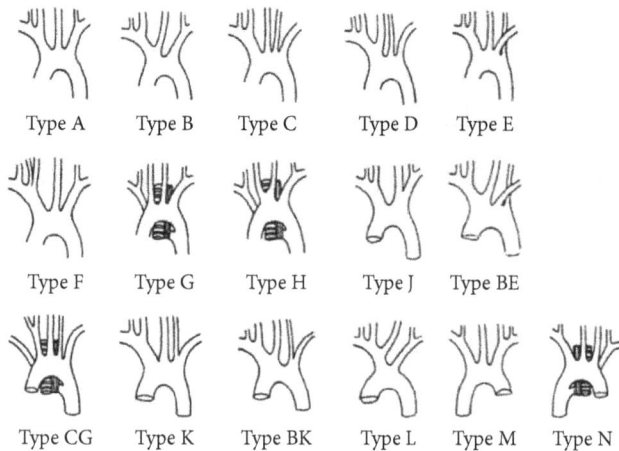

FIGURE 5: A schematic drawing of aortic arch branch classifications by Adachi, Williams, and Nakagawa. Cited from Williams et al. [5].

directly after symptom onset, the case was considered to be uncomplicated, and therefore we performed conservative treatment. While operative treatment is recommended for complicated type B dissection, the incidence of complications associated with operative treatment is high, and the indications for operative treatment and surgical methods remain controversial. In recent years, TEVAR has been reported as effective. In our department, operative treatment is generally only performed in patients whose findings reveal the appearance or exacerbation of symptoms such as the emergence of pain, enlargement of ULP, or enlargement of arterial diameter. There is no consensus concerning the intervention period for performing TEVAR.

We administer antihypertensives, order bed rest, and continue conservative management of symptoms because, during the postoperative acute phase (within 2 weeks after onset), the arterial wall that has dissected is inflamed and fragile, even in cases where findings associated with the abovementioned complicated type are present. After the acute phase has passed, we then perform TEVAR. In exceptional cases when the risk of rupture is determined to be high based on the findings, the surgeon may perform TEVAR during the acute phase.

Our patient received conservative treatment and rehabilitation during the 2-week period of hospitalization after the onset of symptoms, and contrast-enhanced CT findings during follow-up were stable. The patient was discharged with only conservative treatment. However, because contrast-enhanced CT images taken during outpatient treatment on day 25 after onset revealed the emergence of ULP, we elected to perform urgent TEVAR.

No consensus has been reached concerning the TEVAR sealing zones in cases of Stanford type B aortic dissection. The policy for clinical practice in our department is to take the prevention of paraplegia into consideration and maintain spinal cord perfusion as much as possible by reducing the number of obstructed lumbar and intercostal arteries, limiting entry to a region as small as possible, and performing coverage of entry closure as much as possible. The sealing

zone is specified to be 3 cm or longer, and in cases where the condition of the tunica intima is favorable or space is limited due to the position of the stent graft or the anatomical shape of the aorta, it is possible for the length to be shortened to 2 cm. The smallest stent graft size that can be placed is carefully considered to meet these conditions.

In the present patient, a proximal sealing zone of 3 cm would mean that the tip of the bare stent came into contact with the arterial wall of the distal region of the greater curvature of the aortic arch. For this reason, in order to obtain a sealing zone of 3 cm or longer, it was necessary to place the stent from a position on the top of the aortic arch to the median side. However, to shorten the length of long-term treatment, it was necessary to place the stent in a more distal position so that the tip of the bare stent did not come into contact with the distal wall of the curve.

In order to place a stent in the center, it was necessary to obstruct the right subclavian artery. When performing obstruction, coil embolization was necessary to prevent type II endoleaks. It has been reported that, in this variation, the right subclavian artery puts pressure on the esophagus [8]. Moreover, it has been reported that placement of stent grafts from the right subclavian artery to the aorta in this type of patient has led to esophageal perforation [9]. For this reason, we thought that, by placing a coil in the right subclavian artery, the risk of esophageal perforation could be avoided, and therefore we considered distal placement to be preferable. When placing a stent in the periphery of the distal region of the arch, the expected landing zone was 25 mm, shorter than the desired 30 mm, but the condition of the arterial wall was favorable and sealing seemed to be possible. Indeed, angiographic findings after placement of the stent grafts revealed that the ULP had disappeared, and entry closure could be sufficiently performed.

There is a high incidence of pulmonary, renal, and neural complications and early postoperative mortality associated with the conventional operative treatment of Stanford type B acute aortic dissections through thoracotomy [10]. Furthermore, many studies have reported a high risk of damage to the aberrant artery in patients who present with aberrant branching of the aortic arch. By utilizing TEVAR, there was no large difference in risks associated with operative treatment between patients with ordinary branching and the present patient. Even when guiding the wire, there were no adverse events such as migration of the wire into the right subclavian artery, and the procedure could be safely completed.

This case indicates that TEVAR is an effective treatment method for aortic dissection in patients who have ARSCA. However, the long-term prognoses of patients who have B-type aortic dissection have not been elucidated, and future observations and examination are needed.

4. Conclusion

It is the authors' opinion that TEVAR is an effective treatment for Stanford type B (complicated type) acute aortic dissection in patients who have ARSCA. As far as we pay attention to the aberrant anatomy preoperatively and during the operation, we can perform straightforward procedure in a patient with a type B dissection that is complicated and has abnormal rare anatomy. Future observations and examination of long-term prognoses are needed.

References

[1] E. Kieffer, "Dissection of the descending thoracic aorta," in *Vascular Surgery*, R. B. Rutherford, Ed., pp. 1326–1345, WB Saunders, Philadelphia, Pa, USA, 5th edition, 2000.

[2] L. F. Hiratzka, G. L. Bakris, J. A. Beckman et al., "ACCF/AHA/AATS/ACR/ASA/SCA/SCAI/SIR/STS/SVM guidelines for the diagnosis and management of patients with Thoracic Aortic Disease: a report of the American College of Cardiology Foundation/American Heart Association Task Force on Practice Guidelines, American Association for Thoracic Surgery, American College of Radiology, American Stroke Association, Society of Cardiovascular Anesthesiologists, Society for Cardiovascular Angiography and Interventions, Society of Interventional Radiology, Society of Thoracic Surgeons, and Society for Vascular Medicine," *Circulation*, vol. 121, no. 13, pp. e266–e369, 2010.

[3] J. L. Cronenwett, K. W. Johnston, and R. B. Rutherford, *Rutherford's Vascular Surgery*, Saunders Elsevier, Philadelphia, Pa, USA, 7th edition, 2010.

[4] A. Farber, W. H. Wagner, D. V. Cossman et al., "Isolated dissection of the abdominal aorta: clinical presentation and therapeutic options," *Journal of Vascular Surgery*, vol. 36, no. 2, pp. 205–210, 2002.

[5] G. D. Williams, H. M. Aff, M. Schmeckebier, H. W. Edmonds, and E. G. Graul, "Variations in the arrangement of the branches arising from the aortic arch in American whites and negroes," *The Anatomical Record*, vol. 62, pp. 139–146, 1935.

[6] G. Weinberger, P. A. Randall, F. B. Parker, and S. A. Kieffer, "Involvement of an aberrant right subclavian artery in dissection of the thoracic aorta," *American Journal of Roentgenology*, vol. 129, no. 4, pp. 653–655, 1977.

[7] S. Kawamoto, D. A. Bluemke, and E. K. Fishman, "Aortic dissection involving an aberrant right subclavian artery. CT and MR findings," *Journal of Computer Assisted Tomography*, vol. 22, no. 6, pp. 918–921, 1998.

[8] L. F. Donnelly, R. J. Fleck, P. Pacharn, M. A. Ziegler, B. L. Fricke, and R. T. Cotton, "Aberrant subclavian arteries: cross-sectional imaging findings in infants and children referred for evaluation of extrinsic airway compression," *American Journal of Roentgenology*, vol. 178, no. 5, pp. 1269–1274, 2002.

[9] A. Morisaki, H. Hirai, Y. Sasaki, K. Hige, Y. Bito, and S. Suehiro, "Aortoesophageal fistula after endovascular repair for aberrant right subclavian artery aneurysm," *Annals of Thoracic and Cardiovascular Surgery*, vol. 20, supplement, pp. 790–793, 2014.

[10] J. Y. Won, D. Y. Lee, W. H. Shim et al., "Elective endovascular treatment of descending thoracic aortic aneurysms and chronic dissections with stent-grafts," *Journal of Vascular and Interventional Radiology*, vol. 12, no. 5, pp. 575–582, 2001.

27

Critical Limb Ischemia in a Young Man: Saddle Embolism or Unusual Presentation of Thromboangiitis Obliterans?

Federico Bucci,[1] Adriano Redler,[2] and Leslie Fiengo[2]

[1] *Vascular Surgery Department, Sud Gironde Community Hospital, rue Langevin, 33210 Langon, France*
[2] *General and Vascular Surgery Department, "Umberto I" University Hospital, Viale del Policlinico, 00186 Rome, Italy*

Correspondence should be addressed to Federico Bucci; federicobucci@hotmail.fr

Academic Editors: H. Naess and J. L. Ruiz-Sandoval

Thromboangiitis obliterans (TAO), also known as Buerger's disease, is a rare cause of peripheral arterial disease in western countries. Tobacco smoking is strongly correlated to the pathogenesis of this inflammatory vascular disease. We report the case of a 32-year-old tobacco and cannabis consumer presenting with right critical limb ischemia. Computerized tomography angiography revealed a bilateral tibioperoneal arterial occlusion and an aortoiliac saddle embolus. The patient was treated with intravenous heparin, transcatheter thrombolysis, and selective Fogarty embolectomy. Instrumental and laboratory examinations revealed that patient's most likely diagnosis was TAO. Arterial embolism is uncommon in Buerger's disease but should be always excluded in these patients.

1. Introduction

Thromboangiitis obliterans (TAO), also known as Buerger's disease (BD), is a rare cause of peripheral arterial disease (PAD) in western countries. Reportedly, annual incidence of TAO is 12.6 per 100,000 representing only 0.5% of all causes of PAD. Tobacco is essential in promoting and maintaining this disease and 95% of patients affected by TAO are smokers [1].

2. Case Report

A 32-year-old man was referred to the emergencies of our hospital because of a right lower limb critical limb ischemia. Past medical history included chronic alcoholism and a three-month history of bilateral intermittent claudication. He did not report any episode of superficial thrombophlebitis. He smoked about 10 cigarettes since the age of ten and 10 cannabis joints daily since the age of twelve. He had no other cardiovascular risk factors. At clinical examination, his right leg was extremely painful and pale. He had absent pedal pulses on both sides, and a mild sensory loss on the right side. Allen's test of upper extremities was negative. Echo Doppler was suggestive of a bilateral common iliac occlusion and of a three-vessel occlusion on the right leg. A computerized tomography (CT) angiography detected the presence of an intraluminal aortic and iliac clot (Figure 1) and a bilateral distal tibial vessels occlusion (Figure 2). The patient was then fully anticoagulated with intravenous heparin. A transthoracic echocardiogram was also performed and did not detect any proximal source of emboli. The patient was then operated on: under general anesthesia, a right iliofemoral embolectomy associated to a selective right popliteal, tibial, and peroneal embolectomy and intraoperative intraarterial thrombolysis of tibial vessels. During the operation, no thrombus was found in the infrapopliteal vessels, but intraoperative arteriography showed a diffuse narrowing associated to total occlusion at the ankle with the typical "corkscrew" collateral arteries suggestive of a chronic vasculitis (Figure 3). BD was then suspected. The postoperative period was uneventful, with complete remission of symptoms. The aortoiliac embolus was sent to bacteriology and some *Micrococci* were found. Subsequently, the patient was treated with medical therapy including full dose low molecular weight heparin, antiplatelets, and pentoxifylline, and a smoking-cessation program was started. A control thoracic and abdominal angio-CT scan, done also in order to detect a proximal source of embolism, showed the absence of residual aortoiliac clot, but the chronic occlusion of the anterior tibial and peroneal arteries bilaterally. The contralateral lower limb did not require any operation. After discharge

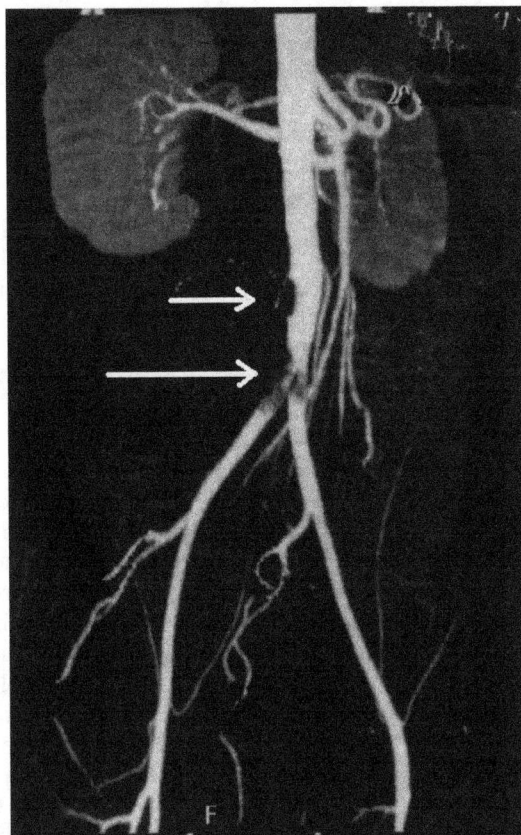

FIGURE 1: CT angiography showing the presence of an intraluminal aortic (short arrow) and iliac (long arrow) saddle embolus.

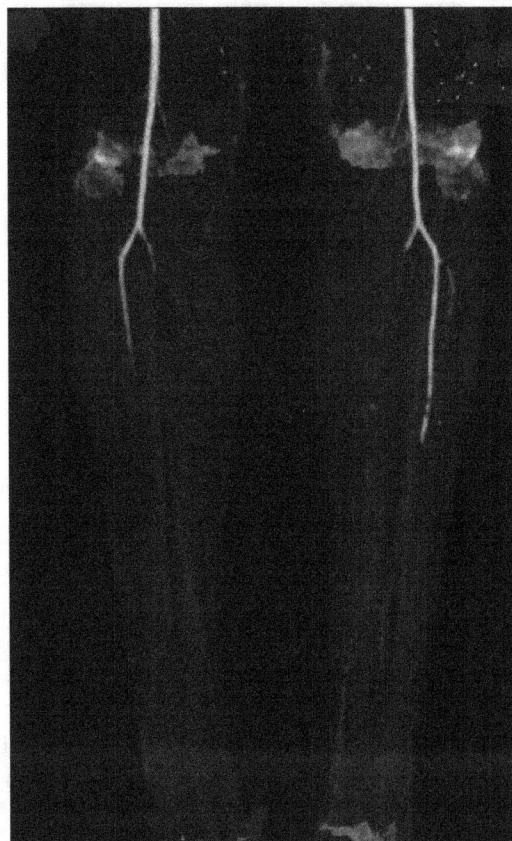

FIGURE 2: CT angiography of the lower limbs showing distal posterior and anterior tibial artery occlusion of the left side and three-vessel occlusion of the right side.

the patient underwent laboratory tests looking for diabetes and thrombophilia that were unremarkable. These included factor II and V mutation, disorders of plasminogen activation, ATIII deficiency, protein C and protein S deficiency, and homocysteine serum levels. Extensive autoimmune testing looking for autoimmune disorders potentially responsible for thrombotic events including anti-lupus erythematosus, antinuclear, antimitochondrial, and anti-phospholipids antibodies were all negative. We then concluded that the patient was affected by BD.

Anticoagulation was stopped. On the last visit at 12 months, the patient has recently restarted smoking about five cannabis joints every day; he still presents a right-sided intermittent claudication with long walking distances. Control angio-CT scan was unchanged if compared to the last one realized at hospital.

3. Discussion

TAO is a nonatherosclerotic inflammatory occlusive disease that affects small and medium-sized arteries and veins of upper and lower extremities. The role of tobacco as the most important etiopathogenic factor of TAO is well established, probably because of an idiosyncratic autoimmune response to some of its components [1]. Some authors suggest that addictions such as cannabis and cocaine may be coresponsible for Buerger's disease, accelerating its clinical presentation and aggravating its extension [2, 3]. Genetic predisponding factors are probably relevant as well. In fact, this vasculitis is more frequent in East Europe, Middle East, and Asia, with the highest prevalence documented in the Ashkenazi Jews population [4, 5]. Recurrent periodontal infections could play a role [6]. In our patient's case bacteriological tests of the removed thrombus revealed the presence of some bacteria belonging to the former genus *Micrococcus*, but we cannot exclude that it was a contamination of the thrombus during the operation.

TAO usually concerns young men, but its prevalence is increasing in women because patterns in smoking are changing, with an increasing number of female smokers. The most common age of presentation is during the fourth decade. TAO usually affects the distal infrapopliteal arteries, but iliac and femoral localization of the disease have also been described. Clinical presentation of TAO usually starts with coldness, pallor, and paraesthesia of the extremities. Intermittent claudication, whenever present, usually lasts for a short period. Critical limb ischemia occurs at a more advanced stage of the disease and is the most common clinical presentation of TAO on admission. Episodes of superficial migratory thrombophlebitis may also be referred

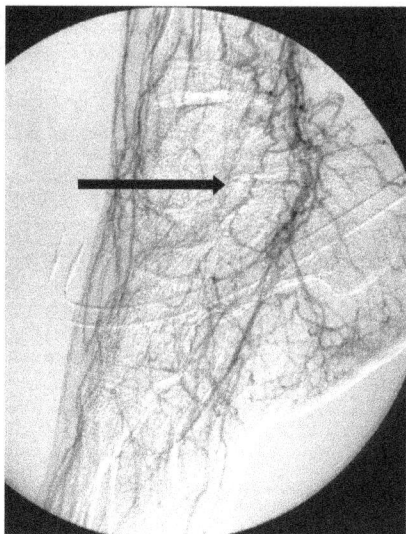

FIGURE 3: Intraoperative arteriography showing the distal occlusion of right tibial and peroneal arteries, with the typical "corkscrew" collateral arteries (black arrow), suggestive of a vasculitis.

[1, 3]. Thromboembolism is uncommon in TAO and differential diagnostics with diabetes, hypercoagulable states, and autoimmune abnormalities predisposing to thrombosis such as lupus erythematosus, antiphospholipid syndrome, and sclerodermia are strongly recommended [7]. The presence of a proximal or a cardiac source of embolism should always be excluded as well.

The occlusion of infrapopliteal vessels is a potentially limb-threatening event that can be particularly dramatic in this population as TAO usually presents on young patients. Long-term outcome is very poor with an amputation risk of 38% at ten years if smoking is not discontinued [8]. Because of this, the use of psychological support should be considered.

Diagnostic workup can include Doppler US, computerized tomography, magnetic resonance imaging, and standard angiography. In our opinion, standard arteriography is still an excellent tool, especially in cases where there is diagnostic doubt.

Most of uncomplicated TAO patients are currently managed with antiplatelets and vasodilators, such as calcium-channel blockers and alpha-blockers. In a recent small study, Bosentan, an orally administered molecule normally used to treat pulmonary arterial hypertension in systemic sclerosis patients, showed good short and mid-term results to treat TAO [9]. Another option is represented by prostanoids such as Iloprost, a strong vasodilator that is administered intravenously on an inpatient basis. Iloprost seems to be safe and effective to relief rest pain and increase wound healing in case of critical limb ischemia [10]. Percutaneous interventions could theoretically play a role for TAO patients in case of desperate limb salvage, but long-term results are still unclear [11]. The role of bypass surgery is very controversial and rarely possible, with poor results at medium and long-term because of the absence of a viable distal vascular bed [12]. Intra-arterial thrombolytic agents such as urokinase

or recombinant tissue plasminogen activator (rtPA) may occasionally be used in the acute phase of the disease and whenever, as in our patient's case, there is evidence of fresh thrombus.

Other typologies of treatment such as peripheral sympathectomy, hyperbaric oxygen therapy, and spinal cord stimulation seems to be effective especially to treat rest pain, but to this day have not clearly proved their efficacy [5, 13]. Therapeutic neoangiogenesis with autologous bone marrow mononuclear cell implantation showed promising short- and mid-term results [14, 15], but its value remains to be demonstrated in the long period.

Regarding our reported case, the presence of an aortoiliac fresh thrombus and of a consequent distal embolization made the diagnosis quite challenging. According to Olin's criteria [1] elements suggestive of TAO were first of all patient's history of a heavy smoker since extremely young age. Secondly, the angiographic finding of a total occlusion of tibial and peroneal vessels at the ankle with abundant collaterals, described as "corkscrew," suggestive of a chronic occlusive process (Figure 3). The suspicion of BD was basically confirmed by the differential diagnostic work up: a transthoracic echocardiogram and a thoracoabdominal CT angiography were performed and did not detect any proximal source of emboli. Once clot's removed a postoperative angio-CT confirmed that the abdominal aorta, the bifurcation and the iliacs were totally normal. All the laboratory blood tests (diabetes mellitus, hypercoagulability states, autoimmune diseases, and connective tissue disorders) were unremarkable as well. In the authors' opinion the most likely is the coexistence of two separate entities, the vasculitis, and the thromboembolic phenomena, in the same patient, rather than a manifestation of BD. Even if theoretically smoking may exacerbate the disease by increasing platelet aggregation and clot's formation [16], the cause of this saddle embolus remains unclarified.

References

[1] J. W. Olin, "Thromboangiitis obliterans (Buerger's disease)," *The New England Journal of Medicine*, vol. 343, no. 12, pp. 864–869, 2000.

[2] F. Grotenhermen, "Cannabis-associated arteritis," *The Journal of Vascular Diseases*, vol. 39, no. 1, pp. 43–53, 2010.

[3] G. Martin-Blondel, F. Koskas, P. Cacoub, and D. Sne, "Is thromboangiitis obliterans presentation influenced by cannabis addiction?" *Annals of Vascular Surgery*, vol. 25, no. 4, pp. 469–473, 2011.

[4] M. Kobayashi, N. Nishikimi, and K. Komori, "Current pathological and clinical aspects of Buerger's disease in Japan," *Annals of Vascular Surgery*, vol. 20, no. 1, pp. 148–156, 2006.

[5] E. E. Joviliano, R. Dellalibera-Joviliano, M. Dalio, P. R. Évora, and C. E. Piccinato, "Etiopathogenesis, clinical diagnosis and treatment of thromboangiitis obliterans—current practices," *International Journal of Angiology*, vol. 18, no. 3, pp. 119–125, 2009.

[6] T. Iwai, Y. Inoue, M. Umeda et al., "Oral bacteria in the occluded arteries of patients with Buerger disease," *Journal of Vascular Surgery*, vol. 42, no. 1, pp. 107–115, 2005.

[7] T. Lee, J. W. Seo, B. E. Sumpio, and S. J. Kim, "Immunobiologic analysis of arterial tissue in Buerger's disease," *European Journal of Vascular and Endovascular Surgery*, vol. 25, no. 5, pp. 451–457, 2003.

[8] L. T. Cooper, T. S. Tse, M. A. Mikhail, R. D. McBane, A. W. Stanson, and K. V. Ballman, "Long-term survival and amputation risk in thromboangiitis obliterans (Buerger's disease)," *Journal of the American College of Cardiology*, vol. 44, no. 12, pp. 2410–2411, 2004.

[9] J. de Haro, F. Acin, S. Bleda, C. Varela, and L. Esparza, "Treatment of thromboangiitis obliterans (Buerger's disease) with bosentan," *BMC Cardiovascular Disorders*, vol. 12, article 5, 2012.

[10] J. N. Fiessinger and M. Schäfer, "Trial of iloprost versus aspirin treatment for critical limb ischaemia of thromboangiitis obliterans," *The Lancet*, vol. 335, no. 8689, pp. 555–557, 1990.

[11] L. Graziani, L. Morelli, F. Parini et al., "Clinical outcome after extended endovascular recanalization in Buerger's disease in 20 consecutive cases," *Annals of Vascular Surgery*, vol. 26, no. 3, pp. 387–395, 2012.

[12] T. Sasajima, Y. Kubo, M. Inaba, K. Goh, and N. Azuma, "Role of infrainguinal bypass in Buerger's disease: an eighteen-year experience," *European Journal of Vascular and Endovascular Surgery*, vol. 13, no. 2, pp. 186–192, 1997.

[13] G. Piazza and M. A. Creager, "Thromboangiitis obliterans," *Circulation*, vol. 121, no. 16, pp. 1858–1861, 2010.

[14] K. Miyamoto, K. Nishigami, N. Nagaya et al., "Unblinded pilot study of autologous transplantation of bone marrow mononuclear cells in patients with thromboangiitis obliterans," *Circulation*, vol. 114, no. 24, pp. 2679–2684, 2006.

[15] R. W. Franz, K. J. Shah, J. D. Johnson et al., "Short- to midterm results using autologous bone-marrow mononuclear cell implantation therapy as a limb salvage procedure in patients with severe peripheral arterial disease," *Vascular and Endovascular Surgery*, vol. 45, no. 5, pp. 398–406, 2011.

[16] J. Hung, J. Y. T. Lam, L. Lacoste, and G. Letchacovski, "Cigarette smoking acutely increases platelet thrombus formation in patients with coronary artery disease taking aspirin," *Circulation*, vol. 92, no. 9, pp. 2432–2436, 1995.

28

Surgical Treatment of Cystic Adventitial Disease of the Popliteal Artery

Kimihiro Igari, Toshifumi Kudo, Takahiro Toyofuku, and Yoshinori Inoue

Division of Vascular and Endovascular Surgery, Department of Surgery, Tokyo Medical and Dental University,
1-5-45 Yushima, Bunkyo-ku, Tokyo 113-8519, Japan

Correspondence should be addressed to Kimihiro Igari; igari.srg1@tmd.ac.jp

Academic Editor: Muzaffer Sindel

Cystic adventitial disease (CAD) is a rare cause of intermittent claudication and nonatherosclerotic conditions in middle-aged men without cardiovascular risk factors. The etiology of CAD is unclear; however, the direct communication between a cyst and a joint is presumed to be a cause. We herein report a case series of CAD of the popliteal artery (CADPA), in which patients were treated with surgical resection and vascular reconstruction. Although less invasive treatment modalities, including percutaneous cyst aspiration and percutaneous transluminal angioplasty, have been the subject of recent reports, these treatments have had a higher recurrence rate. Therefore, all of the CAPDA cases in the present series were treated surgically, which lead to good outcomes.

1. Introduction

Cystic adventitial disease (CAD) is a rare nonatherosclerotic condition in which fluid accumulates subadventitially and compresses the lumen of the arteries and veins. In 80–90% of cases, CAD is located in the popliteal artery, where it may cause intermittent claudication and critical limb ischemia [1, 2]. The etiology of CAD has not been completely elucidated. It is hypothesized that a direct connection in the adventitia between the joint and the affected vessel grows into an abnormal cyst [3]. Due to this hypothesis, it is thought that CAD mainly affects the popliteal artery, which is located adjacent to the knee joint. CAD of the popliteal artery (CADPA) predominantly affects men of the ages of 40–50 years [4]. CADPA should differ from other peripheral arterial disease without the risk factors of cardiovascular diseases. In this report, we describe the results of our experience in the surgical treatment of CAD of the popliteal artery.

2. Case Presentation

2.1. Patients and Methods. A retrospective review was performed of all patients with a diagnosis of PFAA who underwent surgical treatment at Tokyo Medical and Dental University Hospital between January 2004 and December 2014. All subjects provided informed consent, and approval was obtained from our Institutional Review Board for a retrospective review of the patients' medical records and images. The diagnosis of CADPA was made by imaging methods including ultrasonography (US), computed tomography (CT), magnetic resonance imaging (MRI), and angiography. The medical records were abstracted to include basic demographic information, preoperative symptoms, surgical procedures, intraoperative findings, and long-term imaging findings. The characteristic features of the patients are listed in Table 1.

2.2. Case 1. A 47-year-old male presented with a sudden-onset pain in his left leg and was admitted to another hospital. Angiography showed a 90% stenosis of the left popliteal artery, and he was transferred to our hospital. On physical examination, his left popliteal and pedal pulses were diminished, and his ankle brachial pressure index (ABI) on the left side was 0.5. US and MRI showed a severe stenosis of the left popliteal artery, which was compressed by a cystic mass. He was therefore diagnosed with CADPA. We decided to perform a surgical resection of the affected popliteal artery with vascular reconstruction. Under general anesthesia, his right great saphenous vein was harvested,

TABLE 1: Patients characteristics.

Pt	Gender	Age	Laterality	Clinical symptoms	Diagnostic modality	Comorbidity
1	M	47	Lt	Rest pain, coldness	Angiography, US, MRI	DL, smoker
2	M	36	Lt	IC	CT	Smoker
3	M	58	Rt	IC	CT	HT
4	F	63	Lt	IC	US, CT	HT, smoker
5	M	68	Rt	IC	US, CT	None

*Pt, patient; M, male; F, female; Rt, right; Lt, left; IC, intermittent claudication; US, ultrasonography; MRI, magnetic resonance imaging; CT, computed tomography; DL, dyslipidemia; HT, hypertension.

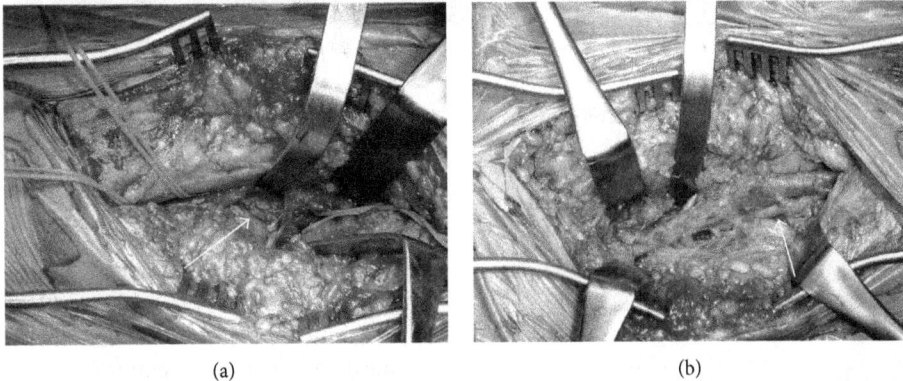

(a)   (b)

FIGURE 1: Intraoperative findings show (a) the controlled affected popliteal artery (white arrow) and (b) the resection being performed with an interposition graft (white arrow). The patient's head was to the right.

and he was positioned prone for a posterior approach. The affected popliteal artery, including the cyst, was exposed and resected (Figure 1(a)), with revascularization using a harvested autologous vein graft (Figure 1(b)). The patient's postoperative course was uneventful. His postoperative ABI increased to 0.8. The histopathological findings showed fibrin and clots within the mucoid gel in the adventitia of the arterial wall, with an intact intima and media.

2.3. Case 2. A 36-year-old male presented with an approximately one month history of intermittent claudication in his left calf with a symptom-free walk interval of 300 meters without rest pain. On physical examination, his left popliteal and pedal pulses were diminished, and his left ABI was 0.66. CT angiography showed an occlusion of the left popliteal artery (Figure 2(a)), compressed by a low density cystic mass (Figure 2(b)). Under general anesthesia, he was positioned prone to harvest the left great saphenous vein below the knee and expose the affected popliteal artery through a posterior approach. The occluded popliteal artery, with a compressing cystic lesion, was resected and the patient was interposed with great saphenous vein graft. The patient's postoperative course was uneventful without any evidence of lower limb ischemia. His postoperative ankle brachial pressure increased to 1.2.

2.4. Case 3. A 58-year-old male presented with one year history of intermittent claudication in his right calf with a symptom-free walk interval of 500 meters without rest pain. On physical examination, his right popliteal and pedal pulses

were palpable, and his right ABI was within the normal range (1.1) at rest. However, after long-distance walking, his right popliteal pulse diminished. CT showed a stenosis of the right popliteal artery, compressed by a low density cystic mass. Under general anesthesia, he was positioned supine to harvest the ipsilateral great saphenous vein and expose the affected popliteal artery through a medial approach. The stenotic popliteal artery with a compressing cystic lesion was resected and the patient was interposed with a great saphenous vein graft. The patient's postoperative course was uneventful without any evidence of lower limb ischemia. His claudication after long-distance walking improved. CAD was confirmed by the histopathological findings, based on the presence of multiple mucinous foci of degeneration in the adventitia of arterial wall (Figure 3).

2.5. Case 4. A 63-year-old female presented with intermittent claudication in her left calf with a symptom-free walk interval of 100 meters without rest pain. On physical examination, her left popliteal and pedal pulses were diminished, and her left ABI was 0.87. CT showed a stenosis of the left popliteal artery, compressed by a low density cystic mass. Under general anesthesia, her right great saphenous vein was harvested, and she was positioned prone for a posterior approach. The affected popliteal artery, including the cyst, was exposed and resected (Figure 4(a)), with revascularization using a harvested autologous vein graft (Figure 4(b)). The patient's postoperative course was uneventful. Her postoperative ABI increased to 1.2.

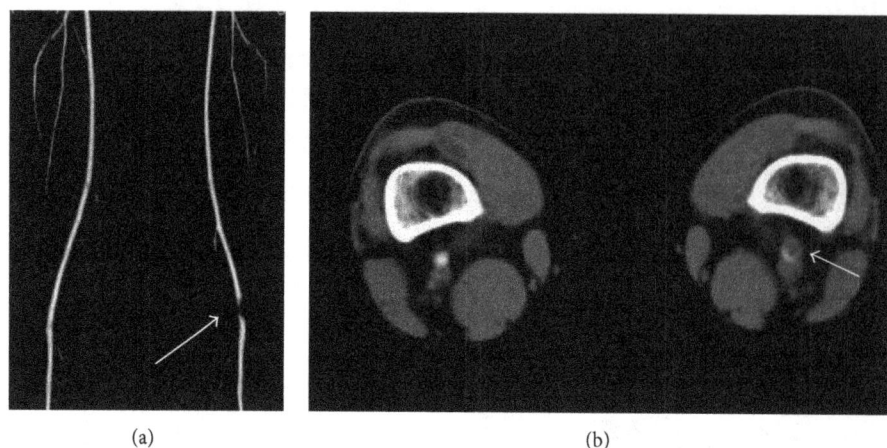

FIGURE 2: Computed tomography shows (a) the occlusion of the left popliteal artery (white arrow) and (b) a cystic mass compressing the popliteal artery (white arrow).

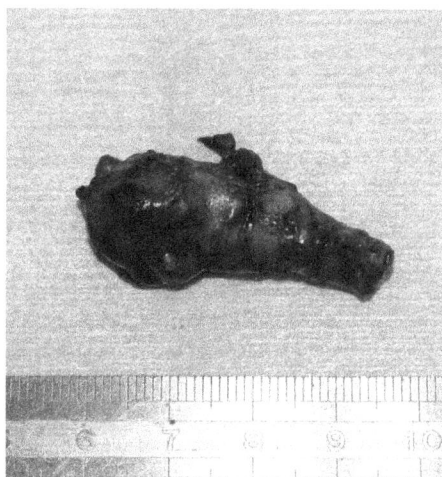

FIGURE 3: A resected specimen showing the popliteal artery with an adventitial cyst.

2.6. Case 5.

A 68-year-old male presented with intermittent claudication in his right calf with a symptom-free walk interval of 200 meters without rest pain. On physical examination, his right popliteal and pedal pulses were diminished, and his right ABI was 0.65. CT showed an occlusion of the right popliteal artery with a length of 6 cm (Figure 5(a)) and a cystic lesion which compressed the popliteal artery (Figure 5(b)). Under general anesthesia, he was positioned supine, and the affected popliteal artery was exposed through a medial approach. The occluded popliteal artery, including the cystic lesion, was resected and the patient was interposed with an 8 mm expanded polytetrafluoroethylene graft. The polytetrafluoroethylene graft was used because the patient's veins were small and unsuitable for the creation of an autologous graft. The patient's postoperative course was uneventful without any evidence of lower limb ischemia. His postoperative ABI increased to 1.11.

2.7. Surgical Procedures and Postoperative Results (Table 2).

A total of five CADPA patients were treated surgically. The mean operative time was 222 minutes (range: 200–262 minutes) and the mean amount of intraoperative blood loss was 180 mL (range: 82–432 mL); thus, none of the patients required a blood transfusion. Four of the five CADPA cases were interposed with a great saphenous vein graft. The other patient was interposed with an expanded polytetrafluoroethylene graft. A pathological examination of the resected popliteal arteries (including cysts) confirmed the diagnosis of CAD for each of the patients.

None of the patients exhibited lower limb ischemia after the surgical procedures and all were discharged successfully. During the long-term follow-up period (mean: 44 months, range: 10–124 months), no patients presented with signs of lower limb ischemia, and all of the interposed grafts remained patent.

3. Discussion

CAD remains a rare cause of lower limb ischemia, with a prevalence of 0.1% among the patients with intermittent claudication [4]. CAD mainly affects men, with a male to female ratio of 15 : 1. Patients with CAD first present clinical symptoms, including lower limb ischemia, between the ages of 10 and 70 years; the peak incidence is at 40 to 50 years [2]. In the present case series, most patients were male (80%), and the age at presentation ranged from 36 to 68 years. These findings are comparable with previous reports. Since CAD patients have no signs of atherosclerotic disease or cardiovascular risk factors; the diagnosis should be differentiated from popliteal artery entrapment syndrome, fibromuscular dysplasia, Buerger's disease, and popliteal artery aneurysm [5].

There are several hypotheses concerning the etiology of CAD, which is currently unclear. The proposed hypotheses include systemic disorders, repetitive trauma, an embryological origin, and the direct communication between a cyst and

TABLE 2: Surgical procedures, intraoperative findings, and long-term follow-up results.

Pt	Surgical procedure	Conduit	Operative time (min)	Intraoperative blood loss (mL)	Follow-up (month)	Limb ischemia	Graft patency
1	Resection + revascularization	AVG	200	150	124	None	Patent
2	Resection + revascularization	AVG	213	432	52	None	Patent
3	Resection + revascularization	AVG	211	155	22	None	Patent
4	Resection + revascularization	AVG	262	84	16	None	Patent
5	Resection + revascularization	ePTFE	228	82	10	None	Patent

*Pt, patient; AVG, autologous vein graft; ePTFE, expanded polytetrafluoroethylene.

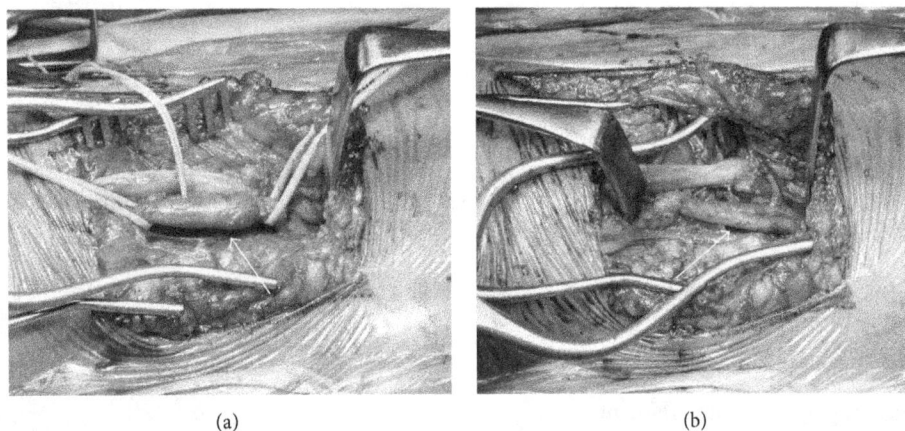

(a)　　　　　　　　　　　　　　　(b)

FIGURE 4: Intraoperative findings showing (a) the controlled left popliteal artery (white arrow) and (b) the performance of resection with graft interposition (white arrow). The patient's head was to the right.

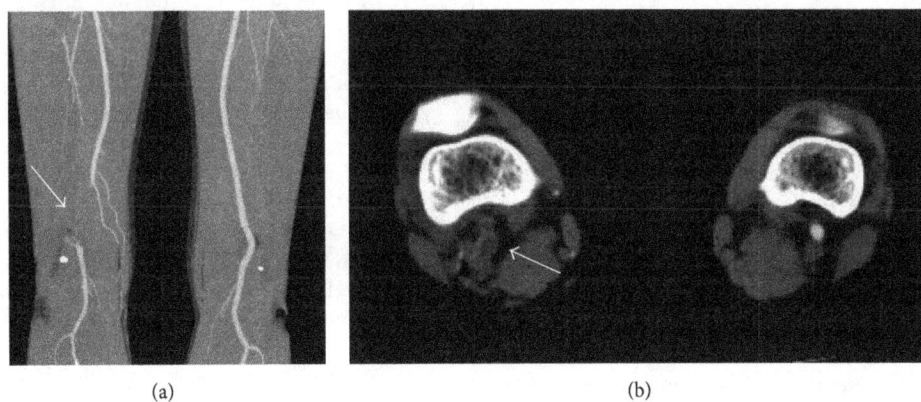

(a)　　　　　　　　　　　　　　　(b)

FIGURE 5: Computed tomography shows (a) the occlusion of the left popliteal artery (white arrow) and (b) a cystic mass compressing the popliteal artery (white arrow).

the adjacent joint (ganglion theory) [6]. Systemic disorders might be associated with generalized disorder, which leads to CAD; however, this hypothesis has failed to gain substantial support since the systemic manifestation of CAD has not been shown in the follow-up examinations of any patients [7]. Even though some authors have shown the traumatic events in patients with CAD, there remains a lack of young patients with CAD who have a history of repeated trauma. There was no history of recurrent trauma in the limbs of the patients in our case series, and it is difficult to decide

the etiology of CAD as trauma. An embryological origin may be explained by the developmental theory, which states that mesenchymal mucin-secreting cell rests become incorporated within the adventitia of arteries during embryonic development [8]. However, this hypothesis is difficult to apply to the explanation of cyst recurrence after total cyst excision [9]. CAD occurs mainly in large arteries and veins which overlie a joint. Since Shute et al. first reported a direct communication between the knee joint and an adventitial cyst in 1973 [10], many authors have reported the same findings. This ganglion theory presumes that an adventitial cyst is the result of capsular synovial structures growing and tracking in the adventitia along the vascular branches. The theory is supported by the fact that the morphology of the cysts is very similar to that of ganglions in that they contain a high concentration of hyaluronic acid [11]. These direct communications have been found on preoperative imaging tests [12], and through intraoperative examinations [3]. This is now the most convincing and best-supported theory. Even though we did not find a pedicle around the cyst connected to the knee joint, the joint connections can be easily missed [13]; therefore, the communications may have been missed in the preoperative images and during intraoperative examination.

A typical clinical symptom of CADPA is the rapid progression of intermittent calf claudication, occasionally with sudden onset [14]. One of the 5 patients in our series presented with sudden-onset claudication; the other four patients presented with claudication that rapidly worsened. In some cases, normal pulses and normal ABI level have been associated with CADPA [15]. The ABI and pedal pulses in the affected side were normal at rest in the third case of our series; however, after exercise, the patient's ABI and pedal pulses diminished. Therefore, patients with a history of intermittent claudication and normal pedal pulses should be checked to differentiate CAD.

US, CT, MRI, and angiography are frequently used to diagnose CAD. MRI seems to be the most helpful of these modalities for detecting the relationship between cysts and vessels or the surrounding structures [16]. Furthermore, MRI can exclude other pathologies included in the differential diagnosis of the popliteal artery, such as atherosclerotic disease, aneurysm, popliteal artery entrapment syndrome, and soft-tissue tumors. MRI has also been demonstrated to be useful in detecting the connection between an adventitial cyst and the knee joint [17]. If MRI is employed more frequently in the diagnosis of CADPA, we might detect these direct connections. At present, however, the direct connection is thought to be too small to be revealed by any imaging techniques.

Several treatment options have been proposed for CAD-PA. These are divided into nonresectional and resectional techniques. Nonresectional techniques include open cyst evacuation with the removal of the cyst wall with or without patch angioplasty [18], percutaneous or open cyst aspiration, and percutaneous angioplasty [19]. Resection techniques consist of the resection of the affected artery and revascularization with direct anastomosis or graft interposition. While the aspiration technique is less invasive, the recurrence rate is high (approximately 40%) [1]. The endoluminal approach has an even higher recurrence rate (67%) [1]. These less invasive approaches are therefore considered to be inadequate for the treatment of CAD. Cyst evacuation has mostly been performed with nonresectional techniques, with an initial success rate of 94% [20]. However, these techniques are not suitable for the treatment of cases with total occlusion of the popliteal artery, which require vascular reconstruction. Therefore, the resectional techniques of cyst resection and vascular reconstruction are generally recommended as the treatment of choice for CADPA, especially in cases of total

occlusion of the popliteal artery [2]. The recurrence rate of CAD treated by this technique is 1% [1], which is lowest rate of all of the treatment modalities. All of the cases in our series were therefore treated by the resection of the affected popliteal artery with autologous vein or prosthetic graft interposition. Furthermore, in resecting the affected popliteal artery, we are able to cut off the direct connection between the cyst and the knee joint, which is thought to create the adventitial cyst. This resectional technique is compatible from the point of view of CAD etiology.

In conclusion, we herein reported a case series of CADPA treated surgically with resection of the affected popliteal artery and vascular reconstruction in which treatment leads to good long-term outcomes. This resectional technique should be considered for the treatment of CAD, especially in cases in which there is an occlusion of affected vessels. Although CAD is a rare condition, it should be included in the differential diagnosis of young patients with intermittent claudication and no or poor comorbidities.

References

[1] N. M. Desy and R. J. Spinner, "The etiology and management of cystic adventitial disease," *Journal of Vascular Surgery*, vol. 60, no. 1, pp. 235–245, 2014.

[2] P. W. J. van Rutte, E. V. Rouwet, E. H. J. Belgers, R. F. Lim, and J. A. W. Teijink, "In treatment of popliteal artery cystic adventitial disease, primary bypass graft not always first choice: two case reports and a review of the literature," *European Journal of Vascular and Endovascular Surgery*, vol. 42, no. 3, pp. 347–354, 2011.

[3] N. Tsilimparis, U. Hanack, S. Yousefi, P. Alevizakos, and R. I. Rückert, "Cystic adventitial disease of the popliteal artery: an argument for the developmental theory," *Journal of Vascular Surgery*, vol. 45, no. 6, pp. 1249–1252, 2007.

[4] M. M. Hernández Mateo, F. J. Serrano Hernando, I. Martínez López et al., "Cystic adventitial degeneration of the popliteal artery: report on 3 cases and review of the literature," *Annals of Vascular Surgery*, vol. 28, no. 4, pp. 1062–1069, 2014.

[5] E. C. Korngold and M. R. Jaff, "Unusual causes of intermittent claudication: popliteal artery entrapment syndrome, cystic adventitial disease, fibromuscular dysplasia, and endofibrosis," *Current Treatment Options in Cardiovascular Medicine*, vol. 11, no. 2, pp. 156–166, 2009.

[6] L. Zhang, R. Guzman, I. Kirkpatrick, and J. Klein, "Spontaneous resolution of cystic adventitial disease: a word of caution," *Annals of Vascular Surgery*, vol. 26, no. 3, pp. 422.e1–422.e4, 2012.

[7] G. Asciutto, A. Mumme, B. Marpe, T. Hummel, and B. Geier, "Different approaches in the treatment of cystic adventitial disease of the popliteal artery," *Chirurgia Italiana*, vol. 59, no. 4, pp. 467–473, 2007.

[8] L. J. Levien and C.-A. Benn, "Adventitial cystic disease: a unifying hypothesis," *Journal of Vascular Surgery*, vol. 28, no. 2, pp. 193–205, 1998.

[9] K. Cassar and J. Engeset, "Cystic adventitial disease: a trap for the unwary," *European Journal of Vascular and Endovascular Surgery*, vol. 29, no. 1, pp. 93–96, 2005.

[10] K. Shute and N. G. Rothnie, "The aetiology of cystic arterial disease," *British Journal of Surgery*, vol. 60, no. 5, pp. 397–400, 1973.

[11] M. P. Buijsrogge, S. van der Meij, J. H. Korte, and W. M. Fritschy, "'Intermittent claudication intermittence' as a manifestation of adventitial cystic disease communicating with the knee joint," *Annals of Vascular Surgery*, vol. 20, no. 5, pp. 687–689, 2006.

[12] I. M. Maged, U. C. Turba, A. M. Housseini, J. A. Kern, I. L. Kron, and K. D. Hagspiel, "High spatial resolution magnetic resonance imaging of cystic adventitial disease of the popliteal artery," *Journal of Vascular Surgery*, vol. 51, no. 2, pp. 471–474, 2010.

[13] R. J. Spinner, N. M. Desy, G. Agarwal, W. Pawlina, M. Kalra, and K. K. Amrami, "Evidence to support that adventitial cysts, analogous to intraneural ganglion cysts, are also joint-connected," *Clinical Anatomy*, vol. 26, no. 2, pp. 267–281, 2013.

[14] Y. Inoue, T. Iwai, K. Ohashi et al., "A case of popliteal cystic degeneration with pathological considerations," *Annals of Vascular Surgery*, vol. 6, no. 6, pp. 525–529, 1992.

[15] A. Miller, J.-P. Salenius, B. A. Sacks, S. K. Gupta, and G. M. Shoukimas, "Noninvasive vascular imaging in the diagnosis and treatment of adventitial cystic disease of the popliteal artery," *Journal of Vascular Surgery*, vol. 26, no. 4, pp. 715–720, 1997.

[16] W. R. Ortiz M, J. E. Lopera, C. R. Giménez, S. Restrepo, R. Moncada, and W. R. Castañeda-Zúñiga, "Bilateral adventitial cystic disease of the popliteal artery: a case report," *CardioVascular and Interventional Radiology*, vol. 29, no. 2, pp. 306–310, 2006.

[17] J. Ortmann, M. K. Widmer, S. Gretener et al., "Cystic adventitial degeneration: ectopic ganglia from adjacent joint capsules," *Vasa*, vol. 38, no. 4, pp. 374–377, 2009.

[18] S. Kikuchi, T. Sasajima, T. Kokubo, A. Koya, H. Uchida, and N. Azuma, "Clinical results of cystic excision for popliteal artery cystic adventitial disease: long-term benefits of preserving the intact intima," *Annals of Vascular Surgery*, vol. 28, no. 6, pp. 1567.e5–1567.e8, 2014.

[19] M. Khoury, "Failed angioplasty of a popliteal artery stenosis secondary to cystic adventitial disease: a case report," *Vascular and Endovascular Surgery*, vol. 38, no. 3, pp. 277–280, 2004.

[20] I. A. Tsolakis, C. S. Walvatne, and M. D. Caldwell, "Cystic adventitial disease of the popliteal artery: diagnosis and treatment," *European Journal of Vascular and Endovascular Surgery*, vol. 15, no. 3, pp. 188–194, 1998.

29

The Infrapopliteal Arterial Occlusions Similar to Buerger Disease

Kimihiro Igari,[1] **Toshifumi Kudo,**[1] **Takahiro Toyofuku,**[1]
Yoshinori Inoue,[1] **and Takehisa Iwai**[2]

[1] *Division of Vascular and Endovascular Surgery, Department of Surgery, Tokyo Medical and Dental University,*
1-5-45 Yushima, Bunkyo-ku, Tokyo 113-8519, Japan
[2] *Tsukuba Vascular Center and Buerger Disease Research Institute, 980-1 Tatsuzawa, Moriya, Ibaraki 302-0118, Japan*

Correspondence should be addressed to Kimihiro Igari; igari.srg1@tmd.ac.jp

Academic Editor: Konstantinos A. Filis

We herein present two cases that required the differential diagnosis of Buerger disease. Case 1 involved a 55-year-old male with a smoking habit who was admitted with ulcers and coldness in his fingers and toes. Angiography showed blockage in both the radial and posterior tibial arteries, which led to an initial diagnosis of Buerger disease. However, a biopsy of the right posterior tibial artery showed pathological findings of fibromuscular dysplasia (FMD). Case 2 involved a 28-year-old male with intermittent claudication who was examined at another hospital. Angiography showed occlusion of both popliteal and crural arteries, and the patient was suspected to have Buerger disease. However, computed tomography disclosed an abnormal slip on both sides of the popliteal fossa, and we diagnosed him with bilateral popliteal artery entrapment syndrome (PAES). These cases illustrate that other occlusive diseases, such as FMD and PAES, may sometimes be misdiagnosed as Buerger disease.

1. Introduction

Buerger disease is a nonatherosclerotic inflammatory occlusive disease [1], which most commonly affects the small- and medium-sized arteries and veins of the upper and lower extremities [2]. Most of patients with Buerger disease are young males, typically <50 years of age [3], and are usually heavy cigarette smokers, with no atherosclerotic risk factors other than smoking.

Buerger disease is one of the many diseases presenting with ischemic symptoms that manifest as intermittent claudication, rest pain, ulceration, and/or gangrene. Since the specific clinical features of Buerger disease are characterized by peripheral ischemia, the diagnostic criteria should be discussed from the clinical point of view. However, the clinical criteria used to diagnose Buerger disease remain controversial [4], and some authors have stated that the diagnosis of Buerger disease requires arteriography and biopsy assessments of the affected arteries [5], which makes it difficult to diagnose Buerger disease precisely. We herein

present two cases of lower extremity ischemic symptoms that required a differential diagnosis of Buerger disease.

2. Case Presentation

Case 1. A 55-year-old male with a smoking habit was admitted with ulcers and coldness in his fingers and toes. His medical history was unremarkable, without diabetes mellitus, hyperlipidemia, or hypertension. During the clinical examination, his third and fourth fingers on the left side were observed to be ulcerated, and his fourth right toe was gangrenous. The bilateral radial and posterior tibial arteries were not palpable; however, the ankle brachial index (ABI) was within the normal range on both sides. The laboratory findings failed to show any thrombophilia, autoimmune disorders, or malignant diseases. However, arteriography disclosed blockage in both the radial and posterior tibial arteries, which led to an initial diagnosis of Buerger disease (Figure 1).

With respect to the Shionoya diagnostic criteria [6], the patient had a history of smoking, and the initial onset of

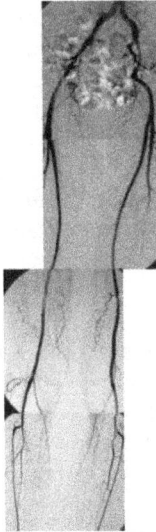

FIGURE 1: Case 1: preoperative arteriography showed that the bilateral iliac, femoral, and popliteal arteries were intact, but the bilateral posterior tibial arteries were occluded.

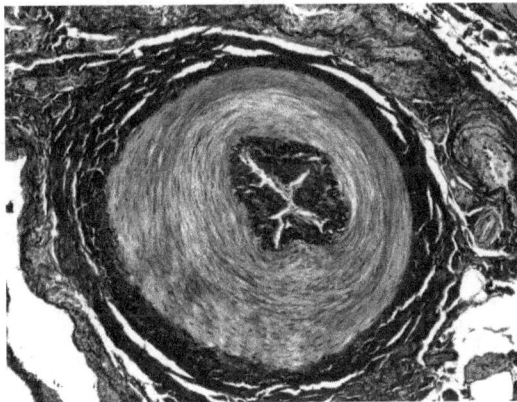

FIGURE 2: A biopsy specimen of the right posterior tibial artery in Case 1. The arterial wall in the media was thickened. There was no evidence of infiltration of inflammatory cells (Elastica van Gieson stain, ×40).

symptoms occurred at 49 years of age. The infrapopliteal and upper extremity arteries were affected, and he had no risk factors for atherosclerosis, except for his smoking habit. Therefore, we diagnosed him as having Buerger disease.

We performed sympathectomy of the left thoracic sympathetic nerve and the right lumbar sympathetic nerve, with a simultaneous biopsy of the right posterior tibial artery. The patient's postoperative course was uneventful, and the ulceration and gangrene healed successfully. On a histopathological examination of the right posterior tibial artery, no organized clotting or venous thrombophlebitis were observed. The resected arterial wall was thickened in the media and hyperplastic in the adventitia and there were no inflammatory cells (Figure 2). These findings suggested that the patient had fibromuscular dysplasia (FMD), rather than Buerger disease. As a result, he was initially diagnosed with

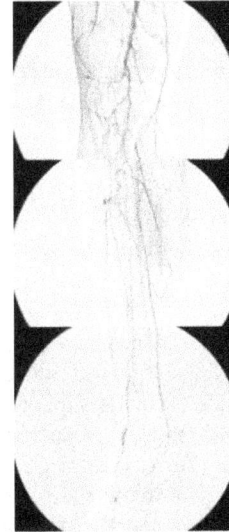

FIGURE 3: Case 2: preoperative arteriography showed that the popliteal artery was occluded, but there were no abrupt interruptions in the tibial or peroneal arteries.

Buerger disease based on the Shionoya diagnostic criteria and then finally diagnosed with FMD based on the pathological findings of the peripheral arteries.

Case 2. A 28-year-old male presented at another hospital with a three-year history of intermittent claudication in the left lower limb and coldness in the toes. He had no cardiovascular risk factors, such as diabetes mellitus, dyslipidemia, or a smoking habit. However, angiography showed occlusion of both popliteal arteries and widespread obstruction of the crural arteries, which led to an initial diagnosis of Buerger disease (Figure 3). The patient was then transferred to our hospital. According to the clinical examinations, the bilateral femoral, popliteal, and brachial arteries were palpable; however, the pedal pulses on the right side were absent. The ABI on the right side was 0.50, while that on the left side was within the normal range.

The laboratory investigations showed no abnormalities, including a hypercoagulable state or autoimmune or infectious diseases. However, computed tomography (CT) revealed compression of the right popliteal artery from the medial head of the gastrocnemius muscle as well as the left popliteal artery due to an accessory slip of the gastrocnemius muscle. The clinical findings did not fulfill the diagnostic criteria for Buerger disease, and the CT results showed that the structure of the bilateral popliteal fossa had caused the ischemia. Therefore, we corrected the diagnosis to popliteal artery entrapment syndrome (PAES) rather than Buerger disease and treated the patient surgically.

We subsequently performed right femoroposterior tibial bypass with autogenous vein and left resection of the accessory slip of the medial head of the gastrocnemius muscle. The patient's postoperative course was uneventful, and the claudication was relieved after the surgery.

3. Discussion

Buerger disease is primarily diagnosed based on clinical symptoms. We use Shionoya's criteria [6] to diagnose Buerger disease at our institution. These criteria include five clinical signs: a history of smoking; onset before 50 years of age; infrapopliteal arterial occlusive disease; upper limb involvement or phlebitis migrans; and the absence of atherosclerotic risk factors other than smoking. Imaging modalities should be used to identify the distribution of arterial involvement. Angiography is essential for making an accurate diagnosis of Buerger disease. Typical arteriographic findings, such as abrupt or tapering occlusion, corkscrew collaterals, and the absence of calcification, provide supporting evidence for a diagnosis of Buerger disease [7]. Biopsy and tissue sampling are rarely needed to confirm the diagnosis of Buerger disease; however, in rare cases with an unusual onset of symptoms, the histopathological findings are useful for making the definitive diagnosis [8].

FMD is a nonatherosclerotic, noninflammatory arterial disease that usually affects the small and medium arteries, followed by luminal narrowing and aneurysm formation [9]. The disease occurs in young patients with few cardiovascular risk factors, and the most distinctive clinical feature of FMD is the distribution of the affected arteries. Notably, the renal arteries (79.7%) and extracranial carotid artery (74.3%) are highly involved in cases of FMD [10]. However, in the current Case 1, the renal and carotid arteries were intact. The onset of FMD in the peripheral arteries, as noted in Case 1, is very rare [11]. FMD is divided histopathologically into five types according to the affected arterial layer: intimal fibroplasia, medial fibroplasia, perimedial fibroplasia, medial hyperplasia, and adventitial fibroplasia [12]. In Case 1, the arterial wall was thickened primarily in the media, and hyperplasia was seen in the adventitia. Therefore, the patient was diagnosed with the perimedial fibroplasia type of FMD. It is interesting that Case 1 was diagnosed as Buerger disease according to Shionoya's clinical criteria and then rediagnosed as FMD based on the histopathological findings. This suggests that FMD may have been present in previous cases of Buerger disease.

In Case 2, Buerger disease was suspected based on the arteriographic findings of diffuse infrapopliteal arterial occlusion. However, the patient had neither a smoking habit nor upper limb involvement. Therefore, we rediagnosed the case as non-Buerger disease, and the CT findings showed abnormal bilateral musculotendinous structures surrounding the popliteal fossa, which led to the correct diagnosis of PAES. The majority of PAES cases have been reported in young males, with over half of patients diagnosed before 30 years of age. Popliteal artery compression by abnormal slips causes intimal damage, thrombosis, and distal embolization [13], which leads to ischemic damage and eventual limb loss. Surgical management requires releasing extrinsic compression and restoring the arterial flow. Myotomy of the abnormal muscle and/or revascularization procedures are required. Sympathectomy is effective for Buerger disease; however, patients with PAES require release of the arterial compression, not sympathectomy, which is the only possible

treatment for relieving the ischemic symptoms. Therefore, PAES should be promptly and accurately diagnosed so that it can be effectively treated in order to prevent the development of severe irreparable ischemic complications. Buerger disease is similar to PAES in the points of the young age of onset and male predominance. However, Buerger disease is strongly correlated with smoking, and the disease generally occurs in young smokers, with episodes of remission being correlated with smoking cessation and relapse being correlated with restarting smoking [14]. In cases such as Case 2, in which the patient did not have a history of smoking, the possibility of peripheral arterial diseases other than Buerger disease should be considered initially because Buerger disease is strongly associated with smoking.

In conclusion, Buerger disease is a clinical diagnosis that requires a compatible history, supportive physical findings, and the presence of diagnostic vascular abnormalities on imaging studies. Laboratory tests, including assessments of the autoimmune system and a hypercoagulable state, are used to exclude alternative diagnoses in patients with suspected Buerger disease. Distal small to medium artery involvement, segmental occlusion, and a "corkscrew" appearance of collaterals are typical angiographic findings in patients with Buerger disease. Diagnosing Buerger disease is not usually difficult in typical cases, although uniform criteria are lacking. Therefore, physicians should be aware that it is possible that other occlusive diseases, such as FMD and PAES, are to be misdiagnosed as Buerger disease in some cases.

References

[1] T. Iwai, Y. Inoue, M. Umeda et al., "Oral bacteria in the occluded arteries of patients with Buerger disease," *Journal of Vascular Surgery*, vol. 42, no. 1, pp. 107–115, 2005.

[2] K. Laohapensang, K. Rerkasem, and V. Kattipattanapong, "Decrease in the incidence of buerger's disease recurrence in northern Thailand," *Surgery Today*, vol. 35, no. 12, pp. 1060–1065, 2005.

[3] G. Piazza and M. A. Creager, "Thromboangiitis obliterans," *Circulation*, vol. 121, no. 16, pp. 1858–1861, 2010.

[4] J. J. Swigris, J. W. Olin, and N. A. Mekhail, "Implantable spinal cord stimulator to treat the ischemic manifestations of thromboangiitis obliterans (Buerger's disease)," *Journal of Vascular Surgery*, vol. 29, no. 5, pp. 928–935, 1999.

[5] J. L. Mills, E. I. Friedman, L. M. Taylor, and J. M. Porter, "Upper extremity ischemia caused by small artery disease," *Annals of Surgery*, vol. 206, no. 4, pp. 521–528, 1987.

[6] S. Shionoya, "Diagnostic criteria of Buerger's disease," *International Journal of Cardiology*, vol. 66, no. 1, pp. S243–S245, 1998.

[7] J. W. Olin and A. Shih, "Thromboangitis obliterans (Buerger's disease)," *Current Opinion in Rheumatology*, vol. 18, pp. 18–24, 2006.

[8] Y. P. Cho, G. H. Kang, M. S. Han et al., "Mesenteric involvement of acute-stage Buerger's disease as the initial clinical manifestation: report of a case," *Surgery Today*, vol. 35, no. 6, pp. 499–501, 2005.

[9] J. W. Olin and B. A. Sealove, "Diagnosis, management, and future developments of fibromuscular dysplasia," *Journal of Vascular Surgery*, vol. 53, no. 3, pp. 826.e1–836.e1, 2011.

[10] J. W. Olin, J. Froehlich, X. Gu et al., "The United States registry for fibromuscular dysplasia: results in the first 447 patients," *Circulation*, vol. 125, no. 25, pp. 3182–3190, 2012.

[11] T. Iwai, S. Konno, K. Hiejima et al., "Fibromuscular dysplasia in the extremities," *The Journal of Cardiovascular Surgery*, vol. 26, no. 5, pp. 496–501, 1985.

[12] C. A. Anderson, K. J. Hansen, M. E. Benjamin, D. R. Keith, T. E. Craven, and R. H. Dean, "Renal artery fibromuscular dysplasia: results of current surgical therapy," *Journal of Vascular Surgery*, vol. 22, no. 3, pp. 207–215, 1995.

[13] T. Iwai, S. Konno, K. Soga et al., "Diagnostic and pathological considerations in the popliteal artery entrapment syndrome," *Journal of Cardiovascular Surgery*, vol. 24, no. 3, pp. 243–249, 1983.

[14] X. Puéchal and J.-N. Fiessinger, "Thromboangiitis obliterans or Buerger's disease: challenges for the rheumatologist," *Rheumatology*, vol. 46, no. 2, pp. 192–199, 2007.

30

Mediastinal B-Cell Lymphoma Presenting with Jugular-Subclavian Deep Vein Thrombosis as the First Presentation

Sherif Ali Eltawansy,[1] Mana Rao,[1] Sidney Ceniza,[1] and David Sharon[1,2]

[1]*Department of Internal Medicine, Monmouth Medical Center, Long Branch, NJ 07740, USA*
[2]*Department of Oncological Medicine, Monmouth Medical Center, Long Branch, NJ 07740, USA*

Correspondence should be addressed to Sherif Ali Eltawansy; seltawansy@barnabashealth.org

Academic Editor: Luca Masotti

Jugular venous thrombosis infrequently could be secondary to malignancy and has seldom been reported secondary to mediastinal large B-cell lymphomas. The postulated mechanisms are mechanical compression that leads to stagnation of blood in the venous system of the neck and/or an increase in the circulating thrombogenic elements that could cause venous thromboembolism as a paraneoplastic phenomenon. We report the case of a middle aged male presenting with right sided neck pain and arm swelling secondary to ipsilateral jugular-subclavian deep vein thrombosis. Investigations revealed it to be secondary to a mediastinal mass shown on CT scan of the chest.

1. Introduction

Malignancies have a causal association with deep vein thrombosis which can be secondary to mechanical pressure of the tumor on the venous system draining blood from the affected part of the body or it could be a systemic phenomenon secondary to thrombogenic material released into the circulation from the tumorigenic tissue. Venous thromboembolism (VTE) is found at autopsy in at least 50% of cancer patients [1, 2]. However, assessment of the true incidence of VTE in cancer patients is difficult because most of these patients receive chemotherapy or hormonal therapy, both of which can precipitate VTE [3]. In addition, many cancer patients have indwelling central venous lines, which can also initiate thrombotic events in relation to the catheter [4]. One of the most common causes of upper extremity vein thrombosis is prolonged central vein catheterization. About 66% of patients with internal jugular vein (IJV) catheters have proof of thrombus formation on ultrasound or at autopsy [5]. Spontaneous internal jugular vein thrombosis (IJVT) without a predisposing cause has been rarely reported [6]. However, IJVT may be secondary to malignancies [7, 8].

2. Case Presentation

A 51-year-old Caucasian male with no significant past medical history presented to the emergency room with a one-week history of right sided acute neck and arm pain associated with progressive swelling in the right upper extremity. He did not have such complaints in the past and had never seen a physician. He was smoking for 30 years (1 pack per year) but quit 5 years ago. His family history was significant only for coronary artery disease. Doppler ultrasound of the right upper extremity showed an occlusive thrombus in the right internal jugular vein; a nonocclusive thrombus in the right subclavian vein with minimal flow is within this vessel. The remaining veins including the axillary and brachial veins are patent. Hypercoagulable status work-up was unrevealing and meanwhile the patient was started on enoxaparin subcutaneously with a 1 mg/kg dose every 12 hours. Computed tomography (CT) scan of the chest and the neck with contrast showed a singular anterior mediastinal mass with persistent thrombosis of the right internal jugular, subclavian and innominate veins (Figures 1(a) and 1(b)). There was questionable extension of the clot into the

(a)

(b)

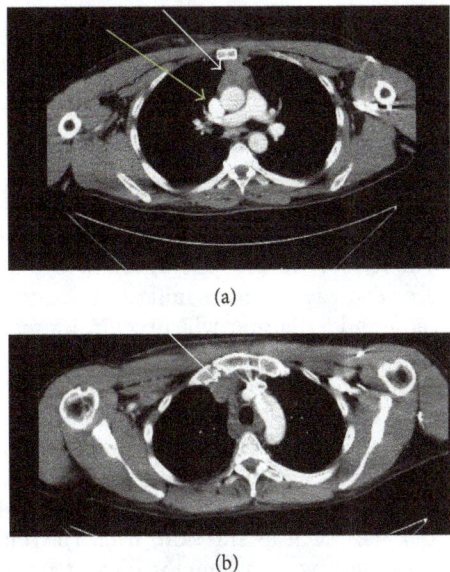

FIGURE 1: CT chest with contrast: 6/29/2014. Technique: contiguous transaxial images were obtained from the thoracic inlet to the upper abdomen with contrast. 125 cc omnipaque 350. (a) Thrombosis of the right internal jugular vein with extension to the right innominate vein and subclavian vein was noted (green arrow). The origin of the great vessels was patent. There was an anterior mediastinal mass (white arrow) present measuring 4.4 × 3.4 cm. Fibrotic changes were noted at the right base. There was no pulmonary mass or infiltrate. The thin cut after contrast series demonstrated no evidence of large pulmonary emboli. Fluid attenuation was noted just superior to the azygos arch likely representing prominence of the pericardial recess. There was a 2.8 × 1.1 cm lymph node in the subcarinal region image. There were prominent right axillary lymph nodes noted. (b) There was prominent soft tissue attenuation in the anterior mediastinum which was abutting the thrombosed jugular and innominate veins (white arrow). This was likely superior extension of the previously mentioned anterior mediastinal mass.

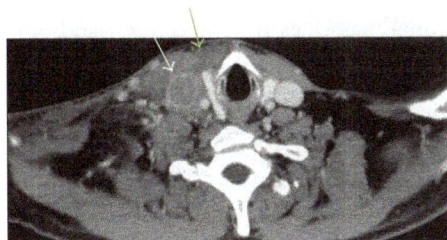

FIGURE 2: Thrombosis of the right internal jugular vein is noted (white arrow). There is hyperemia of the vein wall, and the vein is dilated to 2.9 × 2.4 cm. There is extension of the thrombus into the subclavian vein. There is extension of thrombus into the innominate vein as well. There is a mediastinal soft tissue density measuring 4.1 × 2.8 cm (green arrow). The right vertebral artery is diminutive in size. The basilar artery is patent and the vertebral arteries are patent. The left internal jugular vein is patent. The origins of great vessels are patent. The thrombus in the right jugular vein extends up to the level of the skull base. The extension of the thrombus into the sigmoid sinus on the right is to be noted. The dilated jugular vein is exerting mass effect on the adjacent thyroid gland.

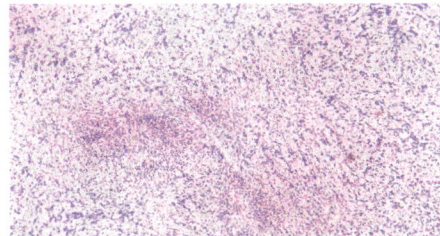

FIGURE 3: Large transformed lymphocytes are identified (low power). They are uniformly CD20+. Having in mind that there is a background sclerosis, the diagnosis is mediastinal large B-cell lymphoma with sclerosis. If the disease is localized to the mediastinum, the prognosis of this lymphoma is excellent. Stains used in this study: CD20, CD3, CD30, and CD10.

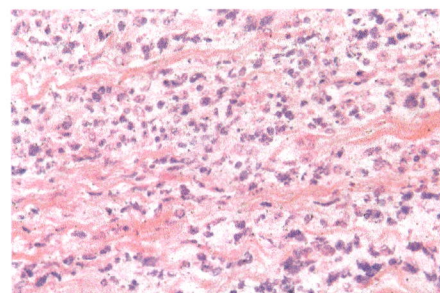

FIGURE 4: Mediastinal large B-cell lymphoma biopsy (high power).

right sigmoid sinus (Figure 2). CT brain and CT abdomen and pelvis were normal. Right video assisted thoracoscopic surgery was done and a biopsy of the anterior mediastinal mass was obtained with no complications. Biopsy showed mediastinal large B-cell lymphoma with sclerosis (Figures 3, 4, 5, and 6). Bone marrow biopsy was obtained and excluded the involvement of bone marrow. Cytogenetics study for lymphoma staging showed an apparently normal 46, XY male complement. No apparent numerical or structural abnormalities were evident. Flow cytometry study showed that the bone marrow was not involved by B-cell lymphoma morphologically and immunophenotypically. Patient started chemotherapy sessions and was continued on enoxaparin subcutaneously. The PET scan was done, showing two large hypermetabolic nodal masses of the mediastinum representing the lymphoma. One component of the lower mass extends into the anterior mediastinum. The patient started chemotherapy with R-CHOP-regimen.

3. Discussion

The internal jugular vein (IJV) drains blood from the transverse, sigmoid, and inferior petrosal sinuses of the brain and originates in the posterior compartment of the jugular foramen at the base of the skull. It also drains blood from the face and courses through the neck in proximity with the carotid artery, ultimately meeting the subclavian vein to form the brachiocephalic (innominate) vein.

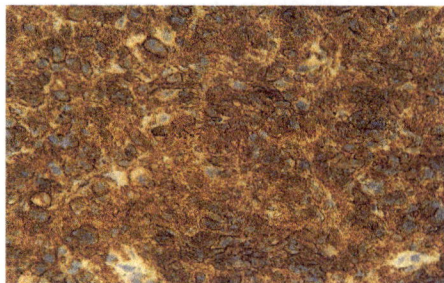

FIGURE 5: CD20 40x. Mediastinal large B-cell lymphoma biopsy CD20 40x.

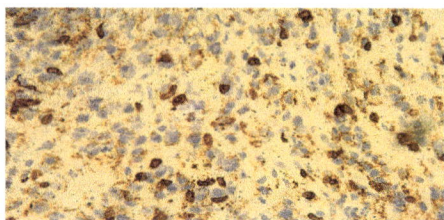

FIGURE 6: CD23 40x. Mediastinal large B-cell lymphoma biopsy CD23 40x.

Internal jugular vein thrombosis (IJVT) may be the result of various conditions of which the most common is maintenance of central venous access devices such as internal jugular vein catheters. The other known and reported reasons for such an occurrence are otolaryngological infections leading to Lemierre syndrome, skin and soft tissue infections around the neck, intravenous drug abuse (direct injection into the IJV), recent head/neck surgery, hypercoagulable states such as protein C or S deficiency, factor V Leiden, antithrombin III deficiency, polycythemia, and hyperhomocysteinemia. Malignant neck masses such as cancers originating in the thyroid or thymus may also precipitate this condition. Ovarian hyperstimulation has also been reported to cause IJVT [9].

The theory behind thrombus formation is the real time interpretation of an archaic concept proposed by Virchow: interruption of blood flow leading to venous stasis, irritation of the blood vessel or its vicinity described as endothelial injury, and phenomena of blood coagulation now known as hypercoagulability.

The way cancers cause venous thrombosis can be either one or both of these: anatomic compression of the blood vessel by tumor bulk or dissemination of prothrombotic material from the tumorigenic tissue (Trousseau's syndrome).

Kunimasa et al. reported a case of spontaneous left sided internal jugular vein thrombosis secondary to a left upper lobe nonsmall cell lung cancer [10]. Serinken et al. reported a case of IJVT secondary to a soft tissue infection in the vicinity of the IJV [11]. Ishida et al. reported a case of IJVT that possibly led to spontaneous spinal epidural hematoma [12]. Chlumský and Havlín encountered a case of IJVT without an obvious cause [13]. Ghatak et al. presented a case of spontaneous pulmonary embolism, IJVT, and subclavian vein thrombosis in a patient with septic shock who was found to have factor V Leiden mutation and activated protein C

resistance and was curiously reported to have dengue IgM positive [14]. Lønnebakken et al. found an internal jugular vein thrombosis incidentally secondary to substernal goiter [15].

Another case with jugular vein thrombosis was reported secondary to a deep neck lipoma [16].

To date, there are no set guidelines for the treatment of internal jugular vein thrombosis. Sheikh et al. report the use of low molecular weight heparin followed by warfarin and superior vena cava filter to mitigate the possibility of clot expansion and extension which could ultimately lead to pulmonary embolism, in a select subset of patients who were not deemed to be candidates for anticoagulation [6]. Lymphoma is a well-known blood/lymphatic malignancy with different clinical presentations that may vary from the occurrence of B symptoms (fever, night sweats, and weight loss) to enlargement of lymph nodes and involvement of extranodal sites such as the skin, liver, gastrointestinal tract, and bone marrow. Less common presentations include but are not limited to symptoms from the primary tumor compressing its surrounding normal tissue. This has been reported in Burkitt's lymphoma causing abdominal pain and fullness, given its predilection for the abdomen. Albeit, it is infrequent to find that superior vena cava syndrome has been reported to occur with tumors that compress the great vessels in the neck and mediastinum [10].

SVC syndrome is even more common in patients with primary mediastinal large B-cell lymphoma with sclerosis, an unusual and aggressive NHL subtype that represents 3 to 7 percent of all diffuse large cell lymphomas. Patients typically present with a rapidly enlarging anterior mediastinal mass, frequently with associated SVC syndrome. In one report of 30 patients, 17 (57 percent) had SVC syndrome at presentation [17].

Our patient was eventually diagnosed with mediastinal large B-cell lymphoma with sclerosis. It is a seldom occurrence and hence as physicians it is imperative to be cognizant about the rare but certainly plausible presentation of mediastinal masses as IJVT and SVC syndrome. A high index of suspicion based on age, history, and appropriate clinical characteristics is vital.

4. Conclusion

It is imperative to be cognizant about the infrequent but certainly plausible presentation of mediastinal masses as jugular vein thrombosis and superior vena cava syndrome. The physician must maintain a high index of suspicion based on age, history, and clinical characteristics.

5. Learning Objective

Internal jugular vein thrombosis is a clinical finding confirmed on the ultrasound in patients presenting with symptoms like arm swelling and neck pain. Mostly it is secondary to clear causes like central venous line catheterization or intravenous drug abuse by history. If source is unidentified, work-up should be initiated to look for rare causes (like malignancy in our case) that may need prompt management.

References

[1] F. W. Peuscher, "Thrombosis and bleeding in cancer patients. A review," *Netherlands Journal of Medicine*, vol. 24, no. 1, p. 23, 1981.

[2] C. M. Thompson and L. R. Rodgers, "Analysis of the autopsy records of 157 cases of carcinoma of the pancreas with particular reference to the incidence of thromboembolism," *The American Journal of the Medical Sciences*, vol. 223, no. 5, pp. 469–478, 1952.

[3] A. Y. Y. Lee and M. N. Levine, "The thrombophilic state induced by therapeutic agents in the cancer patient," *Seminars in Thrombosis and Hemostasis*, vol. 25, no. 2, pp. 137–145, 1999.

[4] M. Verso and G. Agnelli, "Venous thromboembolism associated with long-term use of central venous catheters in cancer patients," *Journal of Clinical Oncology*, vol. 21, no. 19, pp. 3665–3675, 2003.

[5] P. J. S. Hubsch, R. L. Stiglbauer, B. W. A. M. Schwaighofer, F. M. Kainberger, and P. P. A. Barton, "Internal jugular and subclavian vein thrombosis caused by central venous catheters. Evaluation using Doppler blood flow imaging," *Journal of Ultrasound in Medicine*, vol. 7, no. 11, pp. 629–636, 1988.

[6] M. A. Sheikh, A. P. Topoulos, and S. R. Deitcher, "Isolated internal jugular vein thrombosis: risk factors and natural history," *Vascular Medicine*, vol. 7, no. 3, pp. 177–179, 2002.

[7] S. L. Hyer, P. Dandekar, K. Newbold, M. Haq, K. Wechalakar, and C. Harmer, "Thyroid cancer causing obstruction of the great veins in the neck," *World Journal of Surgical Oncology*, vol. 6, article 36, 2008.

[8] G. Panzironi, R. Rainaldi, F. Ricci, A. Casale, and M. de Vargas Macciucca, "Gray-scale and color Doppler findings in bilateral internal jugular vein thrombosis caused by anaplastic carcinoma of the thyroid," *Journal of Clinical Ultrasound*, vol. 31, no. 2, pp. 111–115, 2003.

[9] T. Baba, T. Endo, Y. Kitajima, H. Kamiya, O. Moriwaka, and T. Saito, "Spontaneous ovarian hyperstimulation syndrome and pituitary adenoma: incidental pregnancy triggers a catastrophic event," *Fertility and Sterility*, vol. 92, no. 1, pp. 390.e1–393.e1, 2009.

[10] K. Kunimasa, Y. Korogi, Y. Okamoto, and T. Ishida, "Spontaneous internal jugular vein thrombosis associated with lung cancer," *Internal Medicine*, vol. 52, no. 16, article 1849, 2013.

[11] M. Serinken, O. Karcioglu, and A. Korkmaz, "Spontaneous internal jugular vein thrombosis: a case report," *Kaohsiung Journal of Medical Sciences*, vol. 26, no. 12, pp. 679–681, 2010.

[12] A. Ishida, S. Matsuo, K. Niimura, H. Yoshimoto, H. Shiramizu, and T. Hori, "Cervical spontaneous spinal epidural hematoma with internal jugular vein thrombosis: case report," *Journal of Neurosurgery: Spine*, vol. 15, no. 2, pp. 187–189, 2011.

[13] J. Chlumský and J. Havlín, "Spontaneous jugular vein thrombosis," *Acta Cardiologica*, vol. 64, no. 5, pp. 689–691, 2009.

[14] T. Ghatak, R. K. Singh, and A. K. Baronia, "Spontaneous central vein thrombosis in a patient with activated protein C resistance and dengue infection: an association or causation?" *Journal of Anaesthesiology Clinical Pharmacology*, vol. 29, no. 4, pp. 547–549, 2013.

[15] M. T. Lønnebakken, O. M. Pedersen, K. S. Andersen, and J. E. Varhaug, "Incidental detection of internal jugular vein thrombosis secondary to undiagnosed benign substernal goiter," *Case Reports in Medicine*, vol. 2010, Article ID 645193, 4 pages, 2010.

[16] S. Gallien, F. Rollot, B. Caron, L. Moachon, B. Bienvenu, and P. Blanche, "Pulmonary embolism and deep jugular venous thrombosis resulting from compression by a lipoma," *Dermatology Online Journal*, vol. 12, no. 2, article no. 13, 2006.

[17] M. Lazzarino, E. Orlandi, M. Paulli et al., "Primary mediastinal B-cell lymphoma with sclerosis: an aggressive tumor with distinctive clinical and pathologic features," *Journal of Clinical Oncology*, vol. 11, no. 12, pp. 2306–2313, 1993.

31

Occult Bacteraemia and Aortic Graft Infection: A Wolf in Sheep's Clothing

E. Trautt, S. Thomas, J. Ghosh, P. Newton, and A. Cockcroft

University Hospital of South Manchester, Manchester, UK

Correspondence should be addressed to E. Trautt; elizabethtrautt@yahoo.co.uk

Academic Editors: R. A. Bishara, G. L. Tripepi, and R. Zbinden

We report a case of late-onset aortic prosthetic vascular graft infection. We stress the importance of maintaining a high index of suspicion for any patient presenting with fever on the background of in situ prosthetic material. We present the difficulties in managing these extremely complicated, often life and limb threatening infections and suggest that a multidisciplinary team approach, involving specialist centre referral, may be key to success. We highlight the difficulties in diagnosing late-onset PVGI, where presentation can be subacute with subtle signs and confusing microbiology. In this case the presentation was pyrexia of unknown origin with multiple positive blood cultures isolating a variety of gut-associated organisms; *a wolf in sheep's clothing*.

1. Background

Prosthetic vascular graft infection (PVGI) is a significant complication of arterial reconstructive surgery [1]. The incidence has been reported to vary from 1 percent to 6 percent [2], depending on the site of the graft (infrainguinal 2–5%, aortofemoral 1-2%, and aortic 1%). Although the relative risk of PVGI is low, the clinical consequences of an infected vascular graft can be catastrophic for the patient, with an associated operative morbidity of 40–70% (limb amputation rates of up to 70% for lower extremity grafts [3]) and a recognized mortality rate of 30–50% (up to 75% with intra-abdominal aortic grafts [4]).

We describe an unusual presentation of late-onset aortic graft infection which stresses the importance of maintaining a high index of suspicion in any patient with unexplained fevers and underlying in situ prosthetic material. In management of this case we demonstrate effective clinical use of Daptomycin and highlight the need for national consensus guidelines to guide the management of these complex infections.

2. Case Report

This 79-years-old gentleman was admitted from the Infectious Diseases clinic, in April 2011. He presented to the clinic with night sweats, intermittent fevers, rigors, lethargy, weight loss, poor appetite, and generalised arthralgias. He described a change in the bowel habit over the previous few months with constipation and mild abdominal discomfort. His C-reactive protein was 58. This was his fourth follow-up clinic appointment following a recent hospital discharge.

His past medical history included the following: August 2010 admission for relapsed septic arthritis of a right native knee, joint fluid aspirated at that time isolated *Pseudomonas aeruginosa* and blood cultures repeatedly isolated *Pseudomonas aeruginosa* and *Enterobacter*; July 2010 admission for probable recurrent septic arthritis, blood cultures isolated *Streptococcus constellatus* and *Aerococcus*; December 2009 admission for a primary septic arthritis, culture of synovial fluid isolated *Streptococcus constellatus*. In 1993 he had undergone an aortic aneurysm repair with insertion of an aorto-bi-iliac Dacron surgical graft.

On his admission in December 2009, because of the in situ aortic graft, he had undergone a CT abdomen and pelvis which showed normal appearances of the aorto-bi-iliac graft. The scan was repeated on each subsequent admission, in July 2010 and August 2010, each time showing normal appearances of the graft and no evidence of a fluid or gas collection around the abdominal aorta or iliac arteries. On admission

TABLE 1: Microbiology results.

Date	Clinical situation	Microbiology		Imaging
		Sample site	Culture results	
Dec 2009	Inpatient admission Septic arthritis	Synovial fluid	S. constellatus (enrichment only)	Jan. 2010 CT abdomen with contrast: no acute abnormality detected
Apr 2010	Inpatient admission Relapsed septic arthritis	Blood	S. constellatus Aerococcus urinae	Jul. 2010 CT abdomen and pelvis: no evidence of graft infection
Aug 2010	Inpatient admission Recurrent septic arthritis	Joint fluid Blood (x3)	Pseudomonas aeruginosa Pseudomonas aeruginosa Enterobacter cloacae	Aug. 2010 CT angiogram aorta: no evidence of abdominal aortic stent graft infection
Mar 2011	Outpatient clinic	Blood	Lactobacillus species	
Apr 2011	Outpatient clinic Admitted with PUO	Blood (x4)	Lactobacillus paracasei Lactobacillus species S. oralis	Apr. 2011 CT abdomen and pelvis: at least 2 small droplets of retroperitoneal gas which appear extraluminal and suspicious for sepsis related to the graft

from clinic, he underwent investigation for PUO in which he had multiple sets of blood cultures collected and 3 sets of isolated lactobacillus (Table 1).

He underwent a whole body scan showing a pool of activity in the right knee suggestive of chronic low-grade persistent infection. A transthoracic echocardiogram and a colonoscopy to investigate the altered bowel habit were carried out and were both negative. At this time a fourth repeat CT abdomen and pelvis was requested. This showed small extramural pockets of gas at the level of the graft bifurcation and a further possible tiny pocket of gas at the cranial aspect of the graft, appearances which would be suspicious for sepsis related to the graft.

At this point, there was multidisciplinary team input from vascular surgeons, vascular radiologists, infectious diseases and microbiology and appropriate management options were discussed. The two available options were (1) explantation of the graft with extra-anatomical bypass and (2) long-term suppressive antibiotics with serial CRP and imaging. In view of his age, that the WCC was within normal limits and the CRP was falling, the equivalence of the CT finding, and the fact that the surgery to remove the graft would carry a significant mortality and morbidity risk, the decision was made to start IV antibiotics for a minimum of 6 wks. The caveat to this approach was that in the event of worsening sepsis despite antibiotics and/or CT evidence of worsening perigraft infection or development of aortoenteric fistula, then surgery would be carried out.

IV Daptomycin (6 mg/kg) (plus gentamicin initially) was commenced after confirmatory MIC testing of the lactobacillus to Daptomycin; this was the most recently and most persistently isolated pathogen. Daptomycin was well tolerated by the patient. At 6 weeks, based on good clinical response, this was changed to oral amoxicillin plus clindamycin, and the patient was discharged home. Within 48 hrs of discharge he represented with rigors and fevers. He was readmitted and a repeat CT showed increasing air encircling the right most anterior limb of the aortic graft. At this point the decision was made to carry out surgery to remove the graft.

In July 2011, the infected graft was explanted, the space washed out, and bilateral axillofemoral bypass graft inserted. Intraoperatively, a perforated duodenum was reported, which was the likely source of the multiple bacteraemias isolating the variety of gut organisms seen. This was repaired involving a retrocolic gastrojejunostomy and feeding jejunostomy, in an operation lasting more than 10 hours (Figure 1).

To date, the patient remains well at home, the graft remains patent and perfusing the leg, and he has chosen not to continue oral suppressive antibiotics.

3. Discussion

Diagnosis of PVGI is extremely challenging. It is based on patient history and examination and parameters such as CRP, WCC, blood cultures (which often remain negative in late-onset graft infection), and 8 radiological imaging, which can be extremely difficult to interpret and in this case was repeatedly negative in the early stages. Unlike early-onset PVGI, which is often attributed to contamination of the graft at or soon after insertion [1] and presents mainly as a post-surgical wound infection, the etiology of late-onset graft infections is far less certain. Presentation can be more occult in manner and many patients present with few or no overt symptoms of disease [1]. There may be local signs of infection such as thrombosis or failure of the graft, false aneurysm, or bleeding (aortoenteric fistula formation). In this case the patient presented with occult signs of graft-duodenal erosion, resulting in the translocation of a variety of gut organisms into the blood stream, likely seeding a potentially osteoarthritic knee joint, which was the initial presenting complaint.

Gold standard treatment involves complex surgery to remove the infected graft. For many patients, however, multiple comorbidities often render this an unfeasible option, leaving long courses of often empirical broad spectrum intravenous antibiotics as the only alternative. A lack of data on the effectiveness of some of the newer antimicrobial agents in prosthetic graft infection limits the treatment options

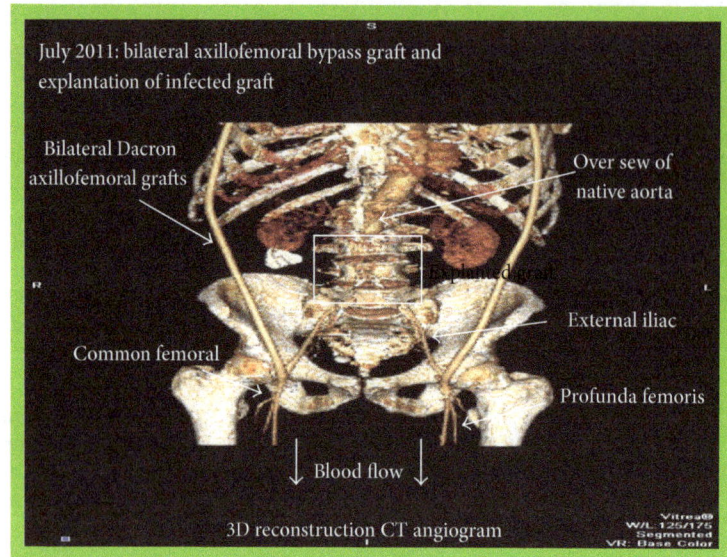

FIGURE 1: 3D-CT angiogram demonstrating removal of the infected aortic graft and extra-anatomical bypass.

available. In this case Daptomycin was used for the suppression of infection. This was an off-licence use of this newer class of antimicrobial agent, and the data to support its use is lacking. Despite the fact that management will often be on a patient-by-patient basis, there is a real and urgent need to develop national consensus treatment guidelines, providing advice on the use of newer antimicrobial agents such as Daptomycin, Linezolid, and Tigecycline in PVGI and on the optimal duration of therapy.

References

[1] C. E. Edmiston Jr., "Vascular graft acute and late-onset infections," *Infectious Diseases in Clinical Practice*, vol. 3, no. 2, pp. 147–150, 1994.

[2] V. S. Antonios, A. A. Noel, J. M. Steckelberg et al., "Prosthetic vascular graft infection: a risk factor analysis using a case-control study," *Journal of Infection*, vol. 53, no. 1, pp. 49–55, 2006.

[3] G. Piano, "Infections in lower extremity vascular grafts," *Surgical Clinics of North America*, vol. 75, no. 4, pp. 799–809, 1995.

[4] G. S. Oderich and J. M. Panneton, "Aortic graft infection: what have we learned during the last decades ?" *Acta Chirurgica Belgica*, vol. 102, no. 1, pp. 7–13, 2002.

32

A Novel Technique of Stenting of the Renal Artery In-Stent Restenosis with GuideLiner® through Radial Approach

Maheedhar Gedela,[1] **Shenjing Li,**[2] **Tomasz Stys,**[2] **and Adam Stys**[2]

[1]*Department of Internal Medicine, University of South Dakota Sanford School of Medicine, Sioux Falls, SD, USA*
[2]*Sanford Cardiovascular Institute, University of South Dakota Sanford School of Medicine, Sioux Falls, SD, USA*

Correspondence should be addressed to Maheedhar Gedela; maheedhargedela@gmail.com

Academic Editor: Hiroyuki Nakajima

In-stent restenosis of the renal arteries is relatively common and its management is not well studied. An 83-year-old female with bilateral renal artery stenosis and balloon angioplasty and stenting bilaterally one year ago was found to have recurrent severe elevations in the blood pressure despite medical management. Renal artery duplex showed 60–99% stenosis of the right renal artery and 20–59% stenosis of the left renal artery. A subsequent angiography of the right renal artery revealed 80% in-stent restenosis at the ostium. We describe a new approach of balloon angioplasty and stenting through radial access site with the assistance of a GuideLiner in a complex in-stent restenosis of the renal artery.

1. Introduction

The estimated prevalence of renal artery stenosis (RAS) is more than 5% in people older than 50 years in the US [1]. Currently, there are no formal guidelines outlining the management of RAS for refractory hypertension. Although percutaneous transluminal renal artery angioplasty had good short-term outcomes, the restenosis rates were high, especially for ostial disease [2]. The stented vessel diameter of <5 mm and stents > 20 mm long increase the risk for restenosis [3, 4]. The available treatment options for recurrent RAS are percutaneous transluminal angioplasty and/or placement of a second stent, use of polytetrafluoroethylene- (PTFE-) covered stents, cutting balloon angioplasty, endovascular brachytherapy, excimer laser-assisted angioplasty, and surgical atherectomy [5, 6].

2. Case Presentation

An 83-year-old female with bilateral renal artery stenosis and balloon angioplasty and stenting bilaterally one year ago was found to have recurrent severe elevations in the blood pressure despite medical management. Her past history included hypertension and coronary artery bypass surgery. The laboratory evaluation revealed stable renal function with creatinine at 0.90 mg/dL (normal: 0.50–1.30). Renal artery duplex showed 60–99% stenosis of the right renal artery (RA) and 20–59% stenosis of the left renal artery. Renal arteries angiogram was performed.

3. Procedure Technique

A right radial access was obtained with a 5/6 French-Slender® sheath. A 5-French 125 cm JR4 diagnostic catheter was used for left renal angiography showing a mild mid in-stent restenosis of left renal artery. A Multipurpose 100 cm 5-French catheter was used for right renal angiography but was too short to reach the ostium. Thus, the 6-French 100 cm Multipurpose guide catheter was used and as it was also too short to reach the ostium, a 6-French GuideLiner (GL) extension was used to allow engagement of RA. Angiography of the right RA revealed 80% in-stent restenosis (ISR) at the ostium with hourglass like stent distortion at this site (Figure 1). The GL allowed endovascular intervention on right RA (Figure 2). A 190 cm BMW guidewire was used

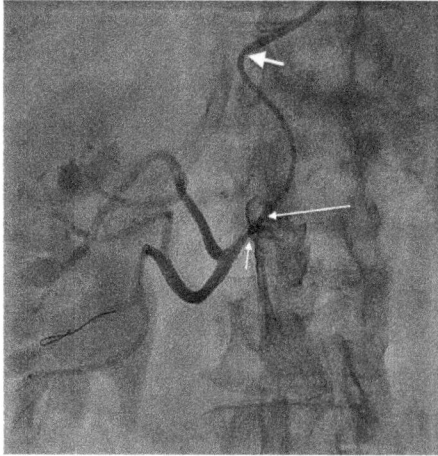

FIGURE 1: Renal artery ostial stenosis with distorted stent (short arrow). Long arrow represents tip of the GuideLiner and thick arrow represents tip of the Multipurpose guide catheter.

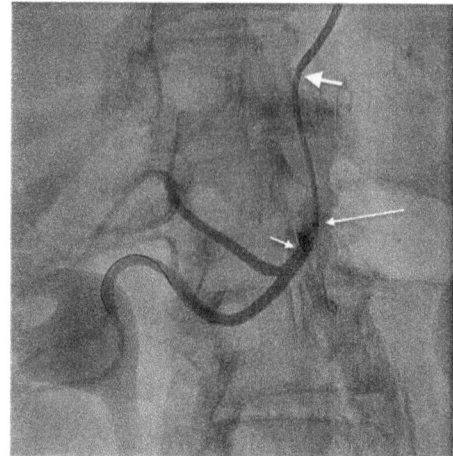

FIGURE 3: Good result after stenting (short arrow). Long arrow represents tip of the GuideLiner and thick arrow represents the tip of Multipurpose guide catheter.

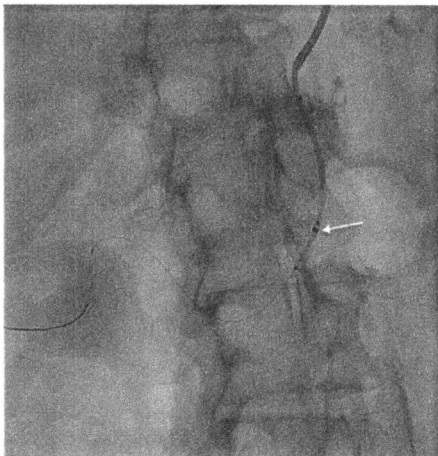

FIGURE 2: Delivery of the drug-eluting stent with the assistance of GuideLiner (arrow represents tip of the GuideLiner).

and stenosis predilated with a 4 × 15 mm balloon. A drug-eluting stent (DES) Xience 4 × 12 mm was deployed at high pressure covering the ostium of the right RA well. The stent was postdilated proximally and in mid-section with a noncompliant 4.5 × 15 mm balloon at high pressure. The procedure was performed with rapid exchange system. DES was used considering the relatively small renal artery size and ISR, with the hope of reducing restenosis. The result was very good angiographically (Figure 3). The patient tolerated the procedure well without any radial access site complications. At the 6-month follow-up clinic visit, the renal artery duplex showed 20–59% stenosis of the right RA and her blood pressure maintained less than 140/80 mmHg consistently.

4. Discussion

RAS is encountered in 6–18% of patients undergoing cardiac catheterization and 16–40% of patients undergoing

arteriography for aortic and peripheral vascular disease [7]. A randomized controlled study showed 75% primary patency rate in combined angioplasty and stent group versus 29% in angioplasty group at 6 months in patients with ostial atherosclerotic RAS [8]. The true incidence of ISR is unknown due to the paucity of the prospective studies [2]. Based on observational studies, the reported rates of ISR following RA stent placement vary from 6 to 60%. Though early studies described the occurrence of ISR within the first 6–12 months, the subsequent analyses noted ISR occurrence anytime following RA stent placement [2, 4]. The recurrent ISR generally occurs from 4 months to 10 years and it is usually high [2]. In a small cohort study where the majority of interventions were performed through femoral access, the drug-eluting stenting showed 0% recurrence of ISR ($n = 0/4$) after a mean follow-up of 258 ± 163 days [4]. Another retrospective small study noted repeat stenting of recurrent ISR resulted in better patency rates compared to angioplasty alone [9]. Kakkar et al. reported wide patency of the renal artery at 6-month follow-up with paclitaxel-eluting stent implantation in a two-time ISR patient [10].

There is a paucity of data in the literature describing renal artery interventions through radial site access [11]. To the best of our knowledge, this is the first case illustrating the novel technique of percutaneous transluminal balloon angioplasty and DES placement with the assistance of GL through radial access in the complex ISR of the renal artery. Radial approach is beneficial for immediate sheath removal, prompt mobilization of the patients, low rate of access site complications, and a potential for utilization of fewer devices. In our case, the right RA take-off was favorable for radial access. However, radial access for renal artery interventions can be associated with technical difficulties of catheter advancement in the aorta, potential for distal embolization, and dependent on operator experience. In our case, the GL extension allowed reaching RA from radial approach, as guide catheter alone was too short for that. Additionally, we think it improved the precision of stent delivery.

Disclosure

Our institution does not require ethical approval for reporting individual cases.

Authors' Contributions

All authors had access to the data and participated in the preparation of the manuscript and approved this manuscript.

References

[1] J. M. Rimmer and F. J. Gennari, "Atherosclerotic renovascular disease and progressive renal failure," *Annals of Internal Medicine*, vol. 118, no. 9, pp. 712–719, 1993.

[2] F. K. Boateng and B. A. Greco, "Renal artery stenosis: prevalence of, risk factors for, and management of in-stent stenosis," *American Journal of Kidney Diseases*, vol. 61, no. 1, pp. 147–160, 2013.

[3] R. J. Lederman, F. O. Mendelsohn, R. Santos, H. R. Phillips, R. S. Stack, and J. J. Crowley, "Primary renal artery stenting: characteristics and outcomes after 363 procedures," *American Heart Journal*, vol. 142, no. 2, pp. 314–323, 2001.

[4] T. Zeller, A. Rastan, U. Schwarzwalder, C. Mueller, T. Schwarz, and U. Frank, "Treatment of instent restenosis following stent-supported renal artery angioplasty," *Catheterization and Cardiovascular Interventions*, vol. 70, no. 3, p. 454, 2007.

[5] L. Bax, W. P. T. M. Mali, P. J. G. Van de Ven, F. J. A. Beek, J. A. Vos, and J. J. Beutler, "Repeated intervention for in-stent restenosis of the renal arteries," *Journal of Vascular and Interventional Radiology*, vol. 13, no. 12, pp. 1219–1224, 2002.

[6] P. M. Patel, J. Eisenberg, M. A. Islam, A. O. Maree, and K. A. Rosenfield, "Percutaneous revascularization of persistent renal artery in-stent restenosis," *Vascular Medicine*, vol. 14, no. 3, pp. 259–264, 2009.

[7] T. P. Murphy, G. Soares, and M. Kim, "Increase in utilization of percutaneous renal artery interventions by Medicare beneficiaries, 1996–2000," *American Journal of Roentgenology*, vol. 183, no. 3, pp. 561–568, 2004.

[8] P. J. G. Van De Ven, R. Kaatee, J. J. Beutler et al., "Arterial stenting and balloon angioplasty in ostial atherosclerotic renovascular disease: A randomised trial," *Lancet*, vol. 353, no. 9149, pp. 282–286, 1999.

[9] Z. M. N'Dandu, R. A. Badawi, C. J. White et al., "Optimal treatment of renal artery in-stent restenosis: repeat stent placement versus angioplasty alone," *Catheterization and Cardiovascular Interventions*, vol. 71, no. 5, pp. 701–705, 2008.

[10] A. K. Kakkar, M. Fischi, and C. R. Narins, "Drug-eluting stent implantation for treatment of recurrent renal artery in-stent restenosis," *Catheterization and Cardiovascular Interventions*, vol. 68, no. 1, discussion 123-124, pp. 118–122, 2006.

[11] Z. Ruzsa, K. Tóth, Z. Jambrik et al., "Transradial access for renal artery intervention," *Interventional Medicine and Applied Science*, vol. 6, no. 3, pp. 97–103, 2014.

33

Typical Asthmatic Presentation of Congenital Vascular Ring Can Masquerade a General Physician

Naveen Swami,[1] Georgey Koshy,[2] Maan Jamal,[3] Thair S. Abdulla,[4] and Abdulaziz Alkhulaifi[5]

[1] Department of Cardiothoracic Surgery, Heart Care Centre, Al Ahli Hospital, 2nd Floor, Bin Omran, P.O. Box 6401, Doha, Qatar
[2] Department of Cardiology, Heart Care Centre, Al Ahli Hospital, Doha, Qatar
[3] Department of Radiology, Al Ahli Hospital, Doha, Qatar
[4] Department of Pulmonary Medicine & Intensive Care Unit, Al Ahli Hospital, Doha, Qatar
[5] Department of Cardiothoracic Surgery, Heart Hospital, Hamad Medical Corporation, Doha, Qatar

Correspondence should be addressed to Naveen Swami; drnaveenswami@gmail.com

Academic Editors: L. Masotti and E. Minar

A 24-year-old woman was referred to pulmonologist with worsening breathlessness and wheeze. During childhood, she was diagnosed with asthma and subsequent exacerbations were treated with bronchodilators for many years. The chest X-ray and a spirometry testing raised a doubt of extrinsic tracheal compression and a subsequent enhanced chest CT (computerized tomogram) scan confirmed a right-sided aortic arch and a vascular ring anomaly compressing the trachea. Standard surgical division of ligamentum arteriosum was able to relieve the trachea and so the symptoms.

1. Introduction

Vascular rings are congenital malformations that result from abnormal development of the aortic arch complex and can cause encirclement of the trachea and oesophagus [1]. Symptoms tend to occur early in life, mainly as a result in airway compression [2]. There have been few cases in the literature of adult vascular rings presenting with asthma-like symptoms [3] and indeed respiratory arrest on one occasion [4].

We report on an interested case of a young woman who had been treated several years as an asthmatic on clinical background, but, in fact the underlying pathology has been a tracheal compression caused by congenital vascular ring.

2. Case

A 24-year-old woman came first time to the pulmonary clinic complaining of progressive breathlessness on exertion, chest tightness, audible wheezing, and dry cough for the past few months. Since her late childhood, she was diagnosed as being asthmatic with intermittent exacerbations. She had received inhalational bronchodilators, antibiotics, and several courses of corticosteroids over the past few years but, never subjected to any spirometry testing. The worsening symptoms, in spite of aggressive medical treatment, compelled her to consult a pulmonologist.

Her physical examination revealed mild inspiratory and expiratory wheezes over the upper anterior chest with stridor, though her pulse oximetry showed 100% oxygen saturation on room air. Otherwise, the rest of the physical examination was normal. A routine chest roentgenogram showed absent aortic knuckle on the left side with a right-sided aortic arch and an abnormal distal tracheal air shadow (Figure 1). In addition to X-ray findings, the flattening of both inspiratory and expiratory segment of flow-volume loop during spirometry raised a possibility of aortic arch and branch vessel anomaly (Figure 2(a)).

Subsequent, spiral CT of chest with 3-dimensional reconstruction (Figure 3) showed a right-sided aortic arch with 3 branch arteries. The left carotid and right carotid arteries were originating as the first and second branches, respectively, whereas the left subclavian, the 3rd branch with aberrant origin (Kommerell's diverticulum), was originating from the distal portion of the arch and traversing the space behind the

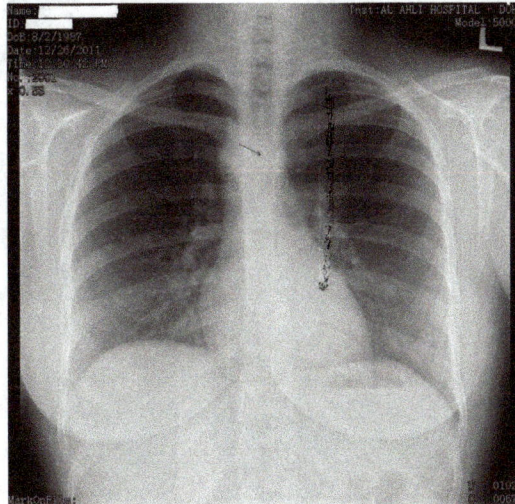

Figure 1: A posteroanterior view of chest X-ray showing an abnormal distal tracheal air shadow (arrow) and the absent left aortic knuckle.

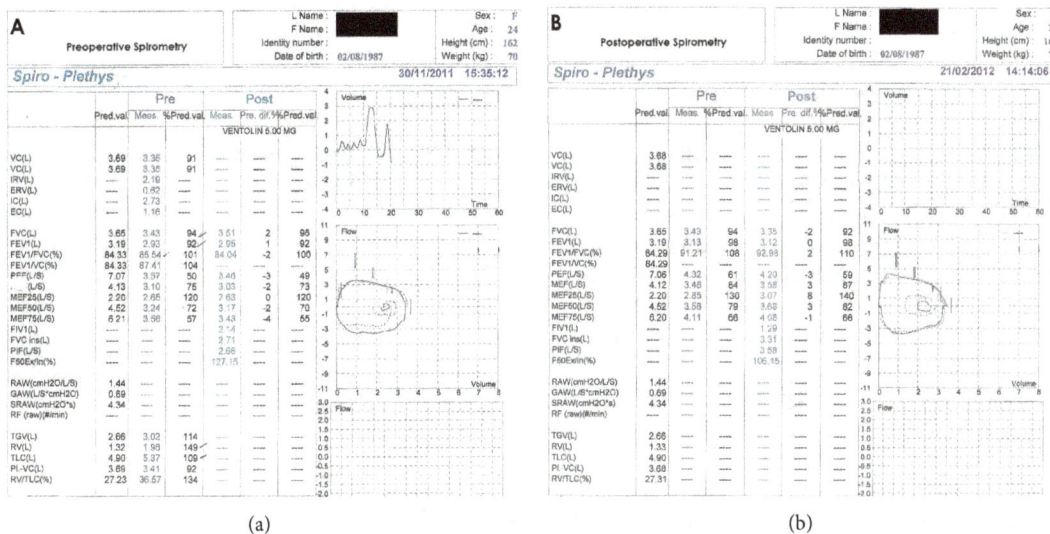

(a) (b)

Figure 2: (a) Preoperative flow-volume loop demonstrating flattening of the inspiratory and expiratory segments (b) Flow-volume loop, after 8 weeks of surgery, showing slightly improved inspiratory and expiratory phases.

esophagus. The descending aorta was only slightly to the right of the midline. A deviation to the left and compression of the trachea and esophagus were seen as a result of the right aortic arch and the anomalous origin and course of left subclavian artery. The ductus arteriosus could not be visualized, possibly due to fibrous obliteration.

She underwent a standard left posterolateral thoracotomy, and through the bed of the 4th rib, chest was entered. The ligamentum arteriosum, connecting the origin of the left subclavian artery and the left pulmonary artery, constituted the majority of compression by culprit vascular ring. Its division, over sewn and with subsequent mobilization of the surrounding structures, successfully relieved the constriction.

(i) The patient made a remarkable improvement after surgery and continued to improve with gradual disappearance of her exertional breathlessness, wheeze, and stridor.

(ii) At 8 weeks, she underwent a repeat Respiratory Function Test which has revealed slight improvement as of increase in FVC and FEV1/FVC% and reshaping of flow-volume loop (Figure 2(b)).

3. Discussion

Vascular rings compressing the trachea and the esophagus are congenital malformations that result from abnormal

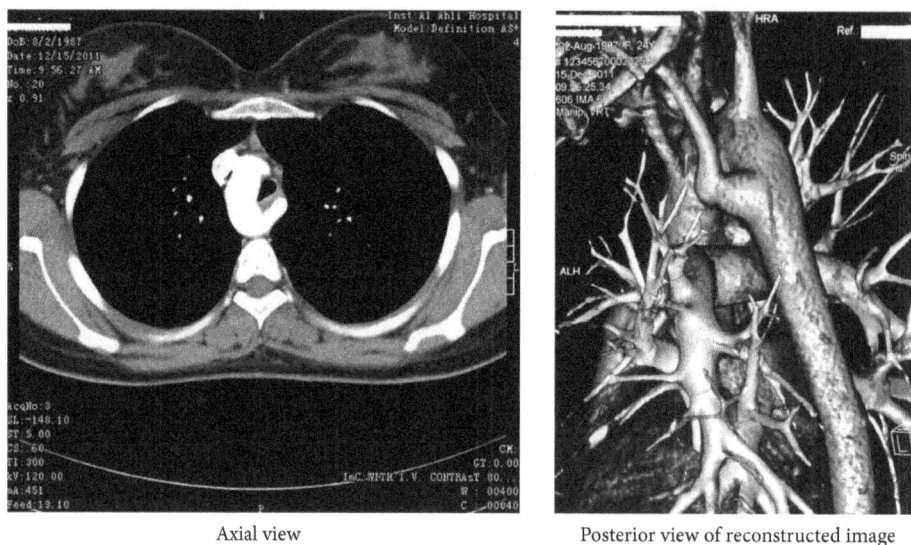

Axial view   Posterior view of reconstructed image

FIGURE 3: A collated picture of chest CT scan with an image of axial view and a reconstructed image with posterior facing showing a right-sided aortic arch, an aberrant origin of left Subclavian artery (Kommerell's diverticulum) behind the oesophagus which was obscured due to compression.

development of the embryonic aortic arch complex. The usual presentation is that of respiratory distress in the neonatal period. However, there have been few cases diagnosed in adulthood with varying modes of presentations, such as asthma [3], dyspnoea, and dysphagia [1, 2]. The commonest two forms of the vascular rings are associated with right aortic arch with either aberrant left subclavian artery or aberrant innominate artery with ligamentum arteriosum completing the vascular ring. Hence, the treatment, when indicated is based on division of the ligament.

In this case, asthma had been diagnosed since childhood and she received several courses of steroids treatment and bronchodilators. One suspect that she had a number of chest X-ray performed, but it is possible that due to the lack of prominence of the right aortic arch and the low index of suspicion, this anomaly could not be suspected. Unfortunately, she did not undergo any pulmonary function testing prior to pulmonologist consultation which could have given a strong suspicion.

It is always imperative to have anatomical details of aortic anomalies as these could determine the surgical approach for correction. As mentioned earlier, in this woman, the anomalous origin and course of left subclavian artery and the ligamentum arteriosum were the main reason for the extrinsic compression of trachea and esophagus. A left thoracotomy was the approach for correction of this anomaly with immediate improvement in symptoms after surgery.

Abbreviations

CT: Computerized tomogram
FEV1: Forced expiratory volume in first second
FVC: Forced vital capacity.

Funding

This work did not require any financial funding from any agency or individual.

Acknowledgments

Thanks to the Department of Pulmonary medicine and Radiology at Al Ahli Hospital, who provided diagnostic modalities to confirm the diagnosis.

References

[1] R. A. Winn, E. D. Chan, E. L. Langmack, C. Kotaru, and E. Aronsen, "Dysphagia, chest pain, and refractory asthma in a 42-year-old woman," *Chest*, vol. 126, no. 5, pp. 1694–1697, 2004.

[2] Y. S. Tjang, J. I. Aramendi, A. Crespo, G. Hamzeh, R. Voces, and M. A. Rodríguez, "Right cervical aortic arch with aberrant left subclavian artery," *Asian Cardiovascular & Thoracic Annals*, vol. 16, no. 4, pp. e37–e39, 2008.

[3] Y. K. Ko, C. L. Hsiao, and Y. J. Lee, "Right aortic arch with a complete vascular ring causing tracheoesophageal compression—a case report," *Journal of Internal Medicine of Taiwan*, vol. 18, no. 2, pp. 104–107, 2007.

[4] R. E. Hardin, G. R. Brevetti, M. Sanusi et al., "Treatment of symptomatic vascular rings in the elderly," *Texas Heart Institute Journal*, vol. 32, no. 3, pp. 411–415, 2005.

34

Iatrogenic IVC Perforation after Successful Catheter-Directed Thrombolysis

Ata Firoozi,[1,2] **Jamal Moosavi,**[1,2] **Omid Shafe,**[1,2] **and Parham Sadeghipour**[1,2]

[1]*Rajaie Cardiovascular Medical and Research Center, Iran University of Medical Sciences, Tehran, Iran*
[2]*Cardiovascular Intervention Research Center, Rajaie Cardiovascular Medical and Research Center,*
Iran University of Medical Sciences, Tehran, Iran

Correspondence should be addressed to Jamal Moosavi; drjamalmoosavi@gmail.com

Academic Editor: Halvor Naess

Central vein perforation as a rare complication of venous interventions is considered a nightmare if occurring in thoracic cage but behaves benignly in abdominal or pelvic region. This is not a rule, as we unfortunately encountered during the procedure of venous intervention in our patient. Although mechanical control of iatrogenic perforation or rupture is the first and most critical step during interventional procedures, the importance of anticoagulant and thrombolytic agents reversal should not be overlooked.

1. Introduction

Venous intervention gradually becomes a major field of cardiovascular interventionists. There are generally four accepted goals for the treatment of lower extremity deep vein thrombosis (LEDVT): (1) diminish the severity and duration of symptoms; (2) prevent pulmonary embolism; (3) minimize the risk of recurrent venous thrombosis; and (4) prevent the postthrombotic syndrome (PTS).

As relief of outflow obstruction is one of the primary goals of therapy for LVEDT, this unfortunately is not accomplished by anticoagulation alone, as thrombus regression occurs in only 50% of patients [1]. According to recent studies, in acute phase of DVT, extensive and centrally located thrombus showed the highest probability in developing severe PTS and disease specific lower quality of life [2].

2. Case Presentation

A 47-year-old hairdresser lady referred to our center with documented diagnosis of extensive vein thrombosis involving the left iliofemoral system according to duplex ultrasound. The patient symptoms including abrupt-onset swelling and crushing pain of left leg began one week ago. Her detailed history lacked any medical admission or consumption of special drugs including hormonal contraceptives. For more delineation of thrombosis propagation we decided to evaluate her precisely using MR venography with gadolinium which revealed "filling defects in the left common and external iliac, common, and superficial femoral and popliteal veins in favor of acute extensive DVT."

Laboratory data was not striking except the level of serum D-dimer (5297 mg/dl). Ongoing and annoying course of patient symptoms and massive burden of thrombosis, in addition to fear of future postthrombotic complications which possibly interfere with our patient occupation, altogether forced the treatment team to choose a definite therapy for her lower extremity DVT.

The access site to the patient left iliofemoral DVT chosen to be ipsilateral popliteal vein with the patient prone on the angiographic table under ultrasound guidance. After successful cannulating the popliteal vein, contrast injection showed totally thrombotic occlusion of left common femoral and iliac veins but obviously patent IVC (Figure 1). The next step was installation of ultrasound-based infusion system, Lysus Infusion System (EKOS corporation, Bothell, WA) which delivered alteplase via a catheter with one central lumen and three separate infusion ports (total dose 1 mg/hour). It combines high-frequency lower-power ultrasound with simultaneous catheter-directed thrombolytics to accelerate clot dissolution [3]. Also heparin was infused (250 U/hour) in conjunction.

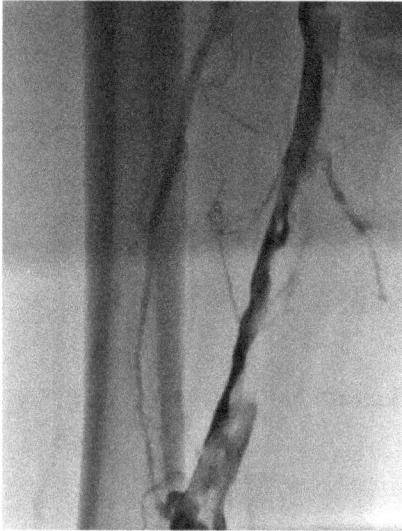

FIGURE 1: Thrombotic occlusion of femoral vein (patient in prone position).

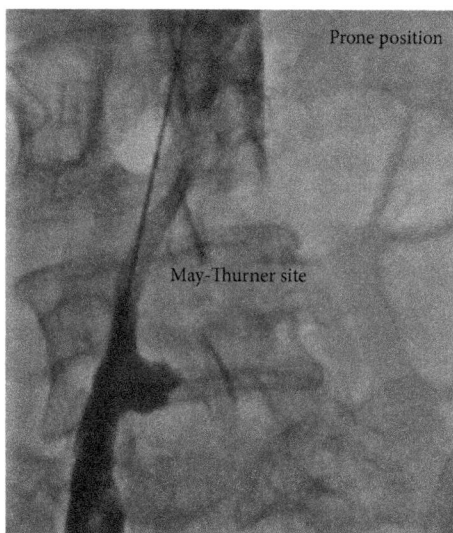

FIGURE 2: Follow-up venography revealed dramatic resolution of clot burden.

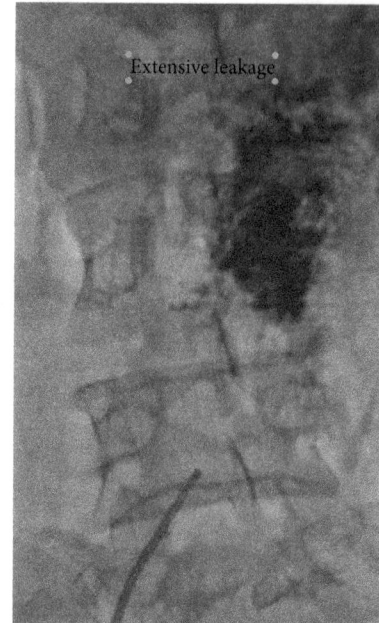

FIGURE 3: Leakage out of caveofemoral junction extensively.

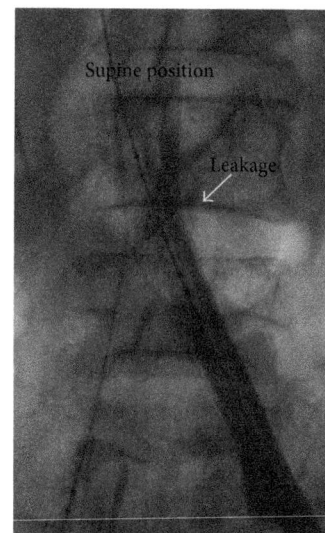

FIGURE 4: Unsuccessful result of balloon inflations forced us to decide to reverse anticoagulant condition of our patient (supine position).

In the following day, the patient was brought back to angiography laboratory to perform follow-up venography which revealed dramatic resolution of clot burden and nice penetration of contrast toward patent IVC (Figure 2). Also, this diagnostic view demonstrated etiologic background of patient nonevoked extensive DVT which was significant stenosis of common iliac vein (May-Thurner syndrome).

During catheter passage and wire exchange, before deploying of stent, unfortunately we encountered leakage out of caveofemoral junction (the distal edge of IVC) extensively (Figure 3). At this critical moment, we decide to complete the stenosis stenting process, with this rational explanation that bleeding in venous system is benign and generally self-limiting. Thereafter, the patient returned to formal access supine position; the right venous femoral access was obtained

quickly. We sent via this new venous route and previous popliteal vein access a BIB of size 24 and inflated it frequently in intervals of 5 to 25 minutes with hope of bleeding site sealing.

In spite of patient stable hemodynamics, hemoglobin level dropped dramatically (6.5 g/dL from 11 g/dL at the beginning). Unsuccessful result of balloon inflations which was showed in subsequent injections (Figure 4) forced us to decide to reverse anticoagulant condition of our patient (due to alteplase and heparin infusion). We did not have aminocaproic acid as a specific antidote to fibrinolytic agents, so for coverage of all aspects of coagulation pathways we

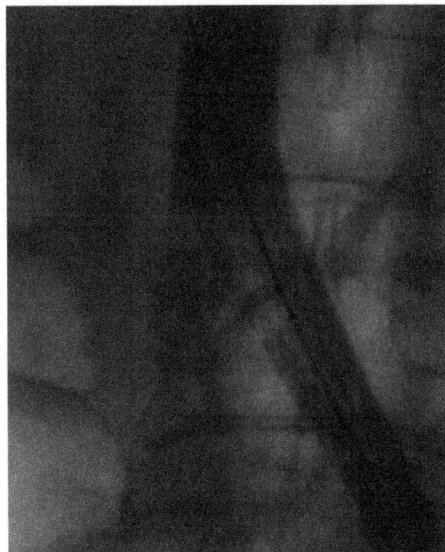

FIGURE 5: Final result of procedure.

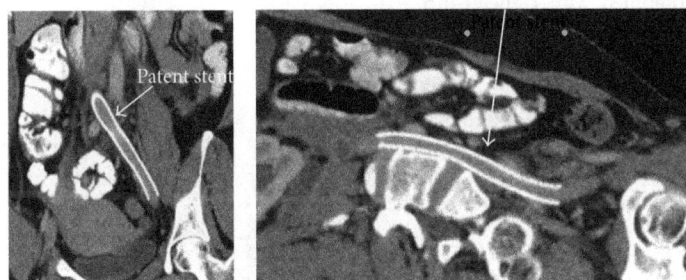

FIGURE 6: Follow-up CT scan showed patent iliac vein stent.

decided to prescribe fresh frozen plasma (FFP) and platelets, in conjunction with protamine sulfate and tranexamic acid.

Fortunately, this courageous strategy in spite of fear of stent thrombosis and even our patient primary pathology itself (acute thrombosis) causes leakage to diminish significantly and in following balloon inflations to stop completely (Figure 5). After this approximately 3-hour stressful process the patient transferred in a stable and satisfactory condition to ICU. Although the next day pelvic and abdominal CT angiography showed the extent of patient bleeding and of course patent iliac vein stent (Figure 6), she passed an uneventful course in following days of admission.

3. Discussion

Intervention in a full anticoagulated milieu is not a safe and free of event procedure as we encountered in this case. Besides, IVC perforation is not a well-known complication, especially after thrombolytic treatment. If a serious bleeding develops in a patient who had received fibrinolytic medications, the first step is the agent cessation. The next step is to institute supportive therapy often including volume repletion and transfusion of blood factors. When possible, direct pressure should be used to control bleeding. If the patient has also been receiving heparin, protamine may be used.

Aminocaproic acid is a specific antidote to fibrinolytic agents. FFP, cryoprecipitate, or both may be used to replenish fibrin and clotting factors. Alteplase has initial half-life of 5 minutes and terminal half-life of 72 minutes but could we wait for this not short period to eliminate the drug itself while the bleeding was active and life-threatening?

4. Conclusion

Venous pharmacomechanical thrombectomy is an attractive technique which may result in a shorter time to vein patency, shorter length of stay, reduction in hemorrhagic risk, and overall cost savings [4, 5]. Catheter-directed thrombolysis trials long term follow-up resulted in a persistent and increased clinical benefit but not quality of life, supporting the use of additional catheter-directed thrombolysis in patients with extensive proximal DVT [6]. Although IVC perforation is not common and seems not to be as threatening as arterial counterparts perforation, this is not true in all situations. Therefore we suggest if IVC perforation occurred especially in an anticoagulated milieu, it is not wise to hesitate in hope of spontaneous stop of bleeding. Sometimes, pharmacomechanical venous intervention needs pharmacomechanical reversal of inadvertent complications.

References

[1] H. K. Breddin, V. Hach-Wunderle, R. Nakov, and V. V. Kakkar, "Effects of a low-molecular-weight heparin on thrombus regression and recurrent thromboembolism in patients with deep-vein thrombosis," *New England Journal of Medicine*, vol. 344, no. 9, pp. 626–631, 2001.

[2] R. H. W. Strijkers, C. W. K. P. Arnoldussen, and C. H. A. Wittens, "Validation of the LET classification," *Phlebology*, vol. 30, pp. 14–19, 2015.

[3] J. V. Braaten, R. A. Goss, and Francis. C. W., "Ultrasound reversibility disaggregates fibrin fibers," *Thromb Haemost*, vol. 78, pp. 1063–1068, 1997.

[4] S. A. Nazir, A. Ganeshan, S. Nazir, and R. Uberoi, "Endovascular treatment options in the management of lower limb deep venous thrombosis," *CardioVascular and Interventional Radiology*, vol. 32, no. 5, pp. 861–876, 2009.

[5] H.-J. Shi, Y.-H. Huang, T. Shen, and Q. Xu, "Percutaneous mechanical thrombectomy combined with catheter-directed thrombolysis in the treatment of symptomatic lower extremity deep venous thrombosis," *European Journal of Radiology*, vol. 71, no. 2, pp. 350–355, 2009.

[6] Y. Haig, T. Enden, O. Grøtta et al., "CaVenT Study Group: Post-thrombotic syndrome after catheter-directed thrombolysis for deep vein thrombosis (CaVenT): 5-year follow-up results of an open-label, randomised controlled trial," *The Lancet Haematology*, vol. 3, no. 2, pp. e64–e71, 2016.

Endovascular Treatment of Infrarenal Abdominal Aortic Aneurysm with Short and Angulated Neck in High-Risk Patient

Stylianos Koutsias,[1] Georgios Antoniou,[1] Christos Karathanos,[1] Vassileios Saleptsis,[1] Konstantinos Stamoulis,[2] and Athanasios D. Giannoukas[1]

[1] Department of Vascular Surgery, University Hospital of Larissa, University of Thessaly Medical School, 41000 Larissa, Greece
[2] Department of Anaesthesiology, University Hospital of Larissa, University of Thessaly Medical School, 41000 Larissa, Greece

Correspondence should be addressed to Stylianos Koutsias; skoutsia@otenet.gr

Academic Editors: A. Iyisoy, L. Masotti, E. Minar, and R. Zbinden

Endovascular treatment of abdominal aortic aneurysms (AAA) is an established alternative to open repair. However lifelong surveillance is still required to monitor endograft function and signal the need for secondary interventions (Hobo and Buth 2006). Aortic morphology, especially related to the proximal neck, often complicates the procedure or increases the risk for late device-related complications (Hobo et al. 2007 and Chisci et al. 2009). The definition of a short and angulated neck is based on length (<15 mm), and angulation (>60°) (Hobo et al. 2007 and Chisci et al. 2009). A challenging neck also offers difficulties during open repairs (OR), necessitating extensive dissection with juxta- or suprarenal aortic cross-clamping. Patients with extensive aneurysmal disease typically have more comorbidities and may not tolerate extensive surgical trauma (Sarac et al. 2002). It is, therefore, unclear whether aneurysms with a challenging proximal neck should be offered EVAR or OR (Cox et al. 2006, Choke et al. 2006, Robbins et al. 2005, Sternbergh III et al. 2002, Dillavou et al. 2003, and Greenberg et al. 2003). In our case the insertion of a thoracic endograft followed by the placement of a bifurcated aortic endograft for the treatment of a very short and severely angulated neck proved to be feasible offering acceptable duration of aneurysm exclusion. This adds up to our armamentarium in the treatment of high-risk patients, and it should be considered in emergency cases when the fenestrated and branched endografts are not available.

1. Introduction

Endovascular treatment of abdominal aortic aneurysms (AAA) is an established alternative to open repair. However lifelong surveillance is still required to monitor endograft function and signal the need for secondary interventions [1].

Endovascular repair (EVAR) may not always be the best treatment option, as not all patients are eligible for EVAR owing to aortoiliac anatomy. Severe infrarenal aortic neck angulation is clearly associated with proximal type I endoleak, while its relationship with stent-graft migration is not clear [2]. Excluder, Zenith, and Talent stent grafts perform well in patients with severe neck angulation, with only a few differences among devices [2]. Aortic morphology, especially related to the proximal neck, often complicates the procedure or increases the risk for late device-related complications [2, 3]. The definition of a short and angulated neck is based on length (<15 mm) and angulation (>60°) [2, 3].

Fenestrated stent grafts crossing the orifices of the renal arteries have been developed to overcome insufficient neck lengths [4]. Its deployment in an angulated neck is considerably more risky than in a straight neck.

Dilatation of the proximal infrarenal aortic neck, which was found to be another predictor for endograft migration in an earlier EUROSTAR report [5], was also associated with severe neck angulation.

However, a challenging neck also offers difficulties during open repairs (OR), necessitating extensive dissection with juxta- or suprarenal aortic cross-clamping. Patients with extensive aneurysmal disease typically have more comorbidities and may not tolerate extensive surgical trauma [6]. It is, therefore, unclear whether aneurysms with a challenging proximal neck should be offered EVAR or OR [7–12].

In this report, a new method for better stent-graft fixation in a short and angulated aortic neck with the use of currently available devices is presented.

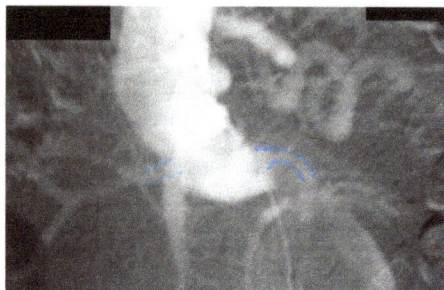

FIGURE 1: DSA arteriography that shows the short and angulated neck of the AAA.

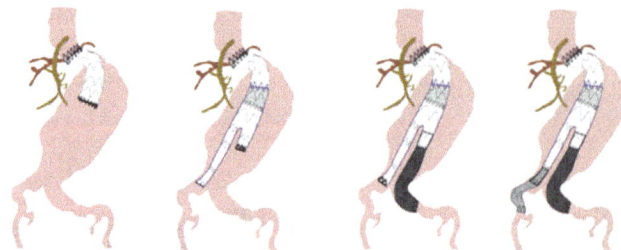

FIGURE 3: The sequence of the graft insertion.

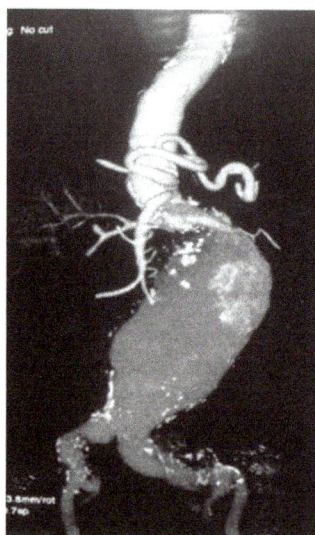

FIGURE 2: CT angiography of the anatomy of the AAA.

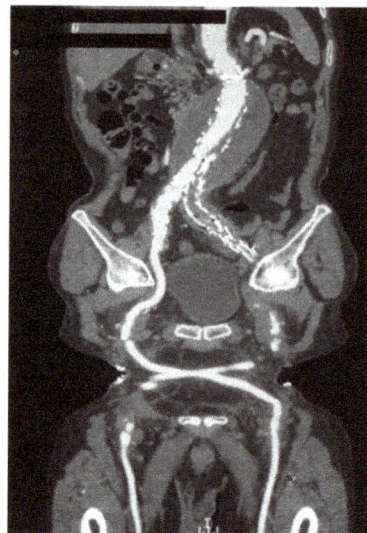

FIGURE 4: Complete exclusion of the aneurysm on CT angiography one month postoperatively.

2. Case Report

A 77-year-old male was admitted from the emergency unit with sudden onset of abdominal pain radiating to lumbar area. On CT scan an infrarenal AAA with maximum diameter of nine (9) cm was discovered. The patient was hypertensive with history of aortocoronary bypass 15 years ago. Shortly after that operation, he had subsequent sternum removal for infection. The coronary grafts were detected and occluded eleven (11) years ago on the occasion of a myocardial infarction that he had suffered. One year later, he had one more episode of myocardial infarction, but since then, he was moderately symptomatic on medical treatment. The patient was considered inoperable for his coronary disease. Anatomic characteristics of the infrarenal aortic neck were unfavourable due to its shortness (~8 mm) and angulation (>60°) (Figures 1 and 2).

It was decided to treat him with EVAR, having his consent. The endovascular procedure was carried out in an operating room (OR) equipped with portable C-arm fluoroscopy device (Philips, Endura) and a radiolucent table.

A 30 mm diameter, free flow thoracic tube endograft (Valiant, Medtronic Vascular, Santa Rosa, CA, USA) was delivered in the proximal neck. Consequently, a bifurcated

Talent (Medtronic Vascular, Santa Rosa, CA, USA) device 32X18X155 was deployed inside the Valiant graft, with adequate overlapping. Two sequential iliac extensions were deployed into the left external iliac artery, and a contralateral limb was placed to the right common iliac artery (Figure 3). CT angiogram at first month documented intact 3-component stent graft, with no endoleak or migration and no increase in aneurysm sac (Figure 4) A month later the left limb was occluded causing intermittent claudication. Endovascular attempt to salvage the left limb of the graft was unsuccessful due to the tortuosity of the external iliac artery. A crossover fem-fem PTFE graft (8 mm) was placed with full restoration of the blood flow to the left lower extremity. Nine (9) months postoperatively, the patient underwent CT angiography that showed no endoleak and good functioning of the thigh-femoral graft (Figure 5).

About a year from the EVAR the patient was admitted from the Emergency Unit with an episode of abdominal pain. On CT scan a type I endoleak was discovered along with mild graft migration (Figures 6(a) and 6(b)). However the abdominal pain was subsided with appropriate control of his hypertension, the patient remained haemodynamically stable, and he decided not to have any further intervention. Then he was discharged with the advice to be on close follow-up and meticulous management of his hypertension.

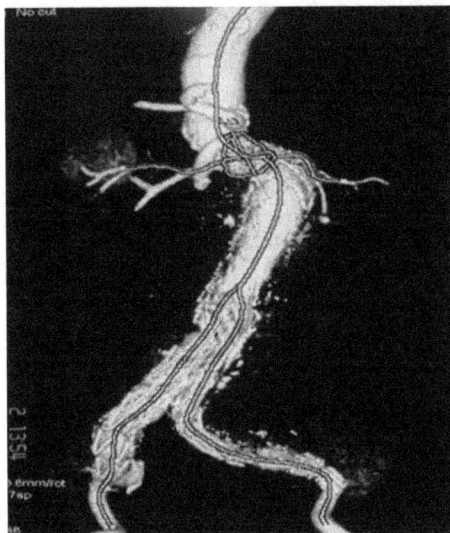

FIGURE 5: No endoleak was detected on CT angiography nine months postoperatively. The left limb of the graft is occluded, and the femorofemoral crossover bypass is patent.

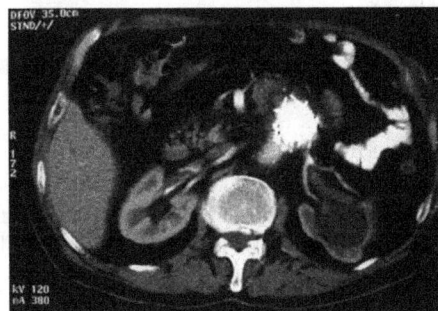

(a)

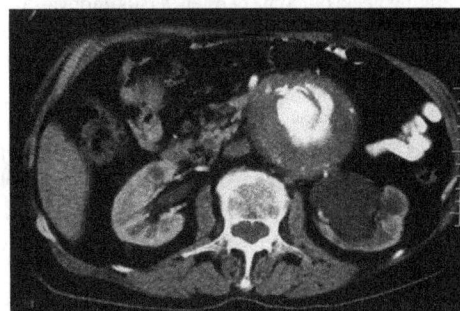

(b)

FIGURE 6: CT scanning one year after EVAR. (a) Migration of the endograft to the straight part of the neck. (b) Endoleak type I detected in the aneurysm.

He remained asymptomatic for another one year when he was admitted with abdominal pain, severe hypotension (systolic BP 60 mm Hg), and oliguria and CT scan showed rupture with contained large retroperitoneal hematoma. The patient was taken urgently to OR and subjected to open repair. The endograft was removed followed by the insertion of a tube 22 mm Dacron. He was transferred to ICU, and the next day he died.

3. Discussion

Conway et al. [13] reported that mortality caused by AAA rupture after a 3-year follow-up in 106 patients considered as high risk for open treatment was 36% in patients with aneurysms between 5.5 and 5.9 cm in diameter, 50% for aneurysms between 6.0 and 7.0 cm, and 55% for aneurysms greater than 7 cm in diameter.

Nonintervention in patients with AAA and high surgical risk is only justified in those with an extremely short life expectancy, in whom the risk of death associated with the surgical procedure is higher than the risk of death caused by aneurysm rupture [14]. In our case the patient was undoubtedly of high risk (ASA IV or Goldman score), but his aneurysm was symptomatic indicating imminent rupture, and having his consent, we proceeded with endovascular repair avoiding OR.

Taking into consideration the study published by Zanchetta et al. [15] ("funnel technique for first-line endovascular treatment of an abdominal aortic aneurysm with an ectatic proximal neck"), we decided to amend the method applied by changing the sequence of endografts inserted. The use of Valiant thoracic endograft was decided on the basis that its free flow design has eight peaks instead of five and has the following properties: allows for the same radial force as

Talent Thoracic Stent Graft with significantly reduced flare and distributes radial force across more points of contact with less force and stress per point. To meet the challenges imposed by our patient's aortic anatomy, we used a composite 3-component stent graft to satisfy the short and angulated aortic neck and optimize graft fixation as well as to ensure adequate sealing.

Primary laparoscopic proximal aortic banding [16] or a fenestrated endograft [16, 17] might also be performed to treat patients with a similar anatomy, but these procedures are, respectively, more invasive and time consuming. Fenestrated and branched endografts also permit the endovascular treatment of juxtarenal and pararenal aneurysms. However, these endografts are not available in emergency cases as the delivery time is about 2-3 months.

In our case the insertion of a thoracic endograft followed by the placement of a bifurcated aortic endograft for the treatment of a very short and severely angulated neck proved to be feasible offering acceptable duration of aneurysm exclusion. This adds up to our armamentarium in the treatment of high-risk patients, and it should be considered in emergency cases when the fenestrated and branched endografts are not available.

Acknowledgment

The authors thank Mrs. Maria Giannouka for her invaluable contribution in the preparation of the drawings.

References

[1] R. Hobo and J. Buth, "Secondary interventions following endovascular abdominal aortic aneurysm repair using current endografts. A EUROSTAR report," *Journal of Vascular Surgery*, vol. 43, no. 5, pp. 896–e1, 2006.

[2] R. Hobo, J. Kievit, L. J. Leurs, and J. Buth, "Influence of severe infrarenal aortic neck angulation on complications at the proximal neck following endovascular AAA repair: a EUROSTAR study," *Journal of Endovascular Therapy*, vol. 14, no. 1, pp. 1–11, 2007.

[3] E. Chisci, T. Kristmundsson, G. de Donato et al., "The AAA with a challenging neck: outcome of open versus endovascular repair with standard and fenestrated stent-grafts," *Journal of Endovascular Therapy*, vol. 16, no. 2, pp. 137–145, 2009.

[4] R. K. Greenberg, S. Haulon, S. O'Neill, S. Lyden, and K. Ouriel, "Primary endovascular repair of juxtarenal aneurysms with fenestrated endovascular grafting," *European Journal of Vascular and Endovascular Surgery*, vol. 27, no. 5, pp. 484–491, 2004.

[5] L. J. Leurs, G. Stultiëns, J. Kievit, and J. Buth, "Adverse events at the aneurysmal neck identified at follow-up after endovascular abdominal aortic aneurysm repair: how do they correlate?" *Vascular*, vol. 13, no. 5, pp. 261–267, 2005.

[6] T. P. Sarac, D. G. Clair, N. R. Hertzer et al., "Contemporary results of juxtarenal aneurysm repair," *Journal of Vascular Surgery*, vol. 36, no. 6, pp. 1104–1111, 2002.

[7] D. E. Cox, D. L. Jacobs, R. L. Motaganahalli, C. M. Wittgen, and G. J. Peterson, "Outcomes of endovascular AAA repair in patients with hostile neck anatomy using adjunctive balloon-expandable stents," *Vascular and Endovascular Surgery*, vol. 40, no. 1, pp. 35–40, 2006.

[8] E. Choke, G. Munneke, R. Morgan et al., "Outcomes of endovascular abdominal aortic aneurysm repair in patients with hostile neck anatomy," *CardioVascular and Interventional Radiology*, vol. 29, no. 6, pp. 975–980, 2006.

[9] M. Robbins, B. Kritpracha, H. G. Beebe, F. J. Criado, Y. Daoud, and A. J. Comerota, "Suprarenal endograft fixation avoids adverse outcomes associated with aortic neck angulation," *Annals of Vascular Surgery*, vol. 19, no. 2, pp. 172–177, 2005.

[10] W. C. Sternbergh III, G. Carter, J. W. York, M. Yoselevitz, and S. R. Money, "Aortic neck angulation predicts adverse outcome with endovascular abdominal aortic aneurysm repair," *Journal of Vascular Surgery*, vol. 35, no. 3, pp. 482–486, 2002.

[11] E. D. Dillavou, S. C. Muluk, R. Y. Rhee et al., "Does hostile neck anatomy preclude successful endovascular aortic aneurysm repair?" *Journal of Vascular Surgery*, vol. 38, no. 4, pp. 657–663, 2003.

[12] R. K. Greenberg, D. Clair, S. Srivastava et al., "Should patients with challenging anatomy be offered endovascular aneurysm repair?" *Journal of Vascular Surgery*, vol. 38, no. 5, pp. 990–996, 2003.

[13] K. P. Conway, J. Byrne, M. Townsend, and I. F. Lane, "Prognosis of patients turned down for conventional abdominal aortic aneurysm repair in the endovascular and sonographic era: Szilagyi revisited?" *Journal of Vascular Surgery*, vol. 33, no. 4, pp. 752–757, 2001.

[14] R. M. Greenhalgh, "Endovascular aneurysm repair and outcome in patients unfit for open repair of abdominal aortic aneurysm (EVAR trial 2): randomised controlled trial," *The Lancet*, vol. 365, no. 9478, pp. 2187–2192, 2005.

[15] M. Zanchetta, F. Faresin, L. Pedon et al., "Funnel technique for first-line endovascular treatment of an abdominal aortic aneurysm with an ectatic proximal neck," *Journal of Endovascular Therapy*, vol. 13, no. 6, pp. 775–778, 2006.

[16] B. M. Stanley, J. B. Semmens, M. M. Lawrence-Brown, M. A. Goodman, and D. E. Hartley, "Fenestration in endovascular grafts for aortic aneurysm repair: new horizons for preserving blood flow in branch vessels," *Journal of Endovascular Therapy*, vol. 8, no. 1, pp. 16–24, 2001.

[17] J. L. Anderson, M. Berce, and D. Hartley, "Endoluminal aortic grafting with renal and superior mesenteric artery incorporation by graft fenestration," *Journal of Endovascular Therapy*, vol. 8, pp. 3–15, 2001.

Right Aortic Arch and Kommerell's Diverticulum Repaired without Reconstruction of Aberrant Left Subclavian Artery

Hiroshi Osawa,[1] **Daisuke Shinohara,**[1] **Kouan Orii,**[1] **Shigeru Hosaka,**[2] **Shoji Fukuda,**[2] **Okihiko Akashi,**[3] **and Hiroshi Furukawa**[4]

[1] *Division of Cardiovascular Surgery, Shimada General Hospital, Higashi-cho 5-3, Choshi, Chiba 288-0053, Japan*
[2] *Department of Cardiovascular Surgery, National Center of Global Health and Medicine, Shinjuku, Tokyo 162-8655, Japan*
[3] *Division of Cardiovascular Surgery, Ikegami General Hospital, Ota, Tokyo 146-8531, Japan*
[4] *Department of Cardiovascular Surgery, Kawasaki Medical University, Kurashiki, Okayama 701-0192, Japan*

Correspondence should be addressed to Hiroshi Osawa; drosawa@yahoo.co.jp

Academic Editors: A. Iyisoy, N. Nighoghossian, G. Pasterkamp, and G. L. Tripepi

Right aortic arch with Kommerell's diverticulum is a very rare situation. Surgical treatment is recommended for symptomatic patients or asymptomatic patients with a large diverticulum. However planning the strategy of operation is difficult without a 3D imaging. We report a case of a 57-year-old man with right aortic arch, Kommerell's diverticulum, and aberrant left subclavian artery. After a 3D-CT imaging, the patient underwent descending aortic replacement without reconstruction of aberrant left subclavian artery. After operation, there was no signs or symptoms of ischemia of the left arm. If the reconstruction of the aberrant subclavian artery was too difficult, closing its orifice is an acceptable decision. It has been found advantageous because of a decrease blood loss and a shorter cardiopulmonary bypass duration. If an ischemia of the arm is noticed, additional reconstruction will have to be considered. 3D-CT imaging was very useful to have a proper orientation and plan for the operative strategy.

1. Introduction

Right aortic arch with Kommerell's diverticulum (KD) is a very rare situation. Most patients with KD are asymptomatic; however the most serious issue in the course of aneurysm is its marked propensity towards rupture and dissection [1, 2]. As per earlier reports, all the patients who presented with rupture has died [1]. Therefore the surgical treatment of KD is indicated, before KD will rupture. However it is difficult to image and make a strategy of operation. So, we report the operating procedure and the evaluation method of KD using several views of 3D-CT imaging.

2. Case Presentation

A 57-year-old man had abnormal X-ray findings during routine medical checkup and an enhanced computed tomography (CT) showed right aortic arch, Kommerell diverticulum (KD), and aberrant left subclavian artery (ALSA).

The maximum diameter of KD was 38 mm, and the aneurysm of aorta was 63 mm (Figure 1). CT revealed a 50% stenosis of the orifice of ALSA. Cerebral magnetic resonance imaging angiography showed hypoplasty of left vertebral artery. Operation was indicated because the diameter was critical, despite the fact that the patient had no symptoms due to KD.

After consideration of using 3D-CT imaging with the ribs (Figure 2), it was decided to go for a posterolateral thoracotomy approach through a fourth inters costal incision.

All the aneurysm repairs were performed using hypothermic cardiopulmonary bypass and an interval of hypothermic circulatory arrest. Cardiopulmonary bypass was established with descending aortic cannulation and bicaval drainage. The left heart was vented through the right upper pulmonary vein. The right phrenic, vagus, and recurrent laryngeal nerves were identified and protected. After establishing circulatory arrest, the aorta was incised and transected proximally just distal to the orifice of the right subclavian artery. Descending aorta with KD was replaced using one branched graft for

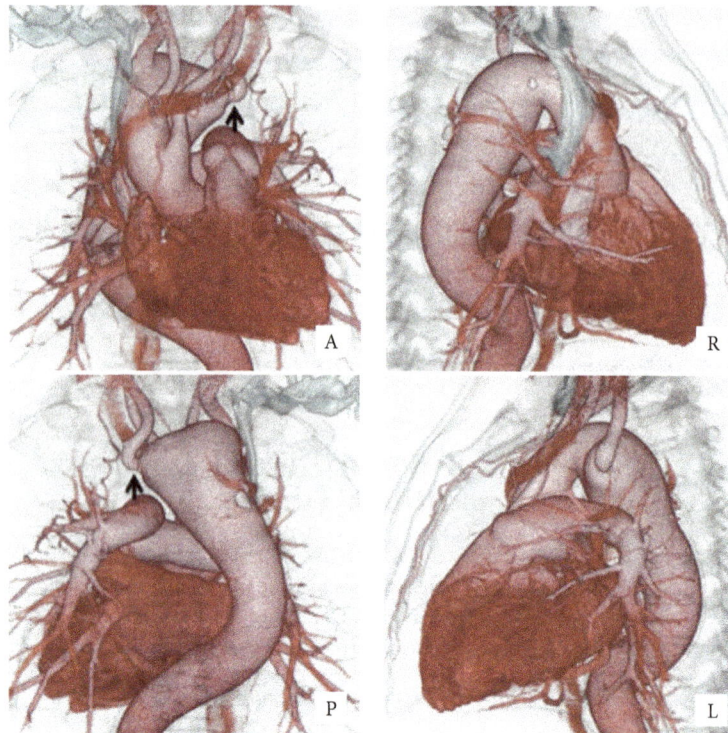

FIGURE 1: Enhanced CT showed right aortic arch, Kommerell diverticulum, and aberrant left subclavian artery. There was a 50% stenosis of the orifice of aberrant left subclavian artery (arrows).

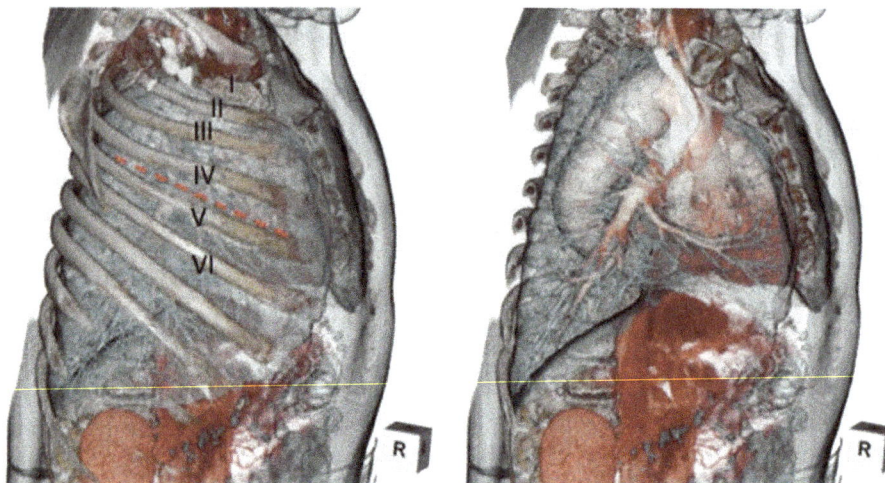

FIGURE 2: 3D-CT imaging, scrolling from superficial to deep layer view with chest wall including the ribs, showed the surgical view and the optimal approach through a posterolateral thoracotomy with the fourth intercostal incision.

the reconstruction of ALSA. However ALSA was not able to be reconstructed anatomically and ligated because ALSA was too deep and difficult to make anastomosis. Rewarming was initiated after completion of the proximal graft to aorta anastomosis. Distal graft to aorta anastomosis was performed under descending aortic clamping and blood supplying from proximal anastomosed graft and descending aorta.

After operation, there were no symptoms of an ischemia of the left arm. The systolic blood pressure of the right arm and the left arm was 110 mmHg and 70 mmHg, respectively. Postoperative CT revealed enhanced ALSA clearly without delay, which was supplied with blood from many branches through the narrow and invisible collateral arteries (Figure 3).

3. Discussion

Kommerell's diverticulum and aberrant subclavian artery can be discovered accidentally in asymptomatic children or

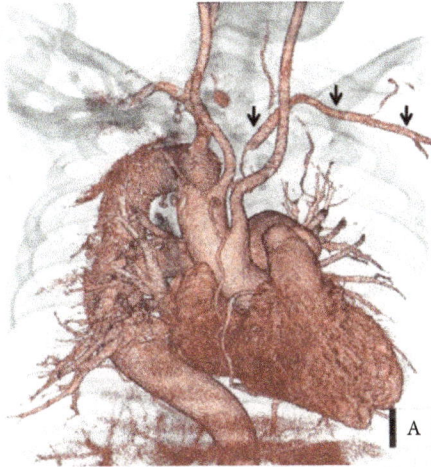

FIGURE 3: Postoperative CT revealed enhanced ALSA (arrows) clearly without delay, which was supplied with blood from many branches through very narrow and invisible collateral arteries.

adults, but sometimes they are associated with complications, such as compression of adjacent structures, dissection or rupture. Standard management of KD has not been established because of the rarity of this anomaly [2]. Generally speaking, surgical intervention is recommended in symptomatic patients or asymptomatic patients with a large diverticulum.

Several reports recommend an operative strategy of descending aortic replacement and anatomical or extra anatomical reconstruction of aberrant subclavian artery [2, 3] for KD. Posterolateral thoracotomy provides excellent exposure of the aortic arch and descending aorta, which allows reconstruction of aneurysm including KD and aberrant subclavian artery repair.

With regard to the reconstruction of the aberrant subclavian artery, in situ repair is optimal. Esposito and colleagues have reported significant ischemic complications such as coldness, rest pain, and fingertip necrosis in 64% of patients treated without restoration of the blood flow to the arm [4].

However, if the reconstruction of the aberrant subclavian artery was too difficult, to close an orifice is acceptable. Because, when the ischemia is noticed after aortic procedure, to make an extra anatomical reconstruction like a subclavian to subclavian artery bypass could be considered. It is one of the options of operation of an aneurysm with KD. It has some advantages, for example, decrease of blood loss and cardiopulmonary bypass time. We recommend this method especially for cases where the orifice of ALSA is noticed over the vertebra. Ota and colleagues reported that ligation of ALSA would be acceptable when a stenosis of orifice of ALSA was noticed, under observation of intraoperative blood pressure of both arm, and confirmation of unchanged blood pressure of left arm [3]. There is a possibility that the stenosis of ALSA might bring a preparation for collateral development. Kouchoukos also recommend a carotid to subclavian artery bypass in patients where direct continuity between the descending thoracic aorta and the distal subclavian artery could not be easily established [2].

To make the right strategy of operation, preoperative 3D-CT identification of anomalous structures is very useful, especially in rare cases such as the one with KD and a right aortic arch [5]. 3D-CT, especially scrolling from superficial to deep layer view with the chest wall including ribs (Figure 2), was very useful for us to have a proper orientation and to make an operative strategy.

4. Conclusion

Kommerell's diverticulum could be repaired without reconstruction of the aberrant left subclavian artery. It was found advantageous because of the decrease of blood loss and the shorter cardiopulmonary bypass time. If an ischemia of arm is noticed, additional reconstruction will have to be considered.

Disclosure

None of the authors have any competing or financial interests to disclosure.

References

[1] E. H. Austin and W. G. Wolfe, "Aneurysm of aberrant subclavian artery with a review of the literature," *Journal of Vascular Surgery*, vol. 2, no. 4, pp. 571–577, 1985.

[2] N. T. Kouchoukos and P. Masetti, "Aberrant subclavian artery and Kommerell aneurysm: surgical treatment with a standard approach," *Journal of Thoracic and Cardiovascular Surgery*, vol. 133, no. 4, pp. 888–892, 2007.

[3] T. Ota, K. Okada, S. Takanashi, S. Yamamoto, and Y. Okita, "Surgical treatment for Kommerell's diverticulum," *Journal of Thoracic and Cardiovascular Surgery*, vol. 131, no. 3, pp. 574–578, 2006.

[4] R. A. Esposito, I. Khalil, A. C. Galloway, and F. C. Spencer, "Surgical treatment for aneurysm of aberrant subclavian artery based on a case report and a review of the literature," *Journal of Thoracic and Cardiovascular Surgery*, vol. 95, no. 5, pp. 888–891, 1988.

[5] T. Nakada, Y. Sakao, A. Gorai, H. Uehara, M. Mun, and S. Okumura, "Two patients of left lung cancer with right aortic arch: review of eight patients," *General Thoracic and Cardiovascular Surgery*, vol. 60, pp. 537–541, 2012.

Sandwich EVAR occludes Celiac and Superior Mesenteric Artery for Infected Suprarenal Abdominal Aortic Aneurysm Treatment

Supatcha Prasertcharoensuk ⓘ,[1] Narongchai Wongkonkitsin ⓘ,[1] Parichat Tunmit,[1] Su-a-pa Theeragul,[1] and Anucha Ahooja ⓘ[2]

[1]*Department of Surgery, Khon Kaen University, Khon Kaen, Thailand*
[2]*Department of Radiology, Khon Kaen University, Khon Kaen, Thailand*

Correspondence should be addressed to Supatcha Prasertcharoensuk; supatcha.p@gmail.com

Academic Editor: Matthew Matson

Introduction. Infected aortoiliac aneurysms are rare, representing only 1% to 2% of all aortic aneurysms; we present a case of infected suprarenal aortic aneurysm with a nearly occluded celiac artery and superior mesenteric artery treated using an endovascular technique to preserve collateral in the retroperitoneal space from the inferior mesenteric artery for supplying visceral organs.

1. Introduction

Infected aortoiliac aneurysms are rare, representing only 1% to 2% of all aortic aneurysms [1]. One study in an Asian population found that infected abdominal aortic aneurysms accounted for 13.6% of cases and were associated with morbidity and mortality rates of 21%–44% [2]. Infected abdominal aortic aneurysm may present in various signs and symptoms that are not specific to infected abdominal aortic aneurysm, which may lead to misdiagnosis and delay treatment [3]. Treatment options for infected suprarenal abdominal aortic aneurysm include medication, open in situ graft repair, and hybrid endovascular repair [4].

There are also several surgical procedures used to treat the condition, including surgical debridement with in situ graft interposition and omental wrapping, aneurysm exclusion and extra-anatomic (axillofemoral) bypass, and aneurysmectomy with polytetrafluoroethylene (PTFE) graft interposition. The main factors associated with outcomes are whether or not appropriate surgical intervention was performed, whether or not the patient was treated with proper antibiotics, and whether or not the IAAA was ruptured. Here, we present a case of infected suprarenal aortic aneurysm with a nearly occluded celiac artery and superior mesenteric artery treated using an endovascular technique to preserve collateral in the retroperitoneal space from the inferior mesenteric artery for supplying visceral organs. We also report on the clinical outcomes of this technique. To our knowledge, this is the first report to describe a total endovascular procedure treatment of the infected suprarenal aortic aneurysm using the sandwich technique without preserved flow to both celiac artery and superior mesenteric artery.

2. Case Report

A 33-year-old woman presented with abdominal pain and having had a low-grade fever for three days. Computed tomographic angiography revealed a saccular aneurysm at the paravisceral aortic region, a nearly occluded celiac artery, and superior mesenteric artery with a large patent inferior mesenteric artery (7.3 mm), which provided a large collateral in the retroperitoneal space for supplying visceral organs, as shown in Figure 1. She had no history of trauma, pancreatitis, diabetes mellitus, recent medical or dental procedures, or drug abuse.

On examination, her blood pressure was 104/64 mmHg and she was febrile. The central abdomen was tender with a four-centimeter palpable pulsatile mass. The patient's pulse at all of the lower limbs was normal. Investigations revealed haemoglobin levels of 12.4 g/dL and a white cell count of 11.9×10^3/uL with neutrophilic change (77.8%) and without band form. Her platelet count was 317×10^3/ml, erythrocyte

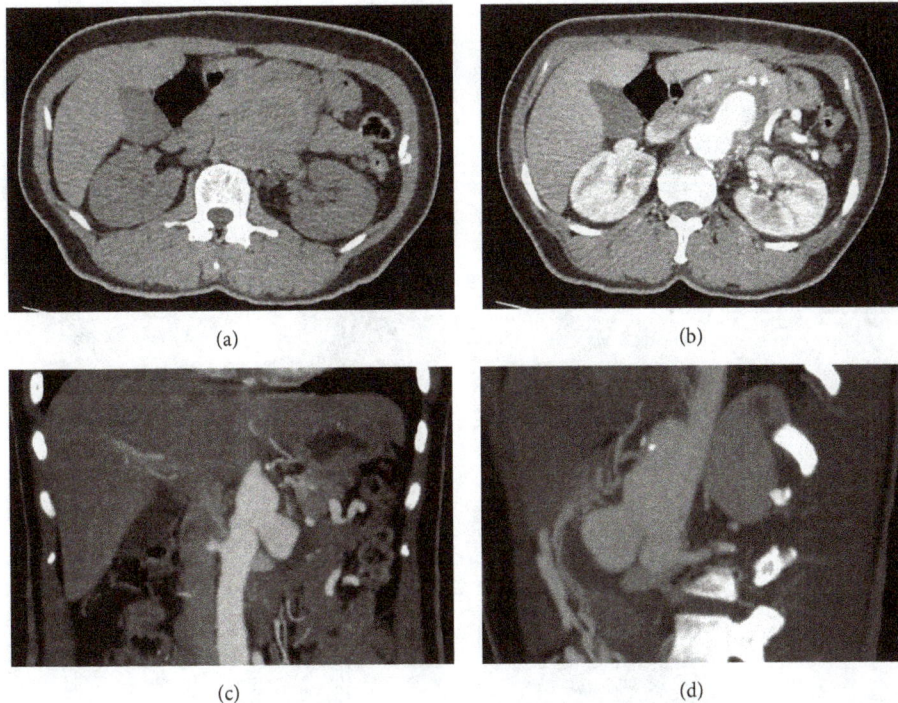

(a)   (b)

(c)   (d)

FIGURE 1: Crescent sign of suprarenal aortic aneurysm (a). A-phase shows saccular aneurysm behind the pancreas (b). Coronal view: suprarenal saccular aneurysm mainly on the left side (c). Sagittal view: aneurysm bulge anteriorly displacing the pancreas (d).

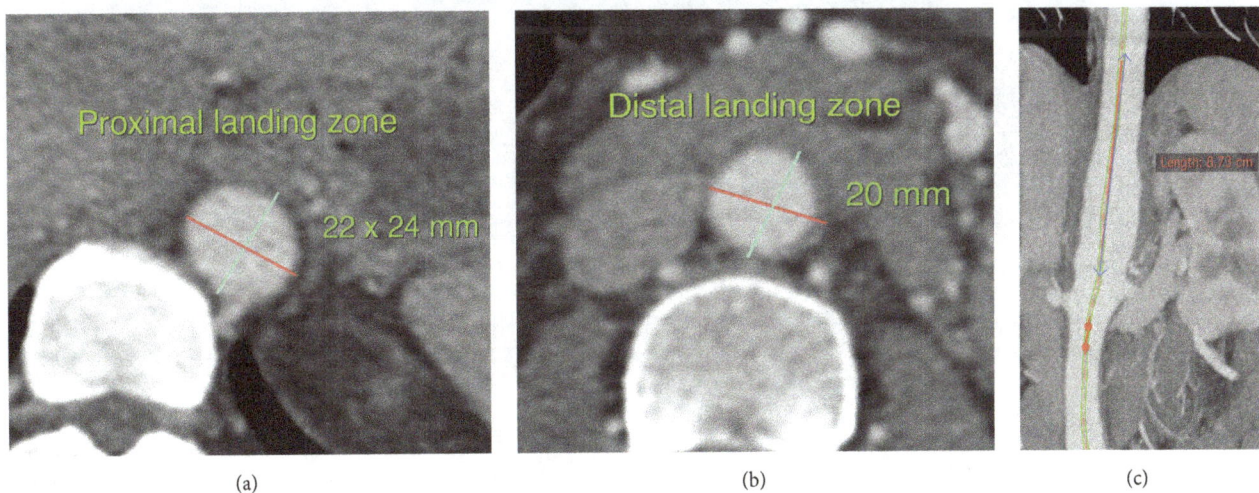

(a)   (b)   (c)

FIGURE 2: Proximal landing zone with diameter of 22 mm (a). Distal landing zone with diameter of 20 mm (b). Coronal view shows inflammatory and saccular aneurysm part (c).

sedimentation rate (ESR) was 90 mm/hr, and C-reactive protein level was 8.9 mg/l. Blood and urine cultures showed no growth. Results of transthoracic echocardiography were normal.

We diagnosed this patient as having an infected suprarenal aortic aneurysm, due to CTA findings showing saccular aneurysm and periaortic inflammation in the visceral segment of the aorta, even though her hemoculture was negative. As such, intravenous ceftazidime and clindamycin were empirical to cover *Burkholderia pseudomallei* and *Salmonella species* which are endemic infections in the Northeast of

Thailand. The patient experienced ongoing pain and developed intermittent pyrexia of up to 38.4°C. Blood cultures remained negative and her white cell count reached $14.5 \times 10^3/uL$ with neutrophilic change (89.7%) and without band form on the fourth day after admission. Measurement of the aorta found the proximal landing zone to be at descending aorta level T10-11 with a diameter of 24 mm and the distal landing zone to be 20 mm in diameter above the IMA. The distance from the proximal landing zone to just above renal arteries was 90 mm, as shown in Figure 2.

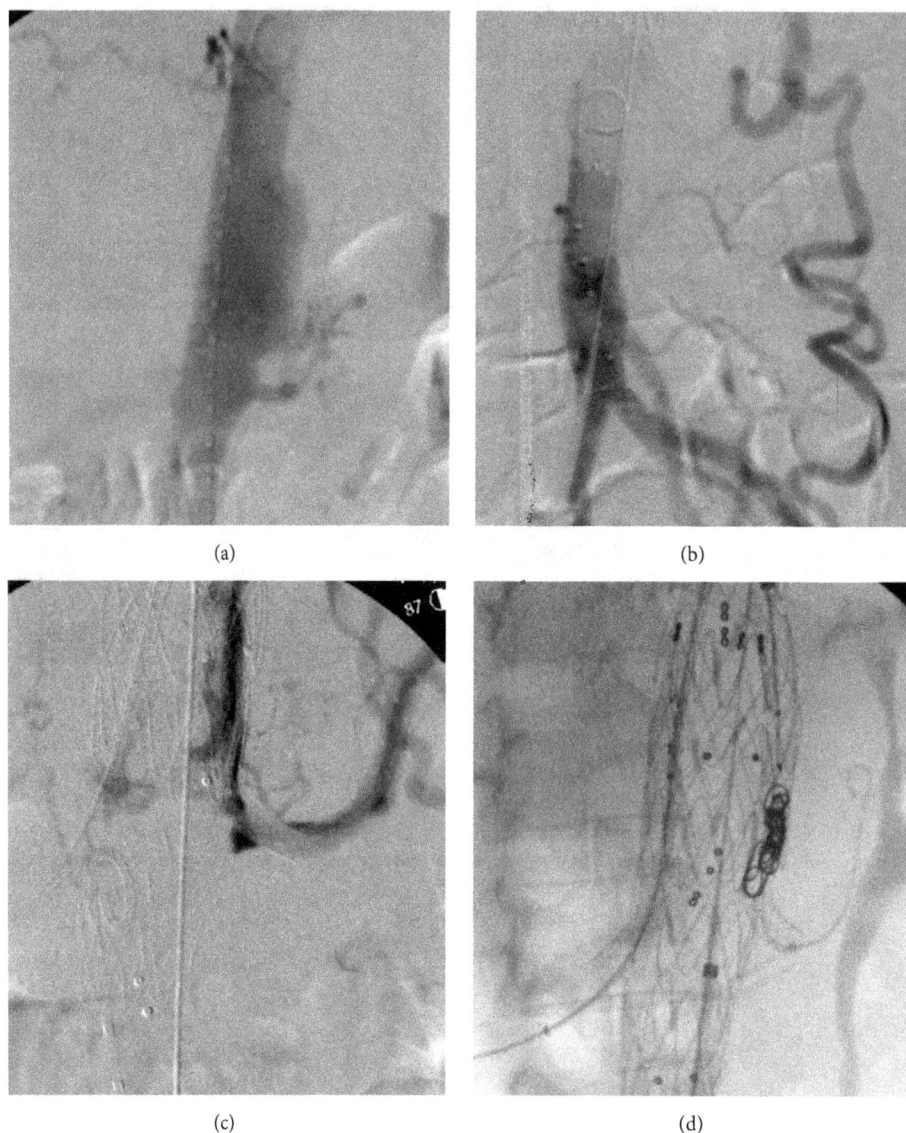

(a)

(b)

(c)

(d)

FIGURE 3: Intraoperative angiogram shows suprarenal saccular aneurysm with nearly occluded celiac and superior mesenteric artery (a). Large patent of inferior mesenteric artery gives blood supply to whole abdomen (b). Endoleak type III from left gutter (c). Extended gutter and coil embolization between left renal stent and aortic stent (d).

The patient underwent EVAR using a sandwich technique; the first aortic stent graft (VAMC2828C100TE) was deployed above left renal artery followed by advance guidewire to select both renal arteries in order to place the balloon covered stents (Begraft 6 × 58) to both sides. Then another endovascular aortic stent (ETTF2828C70EE) was simultaneously deployed to sandwich the renal artery stents. First, in complete aortogram, there was evidence of endoleak type 3 between left renal artery stent and endovascular aortic stent. We extended both renal stents and inner endovascular aortic stent (VAMC2828C100TE) to extend gutter between stents up to 50 mm and coil gutter. In final aortogram, there is only endoleak type 2, as shown in Figure 3. Postoperative management consisted of the prescription of six weeks of intravenous antibiotic (ceftazidime plus clindamycin) and ciprofloxacin and clindamycin orally for the rest of the patient's life. At follow-up after one month and six months, the patient had no abdominal pain and had gained a significant amount of weight. Computed tomographic angiography results revealed that the aneurysm had shrunk, as shown in Figure 4 (three months after surgery). We also found that C-reactive protein (a biomarker) levels were dramatically lower after the aneurysm was repaired and returned to normal after three weeks (Figure 5). At the one-year follow-up, the patient was asymptomatic and had no bowel ischemia.

3. Discussion

Infected abdominal aortic aneurysms account for 2% of abdominal aortic aneurysms. Infected abdominal aortic aneurysms at the suprarenal abdominal aorta are extremely rare according to case reports, reports on small cases series,

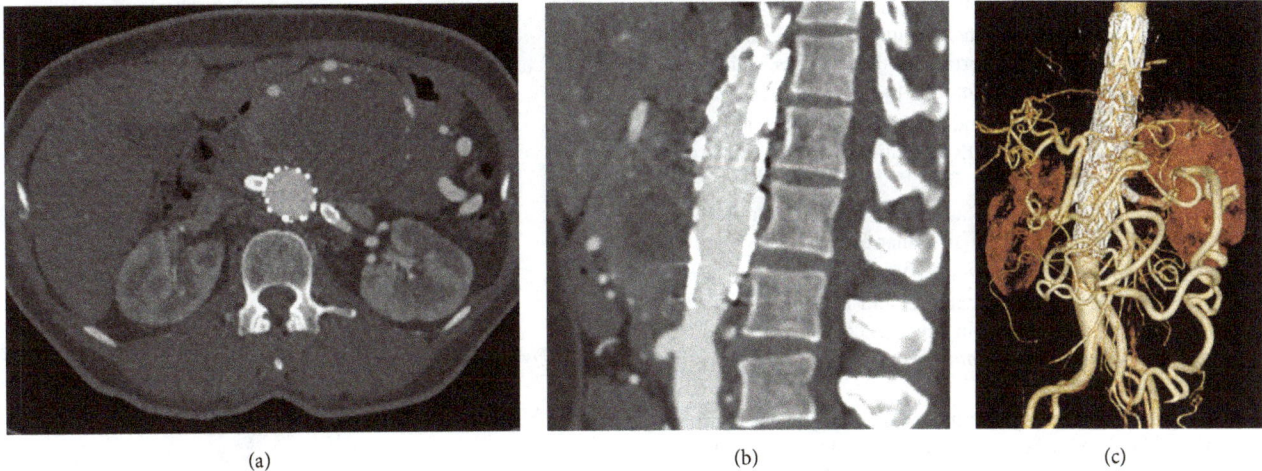

(a)   (b)   (c)

FIGURE 4: CTA: axial view, no endoleak (a). Sagittal view: stent placed superior to inferior mesenteric artery orifice (b). Reconstruction view: adequate flow from the inferior mesenteric artery to supply the celiac artery and superior mesenteric artery.

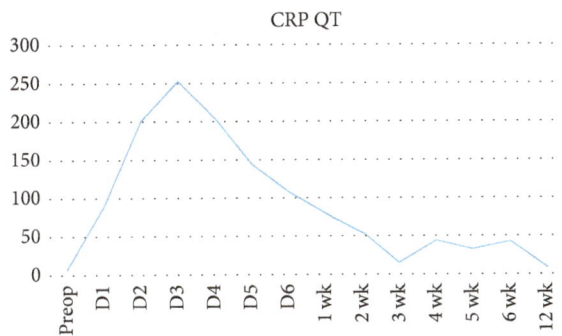

FIGURE 5: C-reactive protein levels from preoperation to 12 weeks after endovascular aneurysm repair (EVAR) by using the sandwich technique.

and literature review [5–8]. The common causative organism is *Salmonella* spp. [9, 10]. Treatment outcomes of IAAA may be associated with an aggressive debridement with in situ prosthetic reconstruction accompanied by prolonged antibiotic therapy and often lifelong suppressive oral antibiotics. However, according to a review based on several case reports, aneurysmectomy with aggressive debridement is reported as having a survival rate that is falsely high [11]. However, this operation is time-consuming, requires a significant number of technically demanding anastomoses to visceral vessels, and is usually associated with bypass-related complications such as renal failure, intestinal ischemia, and paraplegia. Hybrid endovascular repair, combining the open renovisceral debranching and endovascular stenting, is reserved for patients who are in high risk when standard open procedures are approached [12]. In this case, the patient in this study had a large number of collaterals in retroperitoneum, meaning that the debranching procedure may have cut off valuable collaterals that make visceral ischemia, so we abandoned the use of this procedure.

Endovascular repair of suprarenal infected abdominal aortic aneurysm is even more complex because concomitant renovisceral debranching is usually required. There are few clinical cases of total endovascular repair of suprarenal infected abdominal aortic aneurysm. A total of six cases have been reported in the English literature [13–15]. The largest case series by Sörelius et al. in 2009 reported on three cases of endovascular repair of infected suprarenal abdominal aortic aneurysm. Previous studies have reported a mortality rate of 33% (3/9) with two cases of intestinal ischemia (2/9) and one case of sepsis (1/9) [16].

4. Conclusion

Sandwich EVAR can be used safely in cases of complex anatomy, in which emergency intervention is required.

Disclosure

An earlier version of this study has been presented as an oral presentation in LINC 2018.

Acknowledgments

The authors would like to thank (a) Professor Kittisak Sawanyawisuth for assistance with writing this manuscript and (b) Mr. Dylan Southard for assistance with the English-language presentation of the manuscript under the aegis of the Publication Clinic KKU, Thailand.

References

[1] D. J. Reddy, A. D. Shepard, J. R. Evans, D. J. Wright, R. F. Smith, and C. B. Ernst, "Management of Infected Aortoiliac Aneurysms," *JAMA Surgery*, vol. 126, no. 7, pp. 873–879, 1991.

[2] R.-B. Hsu, Y.-G. Tsay, S.-S. Wang, and S.-H. Chu, "Surgical treatment for primary infected aneurysm of the descending thoracic aorta, abdominal aorta, and iliac arteries," *Journal of Vascular Surgery*, vol. 36, no. 4, pp. 746–750, 2002.

[3] M. Bouzas, V. Tchana-Sato, and J. P. Lavigne, "Infected abdominal aortic aneurysm due to Escherichia coli," *Acta Chirurgica Belgica*, vol. 117, no. 3, pp. 200–202, 2017.

[4] K. Laohapensang, S. Aworn, S. Orrapin, and R. B. Rutherford, "Management of the infected aortoiliac aneurysms," *Annals of Vascular Diseases*, vol. 5, no. 3, pp. 334–341, 2012.

[5] M. Alonso, S. Caeiro, J. Cachaldora, and R. Segura, "Infected abdominal aortic aneurysm: In situ replacement with cryopreserved arterial homograft," *Journal of Cardiovascular Surgery*, vol. 38, no. 4, pp. 371–375, 1997.

[6] K. Itatani, T. Miyata, T. Komiyama, K. Shigematsu, and H. Nagawa, "An Ex-Situ Arterial Reconstruction for the Treatment of an Infected Suprarenal Abdominal Aortic Aneurysm Involving Visceral Vessels," *Annals of Vascular Surgery*, vol. 21, no. 3, pp. 380–383, 2007.

[7] D. L. Cull, R. P. Winter, R. T. Wheeler Gregory Jr., S. O. Snyder Jr., and R. G. Gayle, "Mycotic aneurysm of the suprarenal abdominal aorta," *J Cardiovasc Surg (Torino)*, vol. 33, no. 2, pp. 181–184, 1992.

[8] E. A. Suddleson, S. G. Katz, and R. D. Kohl, "Mycotic suprarenal aortic aneurysm," *Annals of Vascular Surgery*, vol. 1, no. 4, pp. 426–431, 1987.

[9] M. N. Gomes, P. L. Choyke, and R. B. Wallace, "Infected aortic aneurysms. A changing entity," *Annals of Surgery*, vol. 215, no. 5, pp. 435–442, 1992.

[10] P. J. Hsu, C. H. Lee, F. Y. Lee, and J. W. Liu, "Clinical and microbiological characteristics of mycotic aneurysms in a medical center in southern Taiwan," *J Microbiol Immunol Infect*, vol. 81, no. 4, pp. 318–324, 2008.

[11] R. G. Atnip, "Mycotic aneurysms of the suprarenal abdominal aorta: Prolonged survival after in situ aortic and visceral reconstruction," *Journal of Vascular Surgery*, vol. 10, no. 6, pp. 635–641, 1989.

[12] R. Patel, M. F. Conrad, V. Paruchuri, C. J. Kwolek, T. K. Chung, and R. P. Cambria, "Thoracoabdominal aneurysm repair: Hybrid versus open repair," *Journal of Vascular Surgery*, vol. 50, no. 1, pp. 15–22, 2009.

[13] M. Soule, I. Javerliat, A. Rouanet, A. Long, and P. Lermusiaux, "Visceral debranching and aortic endoprosthesis for a suspected mycotic pseudoaneurysm of the abdominal aorta involving visceral arteries," *Annals of Vascular Surgery*, vol. 24, no. 6, pp. 825–e16, 2010.

[14] W. C. Liu, B. K. Kwak, K. N. Kim et al., "Tuberculous Aneurysm of the Abdominal Aorta: Endovascular Repair Using Stent Grafts in Two Cases," *Korean Journal of Radiology*, vol. 1, no. 4, pp. 215–218, 2000.

[15] P. Madhavan, C. O. McDonnell, M. O. Dowd et al., "Suprarenal mycotic aneurysm exclusion using a stent with a partial autologous covering," *Journal of Endovascular Therapy*, vol. 7, no. 5, pp. 404–409, 2000.

[16] K. Sörelius, K. Mani, M. Björck, R. Nyman, and A. Wanhainen, "Endovascular repair of mycotic aortic aneurysms," *Journal of Vascular Surgery*, vol. 50, no. 2, pp. 269–274, 2009.

38

Pulmonary Endarterectomy in a Patient with Immune Thrombocytopenic Purpura

Bedrettin Yıldızeli,[1] **Mehmed Yanartaş,**[2] **Sibel Keskin,**[3] **Işık Atagündüz,**[4] **and Ece Altınay**[5]

[1]*Department of Thoracic Surgery, Marmara University School of Medicine, Istanbul, Turkey*
[2]*Department of Cardiovascular Surgery, Kartal Koşuyolu Training and Research Hospital, Istanbul, Turkey*
[3]*Department of Chest Diseases, Muğla Sıtkı Koçman University, Muğla, Turkey*
[4]*Department of Hematology, Marmara University School of Medicine, Istanbul, Turkey*
[5]*Department of Anaesthesia, Kartal Koşuyolu Training and Research Hospital, Istanbul, Turkey*

Correspondence should be addressed to Bedrettin Yıldızeli; byildizeli@marmara.edu.tr

Academic Editor: Paolo Vanelli

Immune thrombocytopenic purpura (ITP) patients are at high risk for bleeding complications regarding surgeries involving cardiopulmonary bypass. We report an ITP patient with chronic thromboembolic pulmonary hypertension who underwent uncomplicated pulmonary endarterectomy with receiving postoperative intravenous immunoglobulin (IVIG) therapy. The positive outcome of this case may suggest that pulmonary endarterectomy surgery is performed safely for ITP patients.

1. Introduction

Immune thrombocytopenic purpura (ITP) is a common hematological disorder which involves immune mediated platelet destruction and impaired platelet production [1]. It is characterized by isolated thrombocytopenia in the absence of other causes or disorders that may be associated with thrombocytopenia [1]. The association of ITP and chronic thromboembolic pulmonary hypertension (CTEPH) represents a complex therapeutic challenge. To our knowledge, no case was reported to describe management of patients with ITP undergoing pulmonary endarterectomy (PEA). We describe our experience of perioperative management in a patient of ITP who underwent surgery.

2. Case Report

A 69-year-old female with shortness of breath (New York Heart Association Class IV) and CTEPH for a 1-year period was referred for PEA. Her medical history revealed that she had hypertension, regulated with oral antihypertensive drugs,

and type II diabetes mellitus. Routine hematological examination was normal with a platelet count of 228,000/mm^3. Her hematologic investigations showed a provisional diagnosis of ITP for 12 years with history of splenectomy 10 years ago. The patient was on chronic corticosteroid and azathioprine therapy on admission.

Her echocardiogram revealed a dilated right ventricle with reduced systolic function and moderate tricuspid regurgitation, but normal left ventricular function with an ejection fraction of 65%. A right heart catheterization revealed slightly elevated pulmonary artery (PA) pressure of 45/16 mm Hg (mean, 28 mm Hg) and cardiac output (CO) of 3.3 L/min. Calculated pulmonary vascular resistance (PVR) was 436 dynes/s/cm^{-5}. Spiral computed tomographic scanning of her chest showed right pleural effusion and web-like filling defects and endoluminal thromboemboli in her pulmonary vasculature on the right and left lower lobe sides consistent with chronic thromboembolic disease (Figure 1). Ventilation perfusion scanning confirmed the diagnosis of CTEPH and the patient was scheduled for pulmonary endarterectomy. The PEA surgery was performed

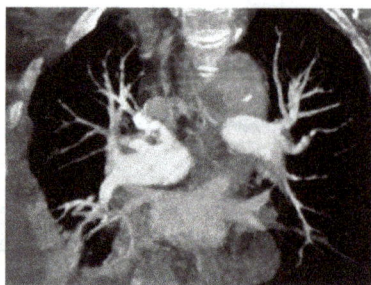

FIGURE 1: Computed tomogram shows right pleural effusion, web-like filling defects, and endoluminal thromboemboli extending into the right and left pulmonary artery.

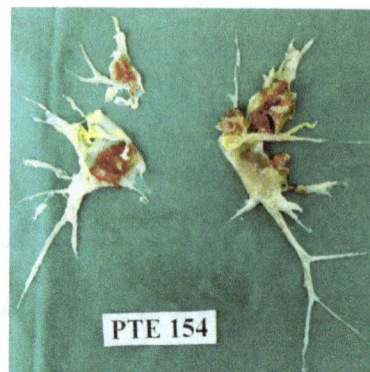

FIGURE 2: Photograph shows the specimen from our patient's pulmonary endarterectomy.

as previously described [2]. In brief, surgery was performed under general anaesthesia through a median sternotomy and using extracorporeal circulation. After anticoagulation with heparin, activated clotting time (ACT) of 480 seconds was attained and cardiopulmonary bypass (CPB) was initiated. The endarterectomy specimen was circumferentially followed down to the segmental and subsegmental branches of the pulmonary artery in each lobe, until a complete endarterectomy of the pulmonary vascular bed was achieved with periods of circulatory arrest under deep hypothermia (20°C) for the right and left pulmonary arteries (Figure 2). Patient weaned from CPB without any difficulty and her PVR was decreased to 250 dynes/s/cm^{-5}. Bleeding was checked thoroughly and heparin was reversed with protamine to normalize ACT. The chest was closed and the patient was transferred to the intensive care unit and put on ventilator with stable hemodynamics. Six hours later, platelets counts were 158,000/mm^3. On the first postoperative day (pod), the patient was put on oral azathioprine 50 mg and oral prednisolone 16 mg daily and subcutaneous injections (s.c.) of low-molecular-weight heparin (LMWH) 0.6 cc twice daily. The platelets counts were 241,000/mm^3. On the 2nd pod platelet counts were decreased to 57,500/mm^3, and, instead of LMWH, an indirect factor Xa inhibitor fondaparinux was initiated 2.5 mg/day s.c. and dose of prednisolone was increased to 100 mg daily. After three days of treatment, a low platelet count of 57,000/mm^3 was observed. Steroid therapy was stopped and intravenous immunoglobulin (IVIG) was started at a dose of 400 mg/kg/day for 5 days. Patient was extubated on 5th pod with stable hemodynamics and blood gases. In the meantime the platelet concentrates were transfused between first and 4th pod. Platelet counts were assessed daily and showed a rising trend. On 7th pod, the platelets counts were 183,000/mm^3. And she was transferred to the ward. IVIG was switched to oral prednisolone treatment, and also azathioprine, fondaparinux, and warfarin therapy was continued. The patient was discharged on 14th pod with a platelet count of 125,000/mm^3 and with substantial functional and hemodynamic improvement and with advice to continue her medications azathioprine 50 mg and prednisolone 16 mg daily and regularly follow up with a hematologist.

3. Discussion

Immune thrombocytopenic purpura is characterized by an abnormally low platelet count of unknown cause. IgG antiplatelet autoantibodies are produced against the platelet glycoprotein IIb/IIIa or GPIb/IX in about 75% of patients causing both platelet destruction and inhibition of thrombopoiesis [1]. The main problem in patients of ITP is an increased risk of bleeding although bleeding symptoms may not always be present. Concomitantly, the ITP patients also present an increased risk of thrombosis related to the presence of hemostatic factors and chronic steroid therapy.

On the other hand, several investigators have recently found in control retrospective and prospective cohort studies that splenectomy is a risk factor of CTEPH [3]. Splenectomy is associated with venous thrombosis in general and, in particular, with nonresolving and recurrent thrombosis and deep vein thrombosis. One late consequence of nonresolution of venous and pulmonary thromboemboli is CTEPH.

Pulmonary endarterectomy is only curative therapy of CTEPH [4]. The technical details of PEA surgery are well established. By using extracorporeal circulation and circulatory arrest under deep hypothermia (20°C), endarterectomy specimen is circumferentially followed down to the segmental and subsegmental branches of the pulmonary artery. Although there is no contraindication for PEA surgery, operability of the CTEPH patient should be determined by an experienced PEA team [4].

Bleeding after CPB surgery is common with about 7% of patients requiring reoperation to control bleeding [5]. Preoperative thrombocytopenia, CPB, deep hypothermia, and induced thrombocytopenia as well as platelet dysfunction and postoperative anticoagulation are expected to increase risk of pericardial effusion and cardiac tamponade. Chowdhry et al. [5] reported a patient with ITP with severe coronary artery disease and mitral regurgitation who underwent CABG and mitral valve replacement. Although early outcome of the surgery was uncomplicated, the patient was dead three weeks later with a diagnosis of pericardial tamponade.

The main treatment of ITP consists of corticosteroids and IVIG. Second and third line therapies, including rituximab, splenectomy, thrombin receptor agonists (TPO-A), and immune-suppressants, are often successful and may cause a long-term increase in the platelet counts [5]. Patients with asymptomatic mild or moderate thrombocytopenia can be followed up with no treatment as platelet counts greater than $5 \times 10^4/mm^3$ are usually not associated with clinically important bleeding. Although platelet transfusion may be short acting, it is useful in instances of severe hemorrhage. Infusion of IVIG has an immediate effect in increasing platelet counts as it blocks the crystallizable fragment (Fc) receptors of macrophages, thus avoiding destruction by phagocytosis.

Jubelirer et al. [6] reported that patients with ITP presenting with mild or moderate thrombocytopenia can be successfully supported to control bleeding during or after coronary artery bypass grafting (CABG) with IVIG and/or platelet transfusions.

The present patient had a diagnosis of ITP and CTEPH disease and underwent successful PEA. To our knowledge, no case of PEA for a patient with a history of ITP has previously been reported. She had an uneventful intraoperative course and there was no difficulty in obtaining surgical hemostasis. In the postoperative period also the patient did not have much bleeding and bleeding related complications. The decrease in the platelet count was managed successfully with platelet transfusion, steroids, and IVIG. Patient was discharged with acceptable platelet counts and with advice about taking anticoagulants, timely INR monitoring, and regular follow-up.

We conclude that PEA surgery can be performed safely to a patient with CTEPH associated ITP. We would recommend that, with an accurate and precise postoperative management, ITP is not contraindicated for PEA surgery.

References

[1] T. Kühne, "Update on the intercontinental cooperative ITP study group (ICIS) and on the pediatric and adult registry on chronic ITP (PARC ITP)," *Pediatric Blood and Cancer*, vol. 60, supplement 1, pp. S15–S18, 2013.

[2] B. Yıldızeli, S. Taş, M. Yanartaş et al., "Pulmonary endarterectomy for chronic thrombo-embolic pulmonary hypertension: an institutional experience," *European Journal Cardio-Thoracic Surgery*, vol. 44, no. 3, pp. e219–e227, 2013.

[3] N. H. Kim and I. M. Lang, "Risk factors for chronic thromboembolic pulmonary hypertension," *European Respiratory Review*, vol. 21, no. 123, pp. 27–31, 2012, Review.

[4] N. H. Kim, M. Delcroix, D. P. Jenkins et al., "Chronic thromboembolic pulmonary hypertension," *Journal of the American College of Cardiology*, vol. 62, no. 25, supplement, pp. D92–D99, 2013.

[5] V. Chowdhry, B. B. Mohanty, and D. Probodh, "Cardiac surgery in a patient with immunological thrombocytopenic purpura: complications and precautions," *Annals of Cardiac Anaesthesia*, vol. 16, no. 2, pp. 147–150, 2013.

[6] S. J. Jubelirer, L. Mousa, U. Reddy, M. Mir, and C. A. Welch, "Coronary artery bypass grafting (CABG) in patients with immune thrombocytopenia (ITP): a community hospital experience and review of the literature," *The West Virginia Medical Journal*, vol. 107, no. 6, pp. 10–14, 2011.

39

Novel Visceral-Anastomosis-First Approach in Open Repair of a Ruptured Type 2 Thoracoabdominal Aortic Aneurysm: Causes behind a Mortal Outcome

Einar Dregelid[1] and Alireza Daryapeyma[2]

[1] *Department of Vascular Surgery, Haukeland University Hospital, Jonas Lies Vei 65, 5021 Bergen, Norway*
[2] *Department of Vascular Surgery, Karolinska University Hospital, 171 76 Stockholm, Sweden*

Correspondence should be addressed to Einar Dregelid; eidreg@yahoo.com

Academic Editors: N. Espinola-Zavaleta, P. Heider, P.-H. Huang, N. Papanas, M. Sindel, and S. Yamashiro

Case reports to analyze causes and possible prevention of complications in a new setting are important. We present an open repair of a ruptured type 2 thoracoabdominal aortic aneurysm in a 78-year-old man. Lower-body perfusion through a temporary extracorporeal axillobifemoral arterial prosthesis shunt was combined with the use of a branch to the permanent aortic prosthesis to enable rapid visceral revascularization using a visceral-anastomosis-first approach. The patient died due to transfusion-induced capillary leak syndrome and left colon necrosis; the latter was probably caused by a combination of back-bleeding from lumbar arteries causing a steal effect, an accidental shunt obstruction, and hemodynamic instability towards the end of the operation. The visceral-anastomosis-first approach did not contribute to the complications. This approach reduces the time when visceral organs are perfused only via collateral arteries to the time needed for suturing the visceral anastomoses. This may be important when collateral perfusion is marginal.

1. Introduction

A subcutaneous axillofemoral bypass has previously been shown to prevent ischemic injury during operations for thoracoabdominal aortic aneurysms [1, 2]. The extracorporeal use of a vascular prosthesis for a temporary shunt has, to our knowledge, only been described in three cases previously [3, 4]. However, the use of a temporary vascular prosthesis shunt has been described without any substantial detail in 10 other cases [5]. A temporary subcutaneous bypass using a vascular prosthesis as opposed to an atrio-arterial bypass eliminates the risk of lower extremity ischemia due to femoral artery cannulation, does not require the same degree of anticoagulation, and causes less activation of blood components [1, 6], but subcutaneous tunneling for the bypass creates a potential bleeding focus and inflicts extra trauma. In the current paper ischemia prevention by lower-body perfusion through a temporary extracorporeal axillobifemoral shunt using a vascular prosthesis was combined with the use of

a branch to the permanent aortic prosthesis to enable rapid revascularization of the visceral territories using a visceral-anastomosis-first approach. The patient contracted severe but well-known complications, not specifically associated with this approach: bleeding, massive transfusions, capillary leak syndrome, and colon necrosis with a deadly outcome. Case reports to analyze causes and possible prevention of complications in a new setting are important.

2. Case Report

A 78-year-old man, an ex-smoker for the last two years was admitted in April 2009 with acute pain in the lower abdomen and back. He was on current medication for chronic obstructive pulmonary disease and hypertension in addition to statin therapy. He could walk between 1 and 2 flights of stairs before being halted by dyspnoea. He had been evaluated for a thoracoabdominal Crawford type 2 aortic aneurysm 2.5 months before admission. Operation was not

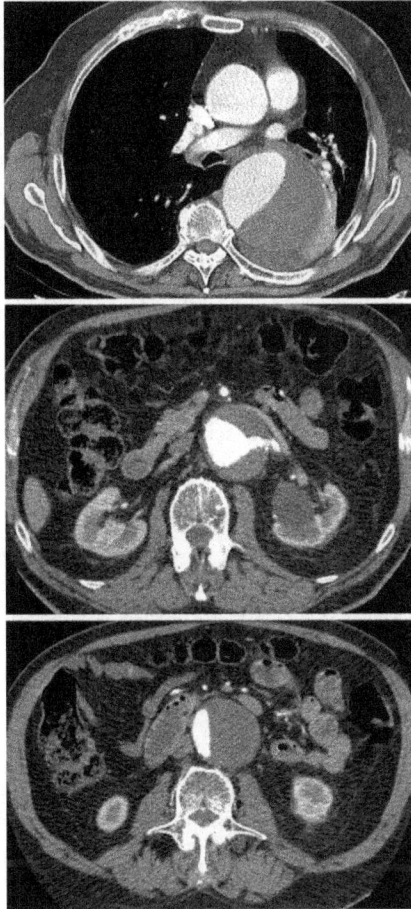

FIGURE 1: Computed tomography sections at the level of the descending aorta (upper panel), at the level of the left renal ostium (middle panel), and at the level of the infrarenal aorta (lower panel).

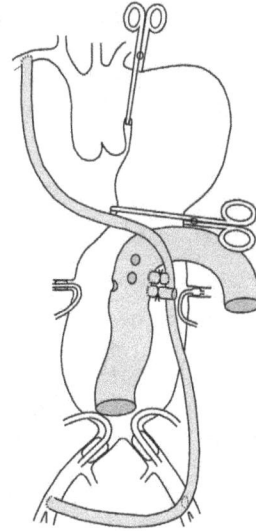

FIGURE 2: The presutured vascular prosthesis construct (shaded grey) consists of a temporary axillobifemoral bypass with a branch to the permanent aortic prosthesis. The drawing depicts an opened abdominal part of the aneurysm. Two Foley catheters are used for iliac occlusion. The left kidney is perfusion-cooled, and occlusion catheters occlude the right renal (shown) and visceral arteries (not shown). Holes in the middle part of the aortic prosthesis, placed after measurements on preoperative computed tomography images, are ready to be anastomosed to the visceral and right renal ostia. After completion of these anastomoses, the ligature on the connection between the temporary bypass and the aortic prosthesis is removed, and the right kidney and intestines are perfused via the middle part of the aortic prosthesis which is isolated using temporary ligatures (not shown), while a side branch with another temporary ligature is anastomosed to the left renal ostium. Finally, the distal and proximal ends of the aortic prosthesis are anastomosed to the aortic bifurcation and to the aorta just distally to the left subclavian artery, respectively.

recommended due to its high risk. Endovascular treatment with branched grafts or combined with thoracic and visceral debranching was still an experimental procedure without proven superiority compared with open repair [7].

On admittance blood pressure was 156/96 mmHg, pulse 81 bpm and regular, and temperature 37.9°C. There was tenderness around the umbilicus. Peripheral circulation and femoral pulses were good. Creatinine was 238 μmol/L, and estimated glomerular filtration rate was 23 mL/min/1.73 m^2. He was given analgesics and labetalol to lower his blood pressure. Computer tomography showed atelectasis of the lower lobe of the left lung and some pleural fluid. Aneurysm diameter was 8.7 cm in the mid-descending part and 5.5 cm at the level of the renal arteries (Figure 1). Imminent aneurysm rupture was suspected. A few hours after arrival, he developed strong chest and back pain and became hypotensive and oliguric. Haemoglobin fell from 140 to 114 g/L. ECG and troponin analysis showed no sign of myocardial infarction. Rupture of the thoracic part of the aneurysm was suspected. He was informed of poor prognosis both without surgical repair and with the planned procedure. He consented and was operated on urgently.

With the patient supine, a presutured vascular prosthesis construct (Figure 2), doubly wrapped in tubular drape, was anastomosed to the right axillary and both femoral arteries after heparinization (5000 IU) by two surgeons working simultaneously. All graft components were made of Dacron. Diameters were 10 mm for the axillobifemoral and connection to aortic graft components, 26 mm for the aortic prosthesis, and 6 mm for the side branch to the left renal ostium. A ring-supported prosthesis for the axillobifemoral bypass of adequate size was not available. The vascular prosthesis was clamped close to each anastomosis. The wounds and clamps were doubly draped, and the patient was turned on his right side. Using double lumen intubation, the aorta was exposed using a thoracoretroperitoneal approach with access in the 7th intercostal space.

There was fresh hematoma in the mid-descending aortic wall. Through another thoracotomy in the 3rd intercostal space, the aorta was clamped distal to the left subclavian artery. Another clamp was applied across the aneurysm proximally to the diaphragm. The abdominal part of the aneurysm was opened, 16 Fr Foley catheters were inserted into both iliac arteries for distal control, and axillobifemoral perfusion initiated. Back-bleeding from the celiac, superior mesenteric, and right renal ostium was prevented by occlusion balloons. Cold Ringer acetate solution was infused into the left renal artery. There was copious bleeding from lumbar arteries which were oversewn.

The openings in the aortic graft were anastomosed to the celiac, superior mesenteric, and right renal arteries which were then perfused while the side branch for the left renal ostium was cut short and anastomosed to the latter. Some residual bleeding, initially misjudged to come from an incomplete occlusion by the clamp just proximal to the diaphragm, was deemed to be irremediable. The bleeding subsequently turned out to be from lumbar arteries which were oversewn. After completing the distal anastomosis, the branch between the axillobifemoral shunt and the aortic graft was clamped, and visceral arteries were perfused via the distal part of the aortic graft.

The thoracic part of the aneurysm was opened, and intercostal arteries were oversewn. Access was somewhat hampered by the intact part of the chest wall between the two thoracotomies resulting in additional blood loss. It was now noted that pulses in the graft just proximal to the left groin could no longer be felt. Pulsation in the distal part of the aortic graft was restored by reopening the branch between the axillobifemoral shunt and the aortic prosthesis. After completion of the proximal anastomosis, this branch was removed. The patient developed consumption coagulopathy with airway and stitch-hole bleeding, necessitating multiple extra sutures, repeated haemostatic packing, and altogether 17.4 L of blood products before satisfactory haemostasis was obtained. In addition 5.7 L of salvaged red blood cells with a haematocrit of 40%–50% were reinfused. The thoracoretroperitoneal and thoracotomy wounds were closed; the patient was again turned to the supine position. The subclavicular and inguinal wounds were closed after removal of the axillobifemoral bypass. Oliguria developed toward the end of the operation. A dialysis catheter was placed in the left femoral vein. The operation lasted 15.5 hours.

Postoperatively, blood gases revealed hypoventilation. Chest X-ray showed no air in the right main bronchus. Ventilation was normalized after retraction of the endotracheal tube. The patient was oedematous and haemodynamically unstable, requiring volume expansion and inotropic support. He subsequently developed a supraventricular tachycardia. Plasma lactate rose to 9.4 mmol/L. Prognosis was considered poor. Life-supportive treatment was stopped, and he died 19 hours postoperatively.

Autopsy showed ischemic gangrene of the left colon. Other organs and lower extremity muscles had been vital until death. There was a horizontal rupture of the mid-descending aortic aneurysm with haemorrhage in the aortic wall and into the mediastinum and 500 mL of bloody fluid in the right pleural cavity. All vessels to the graft were open without any thrombi and with no hematomas around the anastomoses. There were bronchiectases, emphysema, and areas with atelectasis in the lungs.

3. Discussion

A visceral-anastomosis-first approach shortens the time when the intestines are perfused only by collaterals fed by the axillo(bi)femoral shunt. This may be important if collateral perfusion is marginal, although Comerota and White obtained good results with an axillofemoral shunt only [1]. In our patient the axillobifemoral shunt provided adequate collateral blood supply to the torso until the visceral vessels had been revascularized as evidenced by a high pressure in the compartmentalized thoracic aorta, copious back-bleeding from lumbar arteries, and a modest blood pressure drop on visceral reperfusion. It cannot be concluded with certainty that the visceral-anastomosis-first approach prevented a more extensive ischemic injury but it reduced the time when viscera were perfused only via collateral arteries to the time needed for suturing the visceral anastomoses and did not contribute to any of the complications that led to the patient's death.

Although in theory the proximal anastomosis could have been performed first during supraceliac aneurysm clamping and perfusion of the viscera with the axillofemoral shunt, the aneurysm was considered too wide to allow safe supraceliac clamping with full arterial pressure in the abdominal compartment of the aneurysm.

In our patient the right axillary artery was used as an origin for the shunt to allow clamping of the aorta proximally to the left subclavian artery if necessary, and bifemoral perfusion as opposed to unilateral perfusion was elected to optimize collateral supply to torso tissues, to reduce the need for ancillary measures to prevent spinal cord injury and possibly reduce the need for reimplantation of intercostal arteries [8–11]. It turned out that the left axillary artery could have been used in our patient since the aorta could be clamped distally to the left subclavian artery.

The use of the right axillary artery as an origin for the shunt when the patient lies on the right side demands attention to details and meticulous planning with regard to maintenance of sterility. Reapplication of a vascular clamp on the shunt close to the axillary artery is not straightforward in this position. Taylor et al. constructed an extracorporeal shunt between the left axillary and femoral arteries by suturing two grafts to the arteries and only connecting them after turning the patient on the side. Their approach may make logistics easier with regard to maintenance of sterility [3]. It is important to rehearse the entire operation with the whole surgical and anaesthesia team including scrub nurses. The composition of the team should allow change of personnel in case of exertion during such a long operation.

Hypoperfusion of the left colon may have been caused by back-bleeding from segmental arteries causing a steal effect through visceroparietal collaterals [12, 13], by haemodynamic instability towards the end of the operation, and by accidental obstruction of the axillobifemoral graft just proximally to the left groin. Accidental compression of the axillobifemoral graft can be potentially detectable and preventable by femoral pressure or flow monitoring and by the use of externally ring-supported prosthesis [1].

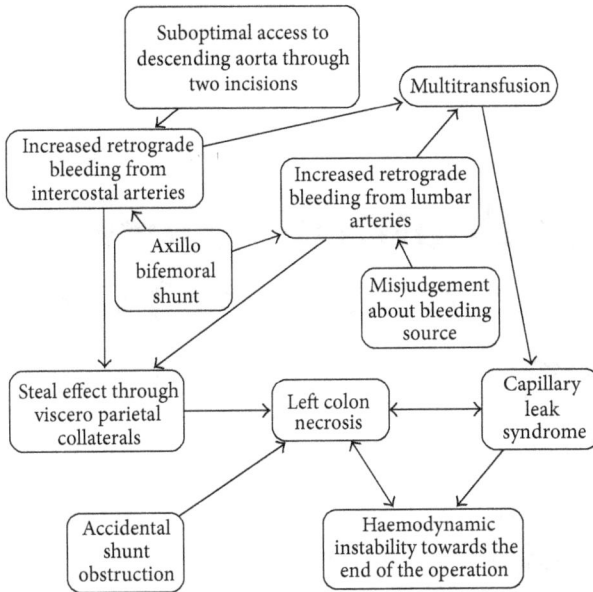

FIGURE 3: The diagram shows probable causalities of the outcome of the case. The axillobifemoral bypass increases visceral perfusion and retrograde bleeding from lumbar and intercostal branch ostia. Prevention of retrograde bleeding increases visceral perfusion further. Hence insufficient prevention of retrograde bleeding contributes to colon necrosis.

Our patient developed a capillary leak syndrome, attributable jointly to massive transfusion and colon necrosis. The latter might have been detected by opening the peritoneum for bowel inspection before wound closure. Also, bleeding from intercostal arteries might have been reduced using a thoracoretroperitoneal incision to give simultaneous access to the entire descending aorta [11, 14]. In our patient, however, access to the aneurysm through two separate incisions was selected because it was believed that it would confer benefit from the reduced trauma compared with one large incision [15]. Figure 3 shows probable causalities.

Although an axillofemoral vascular prosthetic shunt can be expected to stay open at least for the duration of an operation, despite no pressure gradient [1, 16], competing aortic blood flow exposes the temporary bypass to the risk of thrombosis [17]. An extracorporeal vascular prosthesis shunt as opposed to one buried subcutaneously may be clamped close to the anastomoses until it is needed and for short periods while securing haemostasis [3].

4. Conclusion

Visceral and lower limb perfusion via a temporary axillo-femoral or -bifemoral bypass with a branch to the permanent aortic prosthesis using a visceral-anastomoses-first approach may prevent ischemic injury to torso tissues better than only an axillofemoral bypass in operations for thoracoabdominal aortic aneurysms. A meticulously performed haemostasis is essential to avoid consumption coagulopathy and back-bleeding that may cause a steal effect. The colon should be inspected before wound closure after any circulatory

instability. Femoral pressure or flow monitoring may allow timely correction of shunt malfunction.

References

[1] A. J. Comerota and J. V. White, "Reducing morbidity of thoracoabdominal aneurysm repair by preliminary axillofemoral bypass," *American Journal of Surgery*, vol. 170, no. 2, pp. 218–222, 1995.

[2] E. Dregelid, "Operation for an infected thoracoabdominal aneurysm in a patient previously treated with an axillobifemoral bypass for an infected abdominal aortic prosthesis: a case report," *Annals of Thoracic and Cardiovascular Surgery*, vol. 18, no. 1, pp. 75–78, 2012.

[3] P. R. Taylor, Y. P. Panayiotopoulos, A. J. P. Sandison, H. K. Aduful, and C. H. Wood, "Temporary left external axillofemoral bypass during repair of a leaking type B aortic dissection," *British Journal of Surgery*, vol. 84, no. 3, p. 423, 1997.

[4] G. W. Gibbons, P. N. Madras, and F. C. Wheelock, "Aortoiliac reconstruction following renal transplantation," *Surgery*, vol. 91, no. 4, pp. 435–437, 1982.

[5] S. Maeda, T. Miyamoto, H. Murata, and K. Yamashita, "Prevention of spinal cord ischemia by monitoring spinal cord perfusion pressure and somatosensory evoked potentials," *Journal of Cardiovascular Surgery*, vol. 30, no. 4, pp. 565–571, 1989.

[6] C. C. Miller, M. A. Villa, P. Achouh et al., "Intraoperative skeletal muscle ischemia contributes to risk of renal dysfunction following thoracoabdominal aortic repair," *European Journal of Cardio-thoracic Surgery*, vol. 33, no. 4, pp. 691–694, 2008.

[7] M. Wilderman and L. A. Sanchez, "Fenestrated grafts or debranching procedures for complex abdominal aortic aneurysms," *Perspectives in Vascular Surgery and Endovascular Therapy*, vol. 21, no. 1, pp. 13–18, 2009.

[8] S. C. Harrison, O. Agu, P. L. Harris, and K. Ivancev, "Elective sac perfusion to reduce the risk of neurologic events following endovascular repair of thoracoabdominal aneurysms," *Journal of Vascular Surgery*, vol. 55, no. 4, pp. 1202–1205, 2012.

[9] M. S. Bischoff, L. G. Di, E. B. Griepp, and R. B. Griepp, "Spinal cord preservation in thoracoabdominal aneurysm repair," *Perspectives in Vascular Surgery and endoVascular Therapy*, vol. 23, no. 3, pp. 214–222, 2011.

[10] C. W. Acher and M. M. Wynn, "Thoracoabdominal aortic aneurysm. How we do it," *Cardiovascular Surgery*, vol. 7, no. 6, pp. 593–596, 1999.

[11] C. W. Acher and M. M. Wynn, "Technique of thoracoabdominal aneurysm repair," *Annals of Vascular Surgery*, vol. 9, no. 6, pp. 585–595, 1995.

[12] Y. Kawanishi, K. Okada, H. Tanaka, T. Yamashita, K. Nakagiri, and Y. Okita, "The adverse effect of back-bleeding from lumbar arteries on spinal cord pathophysiology in a rabbit model," *Journal of Thoracic and Cardiovascular Surgery*, vol. 133, no. 6, pp. 1553–1558, 2007.

[13] K. Renner, C. Ausch, H. R. Rosen et al., "Collateral circulation of the left colon: historic considerations and actual clinical significance," *Chirurg*, vol. 74, no. 6, pp. 575–578, 2003.

[14] H. J. Safi, "How I do it: thoracoabdominal aortic aneurysm graft replacement," *Cardiovascular Surgery*, vol. 7, no. 6, pp. 607–613, 1999.

Cystic Adventitial Disease of Popliteal Artery with Venous Aneurysm of Popliteal Vein: Two-Year Follow-Up after Surgery

Koki Takizawa,[1] Hiroshi Osawa,[1] Atsuo Kojima,[2] Samuel J. K. Abraham,[3] and Shigeru Hosaka[4]

[1]*Division of Cardiovascular Surgery, Shimada General Hospital, Choshi, Japan*
[2]*Department of Vascular Surgery, Tomei Atsugi Hospital, Atsugi, Japan*
[3]*The Mary-Yoshio Translational Hexagon (MYTH), Nichi-In Center for Regenerative Medicine (NCRM), Chennai, India*
[4]*Department of Cardiovascular Surgery, National Center of Global Health and Medicine, Shinjuku, Japan*

Correspondence should be addressed to Hiroshi Osawa; drosawa@yahoo.co.jp

Academic Editor: Nikolaos Papanas

We report a rare case of cystic adventitial disease of popliteal artery with venous aneurysm of popliteal vein. A 46-year-old woman had sudden-onset intermittent claudication and coldness in her right leg. The right-sided ankle-brachial pressure index (ABI) was 1.01, but peripheral arterial pulsation was decreased at knee venting position. Computed tomography revealed simple cystic lesion of the popliteal artery and stenosis of the arterial lumen in this lesion. The patient was treated by complete resection of the cystic adventitial layer of popliteal artery. A venous aneurysm of popliteal vein was revealed by intraoperative echo and was simply ligated. The patient had uneventful postoperative course and no symptoms of relevance during the two years of follow-up.

1. Introduction

Cystic adventitial disease (CAD) is rare vascular disorder in which a mucinous cystic formation in the adventitial layer of artery disturbs the arterial blood flow and causes intermittent claudication in young-adult patient. CAD was first reported by Atkins and Key in 1947 involving the external iliac artery [1]. CAD of popliteal artery was first described by Ejrup and Hietonn in 1954 [2]. The etiology of CAD is still controversial and several theories have been proposed. We report a case of CAD of popliteal artery with venous aneurysm of popliteal vein. The CAD was simple cystic lesion and resection of the cyst with the adventitia was successful.

2. Case Report

A 46-year-old woman was hospitalized with sudden-onset fatigue and coldness of right leg. She also had intermittent claudication after walking 200 meters. The patient had no risk factors of vascular disease. Diminished popliteal and foot pulses, lost after knee flexion (Ishikawa sign) [3], were found on the affected limb during the clinical examination.

The right ankle-brachial systolic pressure index at rest was 1.01 and the left was 1.1. Computed tomography revealed simple cystic lesion at the popliteal artery and stenosis of the artery in this lesion (Figure 1). Magnetic resonance imaging revealed cystic lesion encompassing the right popliteal artery circumferentially. This cystic lesion exhibited high signal intensity of T2-weighted images (Figure 2).

The patient was diagnosed to have cystic adventitial disease and underwent surgical repair. Surgical exploration was performed through a lateral approach to expose the distal femoral artery and proximal popliteal artery. The circumferential cystic enlargement of popliteal artery was revealed (Figure 3). It was confirmed as a cystic disease by intraoperative echo (Figure 4(a)). Cutting the adventitial layer was done, when clear viscous liquid element flowed out (Figure 5(a)). Complete resection of cystic adventitial layer was made (Figure 5(b)). Arterial pulsation improved immediately (Figure 4(b)). During the procedure, a saccular venous aneurysm of popliteal vein was revealed, just lateral to the popliteal artery (Figure 4(a)), and it was ligated at the orifice (Figure 6). In fact, the venous aneurysm was revealed

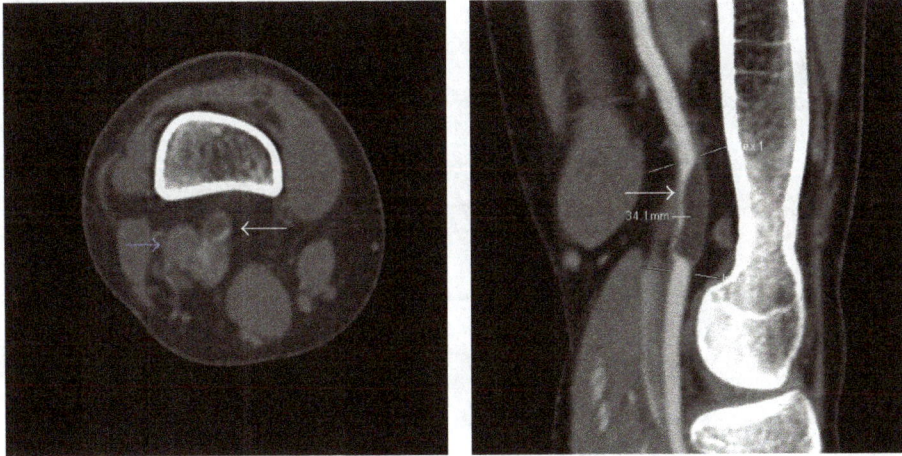

FIGURE 1: Computed tomography revealed simple cystic lesion at the popliteal artery and stenosis of the artery in this lesion. White arrow: cystic lesion of popliteal artery. Blue arrow: venous aneurysm (it was not diagnosed preoperatively).

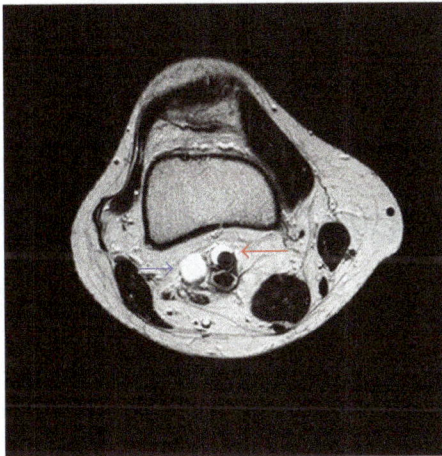

FIGURE 2: Magnetic resonance imaging (T2-weighted images) revealed cystic lesion encompassing the right popliteal artery circumferentially. Red arrow: cystic adventitial disease of popliteal artery. Blue arrow: venous aneurysm of popliteal vein (it was not diagnosed preoperatively).

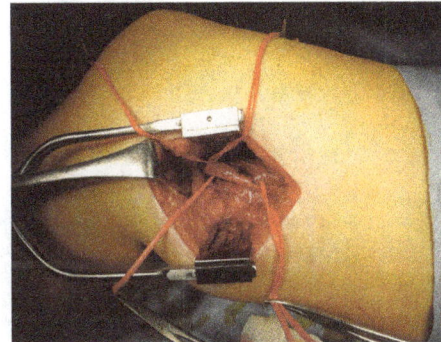

FIGURE 3: The circumferential cystic enlargement of popliteal artery.

by preoperative computed tomography and we confirmed it during the operation (Figure 1).

Postoperative course was uneventful. Postoperative MRI revealed 5 square mm of high intensity adventitial area that is suspected as the remanence of the cystic lesion (Figure 7). However, two years following the surgery, patient is symptom-free with normal ankle pressure with nonchanged MRI findings.

3. Discussion

Cystic adventitial disease (CAD) of the popliteal artery is a rare vascular disorder in which a mucin-containing cyst develops in the adventitial layer of the artery. Several theories about pathogenesis of cystic adventitial disease have been postulated, including trauma, direct anatomic communication with the nearby joint, degeneration, and cyst formation of the adventitial layer and mucin-secretin mesenchymal cells from nearby joint [4]. Desy and Spinner described that the adventitial cyst formation begins with a capsular rent or defect that leads to the tracking of synovial fluid along an arterial articular branch [5]. Motaganahali et al. reported that 71% of patients were either active smokers or ex-smokers, nevertheless there is no relation between smoking and CAD [6].

Color-coded Doppler sonography is the most useful in revealing arterial stenosis and occlusion immediately [7]. Magnetic resonance imaging (MRI) is useful and certain to diagnose CAD. On MRI findings, the cysts are hyperintense on T2-weighted images and have low to intermediate signal intensity on T1-weighted images; it is caused by the existence of mucoid material in the cyst [8]. Multisliced direct computed tomography is very useful in evaluating arteries and planning the operating strategy.

Several treatment methods of CAD have been described following excision of the cysts and arterial segment with interposition bypass grafting, simple resection of the cyst with arterial preservation, CT or ultrasound guided percutaneous aspiration, and endovascular treatment. The treatment method should be selected according to morphology of the cystic disease. It emphasizes that the standard treatment of

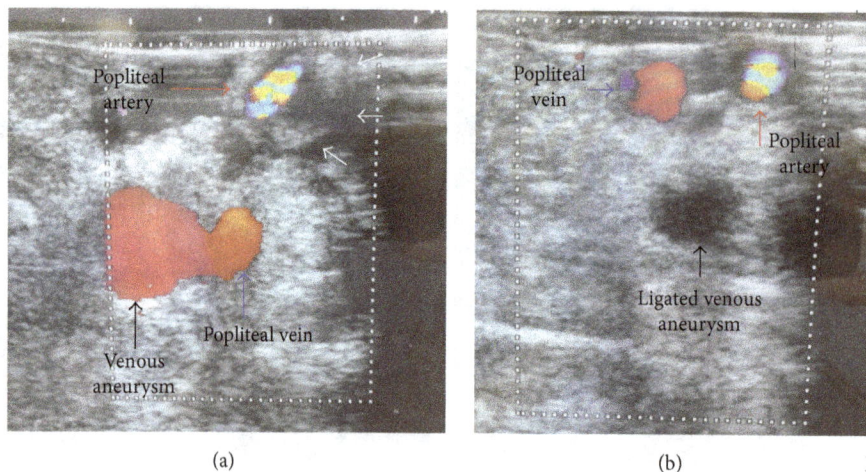

(a)   (b)

FIGURE 4: (a) Intraoperative echo findings revealed cystic adventitial lesion compressed internal lumen of popliteal artery (white arrow). (b) Intraoperative echo findings after resection of adventitial cyst revealed improved arterial compression and ligated venous aneurysm without blood flow (black arrow).

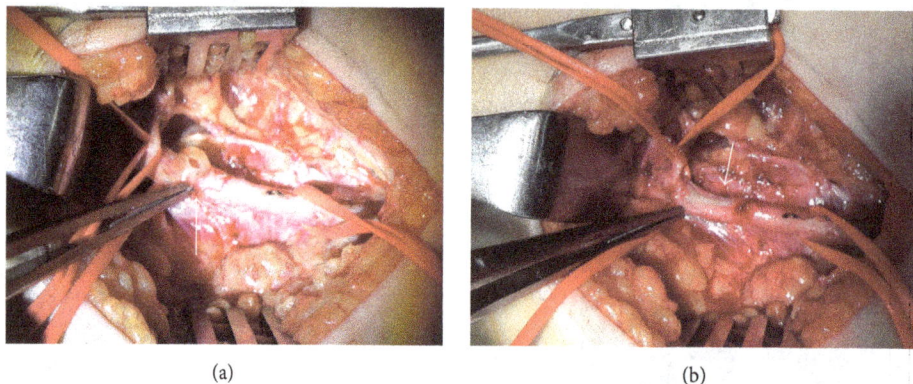

(a)   (b)

FIGURE 5: Clear viscous liquid flowed out after cutting the adventitial layer (arrow). (b) After resection of cystic adventitial lesion (arrow).

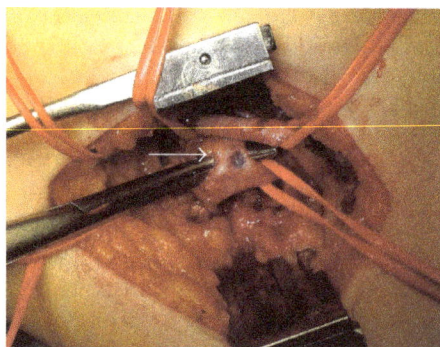

FIGURE 6: The arrow shows the neck of venous aneurysm. Venous aneurysm of popliteal vein was ligated.

CAD is complete resection of the lesion including artery and graft replacement. This method is necessary for multiple cysts with severe arterial stenosis and cyst with direct communication of adjacent joint [4, 9–11]. Nevertheless, the recurrence of cystic disease in the replaced vein graft was reported [12]. Therefore strict follow-up in these patients is indispensable.

Simple resection of the cyst is suitable for simple cystic type without severe arterial stenosis and adhesion between cyst and artery. Because the recurrence is very rare in simple cystic type [8, 13].

Aspiration of cyst is not always possible because the content might be of high viscosity or the cyst is multilocular. A high recurrence rate is reported because the mucin-secretin mesenchymal cells are still present and the fluid may fill again [14].

Endovascular treatment with PTA of the popliteal artery is ineffective with unsatisfactory results. Not only is the recurrence high, but also there is a possibility of developing arterial thrombosis caused by intimal injury [4]. Therefore the endovascular treatment for cystic disease is not recommended.

In our case, cystic disease was simple and the stenosis was not severe. So we chose simple resection of the cyst and preservation of the artery. It is better than graft replacement because it will prevent the graft failure in the future.

Venous aneurysms are also considered to be a rare disease. The most common complication in venous aneurysm is deep vein thrombosis, thrombophlebitis, and recurrent

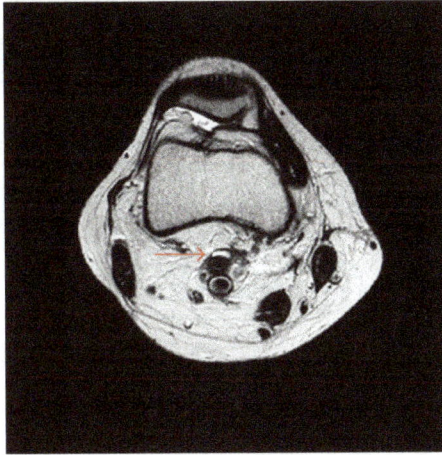

FIGURE 7: Postoperative MRI revealed 5 square mm of high intensity adventitial area (arrow) that was suspected as remaining cystic lesion.

pulmonary embolism [15]. Most venous aneurysms are likely to have a congenital origin [16]; however they may also be a result of degenerative changes or local inflammatory processes such as trauma and infection [17]. Surgical treatment is mandatory of popliteal vein aneurysm for the patient with thromboembolic complication [18]. The indication of surgical treatment in patients with asymptomatic venous aneurysm is controversial. However saccular aneurysm should be treated due to the high potential of future thromboembolic event [19].

About the presence of venous aneurysm nearby cystic disease in this case, there is no past case report of such a combination as far as we searched. We could not describe any comment about relation between adventitial cystic disease and venous aneurysm, but we cannot exclude that there is no relation between adventitial cystic disease and venous aneurysm.

4. Conclusion

Cystic adventitial disease should be suspected in middle-aged female patients who present with sudden-onset intermittent claudication of lower limb without the presence of atherosclerotic disease. Ultrasound, MRI, and CT revealed CAD of popliteal artery with simple cystic lesion and are valuable in diagnosing and deciding the strategy of operation. Simple resection of cyst was successful and the patient has no symptoms after two-year follow-up.

References

[1] H. J. Atkins and J. A. Key, "A case of myxomatous tumor arising in the adventitia of the left external artery; case report," *Br J Surg*, vol. 34, pp. 167–175, 1947.

[2] B. Ejrup and T. Hietonn, "Intermittent claudication; three cases treated by free vein graft," *Acta Chir Scand*, vol. 108, pp. 217–230, 1954.

[3] K. Ishikawa, Y. Mishima, and S. Kobayashi, "Cystic adventitial disease of the popliteal artery: Report of a case," *Angiology*, vol. 12, no. 8, pp. 357–366, 1960.

[4] N. Tsilimparis, U. Hanack, S. Yousefi, P. Alevizakos, and R. I. Rückert, "Cystic adventitial disease of the popliteal artery: an argument for the developmental theory," *Journal of Vascular Surgery*, vol. 45, no. 6, pp. 1249–1252, 2007.

[5] N. M. Desy and R. J. Spinner, "The etiology and management of cystic adventitial disease," *Journal of Vascular Surgery*, vol. 60, no. 1, pp. 235–245, 2014.

[6] R. L. Motaganahali, M. R. Smeds, M. P. Harlander-Locke et al., "A multi-institutional experience in adventitial cystic disease," *J Vasc Surg*, vol. 65, pp. 157–161, 2017.

[7] M. Taurino, L. Rizzo, N. Stella et al., "Doppler ultrasonography and exercise testing in diagnosing a popliteal artery adventitial cyst," *Cardiovasc Ultrasound*, vol. 27, p. 23, 2009.

[8] M. Franca, J. Pinto, R. Machado, and G. C. Fernandez, "Case 157: Bilateral adventitial cystic disease of the popliteal artery," *Radiology*, vol. 255, no. 2, pp. 655–660, 2010.

[9] M. P. Buijsrogge, S. van der Meij, J. H. Korte, and W. M. Fritschy, "'Intermittent claudication intermittente' as a manifestation of adventitial cystic disease communicating with the knee joint," *Annals of Vascular Surgery*, vol. 20, no. 5, pp. 687–689, 2006.

[10] N. Unno, H. Kaneko, T. Uchiyama, N. Yamamoto, and S. Nakamura, "Cystic adventitial disease of the popliteal artery: elongation into the media of the popliteal artery and communication with the knee joint capsule: report of a case," *Surgery Today*, vol. 30, no. 11, pp. 1026–1029, 2000.

[11] K. Igari, T. Kudo, T. Toyofuku, and Y. Inoue, "Surgical treatment of cystic adventitial disease of the popliteal artery: five case reports," *Case Reports in Vascular Medicine*, vol. 2015, Article ID 984681, pp. 1–6, 2015.

[12] T. Ohta, R. Kato, I. Sugimoto, M. Kondo, and H. Tsuchioka, "Recurrence of cystic adventitial disease in an interposed vein graft," *Surgery*, vol. 116, no. 3, pp. 587–592, 1994.

[13] K. Maeda, M. Koh, T. Kawasaki, H. Matue, and Y. Sawa, "A case report of cystic adventitial disease," *Jpn J Vasc Surg*, vol. 16, pp. 571–574, 2007.

[14] K. Sieunarie, M. Lawrence-Brown, and P. Kelsey, "Adventitial cystic disease of the popliteal artery: early recurrence after CT guided perctaneous aspiration," *Cardiovasc Surg*, vol. 32, pp. 702–704, 1991.

[15] H. Ekim, T. Gelen, and G. Karpuzoglu, "Multiple Aneurysms of the Cephalic Vein: A Case Report," *Angiology*, vol. 46, no. 3, pp. 265–267, 1995.

[16] K. Dawson and G. Hamilton, "Primary popliteal venous aneurysm with recurrent pulmonary emboli," *Journal of Vascular Surgery*, vol. 14, no. 3, p. 437, 1991.

[17] S. G. Friedman, K. V. Krishnasastry, W. Doscher, and S. L. Deckoff, "Primary venous aneurysms," *Surgery*, vol. 108, no. 1, pp. 92–95, 1990.

[18] G. D. Grice, R. B. Smith, P. H. Robinson, and J. M. Rheudasil, "Primary popliteal venous aneurysm with recurrent pulmonary emboli," *Journal of Vascular Surgery*, vol. 12, no. 3, pp. 316–318, 1990.

[19] C. Sessa, P. Nicolini, M. Perrin, I. Farah, J.-L. Magne, and H. Guidicelli, "Management of symptomatic and asymptomatic popliteal venous aneurysms: a retrospectve analysis of 25 patients and review of literature," *Journal of Vascular Surgery*, vol. 32, no. 5, pp. 902–912, 2002.

A Case of Successful Coil Embolization for a Late-Onset Type Ia Endoleak after Endovascular Aneurysm Repair with the Chimney Technique

Kimihiro Igari, Toshifumi Kudo, Takahiro Toyofuku, and Yoshinori Inoue

Division of Vascular and Endovascular Surgery, Department of Surgery, Tokyo Medical and Dental University, Tokyo, Japan

Correspondence should be addressed to Kimihiro Igari; igari.srg1@tmd.ac.jp

Academic Editor: Muzaffer Sindel

Juxtarenal aortic aneurysms (JRAAs) are challenging to treat by endovascular aneurysm repair (EVAR) procedures. The chimney technique with EVAR (Ch-EVAR) is one of the feasible and less invasive treatments for JRAAs. However, the main concern of Ch-EVAR is the potential risk of "gutters," which can lead to type Ia endoleak (EL). Most type Ia ELs after Ch-EVAR procedures occurred intraoperatively, and these ELs could be treated using an endovascular technique. However, late-onset type Ia ELs could be extremely rare, which might have a fear of conservative treatment. Type Ia ELs are associated with an increased risk of aneurysm rupture; therefore reintervention is recommended as soon as possible, and we should be aware of the occurrence of type Ia ELs after the Ch-EVAR procedure.

1. Introduction

Endovascular aneurysm repair (EVAR) is a widely accepted procedure in the treatment of infrarenal abdominal aortic aneurysms. However, the conventional EVAR technique is not suitable for treating juxtarenal aortic aneurysms (JRAAs) because it requires a minimum of 10–15 mm of healthy aorta in order to achieve an adequate sealing zone at the proximal neck. To make sure of enough proximal landing zone, some techniques for EVAR procedures have been developed.

Fenestrated and branched endografts (FBEs) have shown promising results with regard to the preservation of visceral perfusion [1]. However, the use of such customized devices mandates strict anatomical requirements, a manufacturing delay, and significant costs, and these devices are not commercially available in Japan. On the other hand, the chimney technique with EVAR (Ch-EVAR) can facilitate the performance of EVAR in the treatment of JRAAs. Ch-EVAR was originally reported by Greenberg et al. [2] as an adjunctive procedure involving visceral artery stenting during intentional endograft coverage of the vessel origin; it can establish an additional proximal fixation zone in patients with JRAAs. Most importantly, the components used in

Ch-EVAR are commercially available, even in Japan. Some articles have therefore reported the operational efficiency of Ch-EVAR [3].

The main problem of Ch-EVAR is the risk of proximal type Ia endoleak (EL) due to so-called gutters. Gutters are channels that may appear between the main aortic endograft and the chimney graft. Gutter leakage after Ch-EVAR is relatively common; however, most ELs are resolved intraoperatively, and late-onset ELs, including type Ia ELs, have been treated conservatively [4]. We herein report the use of coil embolization in the treatment of a late-onset type Ia EL after Ch-EVAR for JRAA, which helped avoid an aneurysmal rupture.

2. Case Presentation

A 77-year-old male with a history of cerebrovascular disease and chronic pulmonary obstructive disease (COPD) was referred to our institution to undergo treatment for a JRAA. A contrast-enhanced computed tomography (CT) scan revealed a JRAA of 59 mm in diameter with a short proximal neck (3 mm to the left renal artery) and a normal neck diameter (24.4 mm) (Figure 1(a)). Ch-EVAR was performed

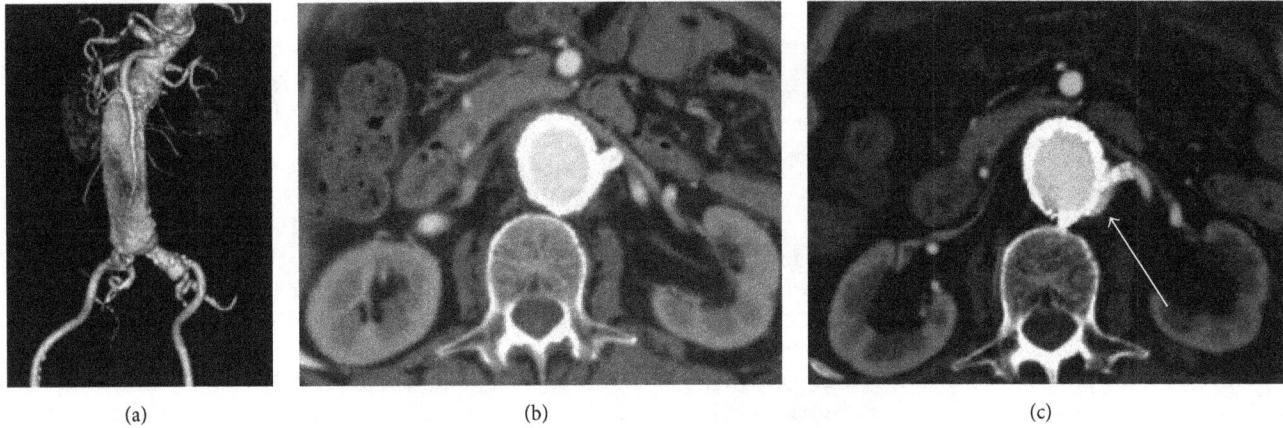

FIGURE 1: (a) Preoperative 3-dimensional computed tomography with the left anterior oblique view showed a juxtarenal aneurysm measuring 59 mm in diameter with a short proximal neck. (b) Early postoperative computed tomography showed a patent endograft and bare stent to the left renal artery without any endoleaks. (c) Two years after endovascular aneurysm repair, computed tomography showed the enlargement of the aneurysmal sac with a type Ia endoleak (white arrow).

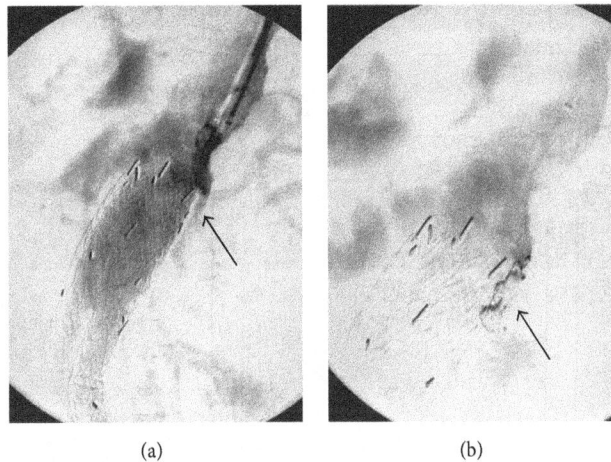

FIGURE 2: (a) Intraoperative angiography showed the origin of the type Ia endoleak (black arrow). (b) Intraoperative angiography after coil embolization showed the disappearance of the origin of type Ia endoleak (black arrow).

because the patient did not appear to be a good candidate for open aneurysmal repair due to his severe COPD. Main bifurcated endografts (Excluder™, W.L. Gore and Associates, Flagstaff, AZ, USA) with a 31 mm sized proximal diameter were positioned just below the ostium of the right renal artery, and a 6 mm bare metal stent (Express SD™, Boston Scientific, Cork, Ireland) was inserted and deployed in the left renal artery. Complete angiography showed a patent left renal artery and a patent endograft without ELs, including type Ia EL or any enhancement of the JRAA. A contrast-enhanced CT scan revealed good results in the early postoperative period (Figure 1(b)).

At the 1-year follow-up, a contrast-enhanced CT scan showed the shrinkage of the aneurysm (45 mm in diameter) with a patent left renal artery stent; however, the 2-year follow-up CT scan showed that the aneurysm diameter had grown (57 mm) and that a type Ia EL (Figure 1(c)) had

occurred due to so-called gutters. He had no pulsation on his abdomen, and CT showed no change of aneurysmal neck (dilatation or shortening). A secondary procedure was therefore performed to treat the type Ia EL, which had caused the extension of the aneurysm. Under local anesthesia, a 4.5 Fr guiding sheath was inserted through the left brachial artery to cannulate the origin of the type Ia EL. Angiography showed a cavity, which caused and the route to the type Ia EL (Figure 2(a)). We thought that it would be impossible to reduce the type Ia EL using the "kissing balloon" technique; thus we attempted to perform coil embolization in the cavity. After gaining brachial access, a microcatheter was positioned into the cavity using a 0.014-inch guidewire. Thereafter, the cavity was embolized with two coils (Ruby™ Coil, Penumbra, Inc., Alameda, CA, USA). After coil embolization, the cavity was diminished. This contributed to the complete exclusion of the type Ia EL (Figure 2(b)). Three months after coil embolization, duplex ultrasonography showed no ELs, including the type Ia EL, and a patent left renal artery without aneurysmal enlargement.

3. Discussion

The current evidence concerning Ch-EVAR procedures shows that their clinical results are promising and that the incidence of perioperative morbidity and mortality, early mortality, and the occurrence of type Ia ELs does not differ to a statistically significant extent from that for FBE [5]. The chimney graft for Ch-EVAR could work well to confirm the endograft in the aortic wall. However, Ch-EVAR technique has a potential risk for the occurrence of type Ia ELs between the main endograft and chimney graft, so-called gutter leakage [6]. Furthermore, the occurrence of type Ia ELs is not always predictable. Coscas et al. [1] reported that 4 of 12 patients (30%) developed type Ia ELs during intraoperative Ch-EVAR procedures. Three of the 4 patients were treated using the kissing balloon technique; the other patient was treated using coil embolization; all type Ia ELs subsequently disappeared. During the follow-up period, 1 patient developed a new type Ia EL, which was carefully monitored. Most type Ia ELs that occurred intraoperatively were therefore treated simultaneously, while most late-onset type Ia ELs were not treated. Most type Ia ELs were observed to occur in the perioperative and early postoperative periods and often appeared to be sealed spontaneously. Even though the conservative management of type Ia ELs might be effective in some cases, we advocated that type Ia ELs should be treated as soon as possible, because they may result in aneurysmal rupture. In our case, the prompt treatment of the patient's type Ia EL led to a good outcome.

Several factors may contribute to the occurrence of type Ia ELs. Balloon-expandable or self-expandable stents with uncovered or covered stents might induce different reactions to lead to gutter leakage. A recent comparison between self-expandable and balloon-expandable stents as chimney stents demonstrated an increased tendency for type Ia ELs when self-expandable stents were used [7]. We therefore used balloon-expandable stents as chimney stents. Many authors have advocated that covered stents are beneficial because they reduce the pressurization of the gutters, lowering the risk of type Ia ELs [8]. However, other authors have suggested that bare stents are not inferior to covered stents with regard to renal patency and protection against type Ia ELs [9]. We have reported good results in the exclusion of AAAs with challenging neck anatomy by EVAR procedures [10] and JRAAs using bare chimney stents [11]. Furthermore, we can only use bare stents for Ch-EVAR because covered stents are not covered by Japanese National Health Insurance. Another factor associated with the occurrence of type Ia ELs is the new neck length. Donas et al. reported that patients with late-onset type Ia EL had a neck length <10 mm [12]. Most reports recommended that a new neck length of >20 mm was necessary in order to avoid type Ia ELs [6, 12]. Thus, we planned a new neck length of >10 mm with a bare stent, which led to the acceptable outcomes of our previous report [11].

The existing data have not provided firm conclusions as to whether these devices and techniques are associated with an increased risk of late-onset type Ia EL. However, type Ia ELs are associated with an increased risk of postprocedural aneurysm rupture; reintervention is therefore recommended as soon as possible after the diagnosis of a type Ia EL. Type Ia ELs after Ch-EVAR can be treated with concomitant ballooning of the stent grafts and visceral stents by the kissing balloon technique [1]. Even though this technique is feasible, it appears to be difficult and it is complicated to perform during the follow-up period. Thus, the simple coiling of the gutters has been described as a potential treatment for patients with gutter endoleaks [13]. In the present case, coil embolization completely resolved the late-onset type Ia EL. However, we should be aware that coils placed at the proximal site of the neck level present a significant hindrance to the interpretation of follow-up CT scans.

In conclusion, we herein described a case of late-onset type Ia EL after a Ch-EVAR operation, which was successfully treated by coil embolization. It is important to remain aware of the higher incidence of type Ia ELs after Ch-EVAR.

Competing Interests

The authors have no competing interests to declare.

References

[1] R. Coscas, J.-P. Becquemin, M. Majewski et al., "Management of perioperative endoleaks during endovascular treatment of juxta-renal aneurysms," *Annals of Vascular Surgery*, vol. 26, no. 2, pp. 175–184, 2012.

[2] R. K. Greenberg, D. Clair, S. Srivastava et al., "Should patients with challenging anatomy be offered endovascular aneurysm repair?" *Journal of Vascular Surgery*, vol. 38, no. 5, pp. 990–996, 2003.

[3] Y. Li, W. Guo, C. Duan et al., "Endovascular chimney technique for juxtarenal abdominal aortic aneurysm: a systematic review using pooled analysis and meta-analysis," *Annals of Vascular Surgery*, vol. 29, no. 6, pp. 1141–1150, 2015.

[4] M. XiaoHui, G. Wei, H. ZhongZhou, L. XiaoPing, X. Jiang, and J. Xin, "Endovascular repair with chimney technique for juxtarenal aortic aneurysm: a single center experience," *European Journal of Vascular and Endovascular Surgery*, vol. 49, no. 3, pp. 271–276, 2015.

[5] K. P. Donas, G. Torsello, T. Bisdas, N. Osada, E. Schönefeld, and G. A. Pitoulias, "Early outcomes for fenestrated and chimney endografts in the treatment of pararenal aortic pathologies are not significantly different: a systematic review with pooled data analysis," *Journal of Endovascular Therapy*, vol. 19, no. 6, pp. 723–728, 2012.

[6] K. P. Donas, J. T. Lee, M. Lachat et al., "Collected world experience about the performance of the snorkel/chimney endovascular technique in the treatment of complex aortic pathologies: the PERICLES registry," *Annals of Surgery*, vol. 262, no. 3, pp. 546–552, 2015.

[7] K. P. Donas, F. Pecoraro, G. Torsello et al., "Use of covered chimney stents for pararenal aortic pathologies is safe and feasible with excellent patency and low incidence of endoleaks," *Journal of Vascular Surgery*, vol. 55, no. 3, pp. 659–665, 2012.

[8] A. Katsargyris, K. Oikonomou, C. Klonaris, I. Töpel, and E. L. G. Verhoeven, "Comparison of outcomes with open, fenestrated, and chimney graft repair of juxtarenal aneurysms: are we ready for a paradigm shift?" *Journal of Endovascular Therapy*, vol. 20, no. 2, pp. 159–169, 2013.

[9] K. J. Bruen, R. J. Feezor, M. J. Daniels, A. W. Beck, and W. A. Lee, "Endovascular chimney technique versus open repair of juxtarenal and suprarenal aneurysms," *Journal of Vascular Surgery*, vol. 53, no. 4, pp. 895–905, 2011.

[10] K. Igari, T. Kudo, T. Toyofuku, M. Jibiki, and Y. Inoue, "Outcomes following endovascular abdominal aortic aneurysm repair both within and outside of the instructions for use," *Annals of Thoracic and Cardiovascular Surgery*, vol. 20, no. 1, pp. 61–66, 2014.

[11] K. Igari, T. Kudo, H. Uchiyama, T. Toyofuku, and Y. Inoue, "Early experience with the endowedge technique and snorkel technique for endovascular aneurysm repair with challenging neck anatomy," *Annals of Vascular Diseases*, vol. 7, no. 1, pp. 46–51, 2014.

[12] K. P. Donas, G. B. Torsello, G. Piccoli et al., "The PROTAGORAS study to evaluate the performance of the Endurant stent graft for patients with pararenal pathologic processes treated by the chimney/snorkel endovascular technique," *Journal of Vascular Surgery*, vol. 63, no. 1, pp. 1–7, 2016.

[13] K. P. Donas, F. Pecoraro, T. Bisdas et al., "CT angiography at 24 months demonstrates durability of EVAR with the use of chimney grafts for pararenal aortic pathologies," *Journal of Endovascular Therapy*, vol. 20, no. 1, pp. 1–6, 2013.

Successful Endovascular Repair of an Iatrogenic Perforation of the Superficial Femoral Artery Using Self-Expanding Nitinol Supera Stents in a Patient with Acute Thromboembolic Limb Ischemia

Tom Eisele, Benedikt M. Muenz, and Grigorios Korosoglou

Department of Cardiology & Vascular Medicine, GRN Hospital Weinheim, 69469 Weinheim, Germany

Correspondence should be addressed to Grigorios Korosoglou; grigorios.korosoglou@grn.de

Academic Editor: Hiroyuki Nakajima

The treatment of acute thromboembolic limb ischemia includes well-established surgical thrombectomy procedures and, in recent times, also percutaneous rotational thrombectomy using Straub Rotarex® system. This modality not only enables efficient treatment of such thrombotic occlusion but also in rare cases may imply the risk of perforation of the occluded artery. Herein, we report the case of a perforation of the superficial femoral artery (SFA) in an elderly female patient with thromboembolic limb ischemia. The perforation was successfully treated by implantation of self-expanding nitinol Supera stents and without the need for implantation of a stent graft.

1. Introduction

Peripheral artery disease (PAD) exhibits increasing morbidity and mortality during the last few decades [1] and is estimated to affect over 200 million people worldwide, including up to 30% of elderly primary care individuals [2, 3]. Patients with symptomatic PAD exhibit a life expectancy of 80% within 5 years of follow-up [4, 5], whereas patients with critical limb ischemia (CLI) show significant poorer outcomes with amputation and death rates of 15–20% and 25%, respectively, within the first year after diagnosis [6].

Especially patients with acute thromboembolic limb ischemia are in high risk of major amputation and death due to sepsis and multiorgan dysfunction. Such patients are usually older than 75 years and show further comorbidities, including atrial fibrillation and history of heart failure [7]. The treatment of this limb- and life-threatening condition includes well-established surgical thrombectomy procedures and, in recent times, also percutaneous rotational thrombectomy procedures using Straub Rotarex system, if required in combination with local thrombolysis [8]. This method enables quick and efficient treatment of peripheral arterial thromboembolic occlusion. Despite the low complication rate of rotational thrombectomy, perforations of the occluded artery have been reported previously. Herein, we report the case of a perforation of the superficial femoral artery (SFA) in an elderly female patient with thromboembolic limb ischemia, which was successfully treated by implantation of self-expanding nitinol Supera stents.

2. Case Presentation

An 85-year-old female patient was referred to our department with new onset of severe pain, paleness, and pulselessness of her left leg since 12 hours. Duplex-sonography revealed thrombotic occlusion of the left common femoral artery (CFA) (Figure 1) and the patient was immediately scheduled for digital subtraction angiography (DSA). The patient had history of arterial hypertension and heart failure but no history of clinically evident PAD. DSA confirmed the thrombotic occlusion of the CFA (Figure 2(a)), and interventional treatment was initiated after injection of 500 mg

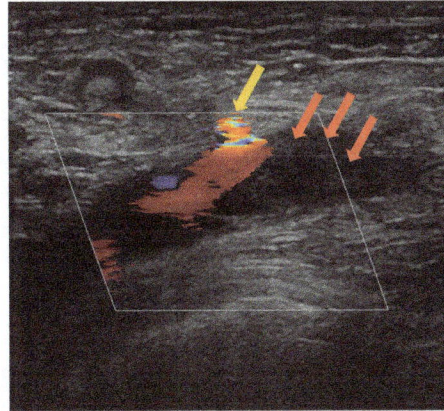

FIGURE 1: Thrombotic occlusion of the left common femoral artery (CFA). Absence of flow can be appreciated in the distal part of the vessel, associated with thrombus formation (red arrows). The origin of a collateral artery can be depicted proximally to the vessel occlusion (yellow arrow).

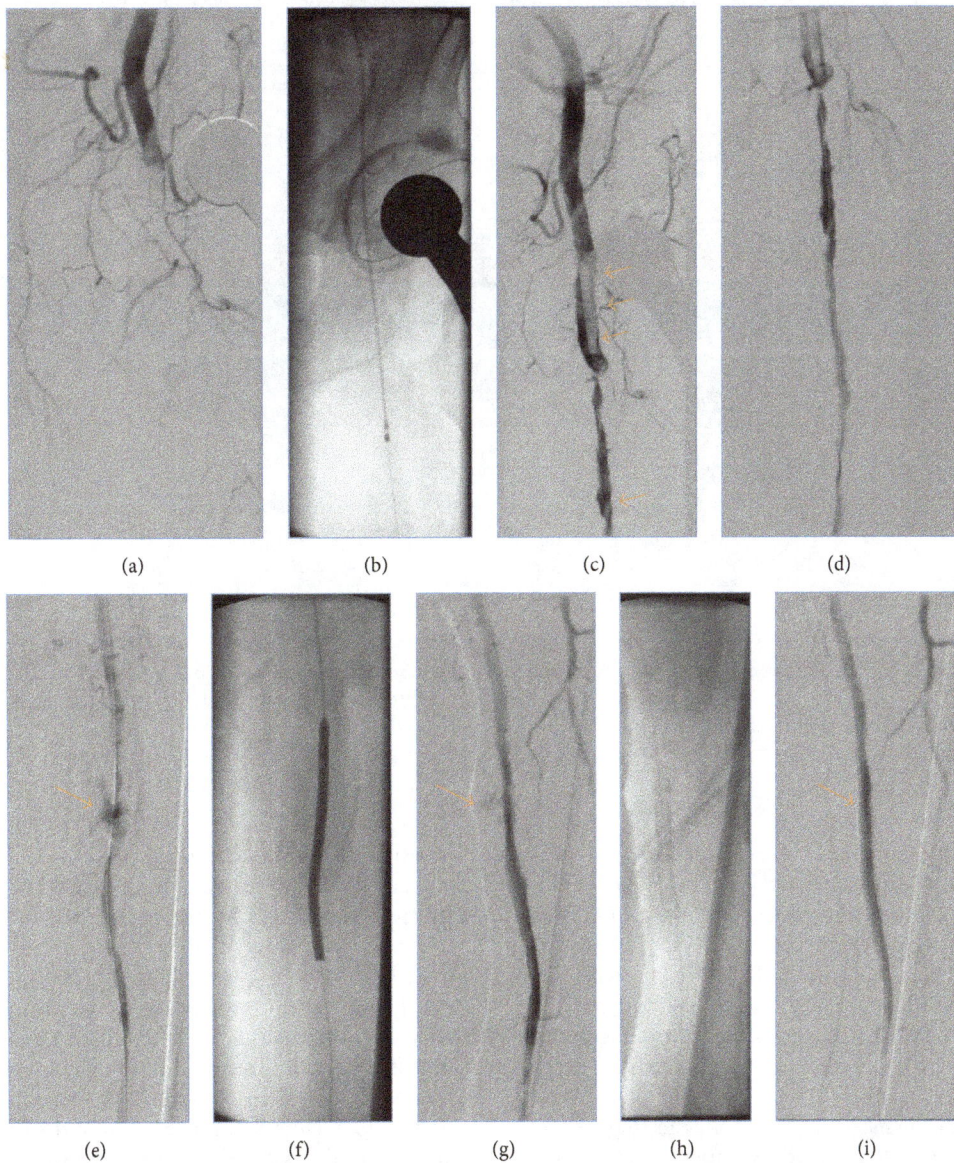

(a)   (b)   (c)   (d)

(e)   (f)   (g)   (h)   (i)

FIGURE 2: Occlusion of the CFA is noticed by DSA (a). Rotarex catheter thrombectomy reestablishes antegrade flow in the CFA and SFA (b), but thrombotic burden remains high as it can be appreciated by the orange arrows in (c). Mid and distal parts of the SFA with thrombus formations can also be appreciated in (d). After repeated Rotarex thrombectomy a perforation of the SFA is noticed, with persistent despite prolonged balloon inflation (orange arrows in (e)–(g)). Subsequently, 2 overlapping nitinol Supera stents are implanted (h), resulting in complete cessation of the bleeding complication (orange arrow in (i)).

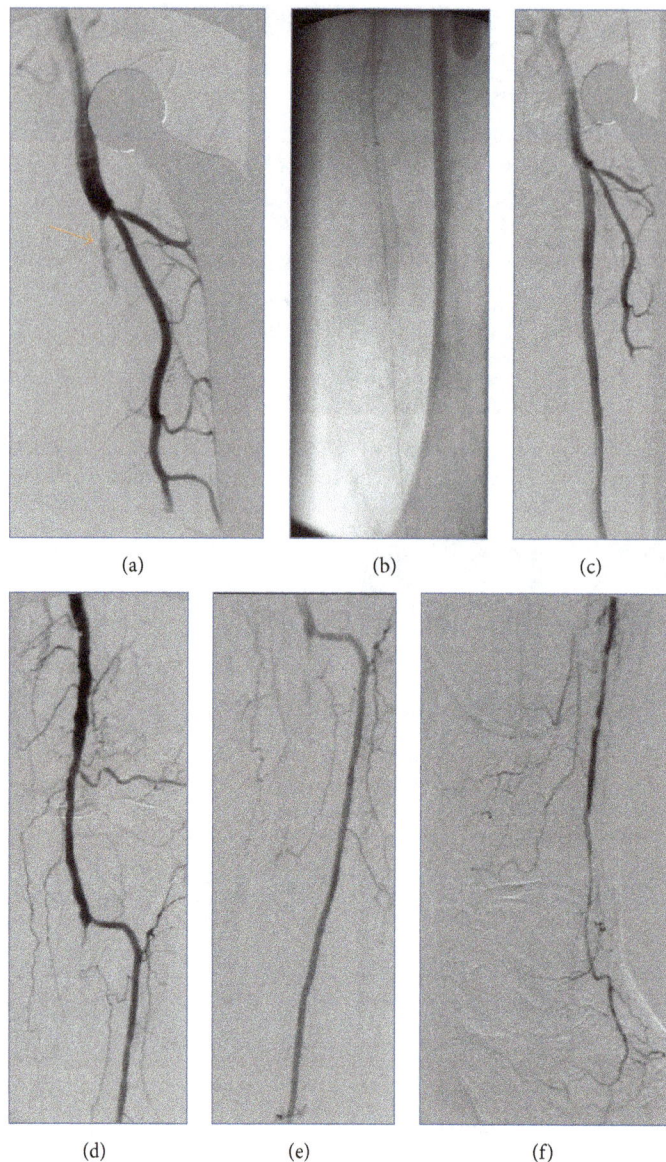

(a)   (b)   (c)

(d)   (e)   (f)

FIGURE 3: During the second angiographic session, DSA reveals not only complete resolution of the thrombus in the CFA (a) but also reocclusion of the SFA (orange arrow in (a)), requiring repeated Rotarex thrombectomy and implantation of further self-expanding nitinol stents (b). Subsequently, good angiographic flow can be achieved in the SFA and in the popliteal artery with a 1-vessel run-off of the anterior tibial artery ((c)–(f)).

aspirin and 5,000 I.U. of heparin. After insertion of an $0.018''$ guide wire, Rotarex catheter (ab medica GmbH, Düsseldorf, Germany) thrombectomy was performed in the CFA and in the proximal superficial femoral artery (SFA) (Figure 2(b)), resulting in antegrade flow in both SFA, but with high remaining thrombotic burden in the CFA (Figures 2(c) and 2(d)). After repeated Rotarex catheter thrombectomy a perforation of the SFA was noticed, which persisted despite prolonged inflation using a $5.0 * 120$ mm balloon (Figures 2(e)–2(g)). Due to persistent perforation, the implantation of 2 overlapping $5.0 * 40$ mm nitinol Supera stents (Abbott Vascular, Illinois, USA) was performed, which resulted in complete repair of the vascular injury of the SFA (Figures 2(h) and 2(i)). Local lysis was subsequently performed due to high

remaining thrombotic burden of the CFA, using 10 mg bolus injection of Actilyse® (recombinant tissue plasminogen activator, Boehringer Ingelheim Pharma GmbH, Ingelheim am Rhein, Germany) and continuous infusion of 1 mg/h for further 16 hours. Repeated DSA was scheduled for the next day. In the mean time, pain symptoms of the patient improved, whereas she recovered from paleness of the lower limb except for the area of her distal foot. The next day, DSA revealed complete resolution of the thrombus in the CFA (Figure 3(a)). However, reocclusion of the SFA was unfortunately noticed (Figure 3(a), orange arrow), requiring repeated Rotarex catheter thrombectomy and implantation of 2 further self-expanding nitinol Innova™ stents ($7.0 * 80$ mm and $6.0 * 120$ mm, Boston Scientific, Ratingen, Germany) in the SFA

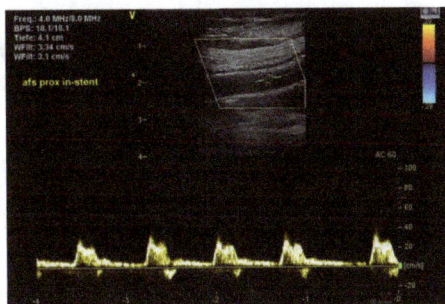

FIGURE 4: Triphasic flow in the SFA at 4 weeks of follow-up.

(Figure 3(b)). Subsequently, good angiographic flow was shown in the SFA and in the popliteal artery with a 1-vessel run-off of the anterior tibial artery (Figures 3(c)–3(f)). After the second angiographic procedure pain symptoms and limb paleness and paresthesia were completely resolved. In addition, holter monitoring revealed the presence of atrial fibrillation and the patient was put on treatment with aspirin (100 mg daily), clopidogrel (75 mg daily), and 5 mg subcutaneous FXa-inhibitor fondaparinux for 4 weeks. Ambulatory Duplex-sonography at 4 weeks of follow-up demonstrated a good triphasic flow pattern in the SFA (Figure 4) and the patient was put on treatment with coumadin.

3. Discussion

To the best of our knowledge this is the first case reporting the placement of self-expanding nitinol Supera stent for the management of a perforation in a peripheral artery.

In the past decades, significant technical developments have occurred with endovascular therapy of acute thromboembolism, which offer several advantages over open surgical embolectomy techniques for the treatment of peripheral arterial thromboembolic occlusion [8]. Although the Straub Rotarex system is widely available and well established for the treatment of such thrombotic lesions, perforations of the occluded artery have been described previously and in our case. In such cases, usually stent grafts are employed. However, such stent grafts are expensive and are usually deliverable using ≥8F sheaths. This may require an additional arterial puncture under full anticoagulation or lead to additional time spent for changing the arterial sheath, which may aggravate bleeding complications. In our case, the SFA perforation could be successfully treated using self-expanding nitinol Supera stents, which are deliverable using a 6F sheath.

4. Conclusion

Herein we report the placement of a self-expanding nitinol Supera stent for the management of a perforation in a peripheral superficial femoral artery. Further novel options of complication management as described in our case may shift the treatment from surgical to even more endovascular treatment procedures in the future.

Competing Interests

The authors declare that they have no competing interests.

References

[1] A. Gallino, V. Aboyans, C. Diehm et al., "Non-coronary atherosclerosis," *European Heart Journal*, vol. 35, no. 17, pp. 1112–1119, 2014.

[2] F. G. R. Fowkes, D. Rudan, I. Rudan et al., "Comparison of global estimates of prevalence and risk factors for peripheral artery disease in 2000 and 2010: a systematic review and analysis," *The Lancet*, vol. 382, no. 9901, pp. 1329–1340, 2013.

[3] A. T. Hirsch, M. H. Criqui, D. Treat-Jacobson et al., "Peripheral arterial disease detection, awareness, and treatment in primary care," *The Journal of the American Medical Association*, vol. 286, no. 11, pp. 1317–1324, 2001.

[4] L. Norgren, W. R. Hiatt, J. A. Dormandy, M. R. Nehler, K. A. Harris, and F. G. R. Fowkes, "Inter-society consensus for the management of peripheral arterial disease (TASC II)," *Journal of Vascular Surgery*, vol. 45, supplement, no. 1, pp. S5–S67, 2007.

[5] P. M. Rothwell, A. J. Coull, L. E. Silver et al., "Population-based study of event-rate, incidence, case fatality, and mortality for all acute vascular events in all arterial territories (Oxford Vascular Study)," *The Lancet*, vol. 366, no. 9499, pp. 1773–1783, 2005.

[6] M. Brooks and M. P. Jenkins, "Acute and chronic ischaemia of the limb," *Surgery*, vol. 26, no. 1, pp. 17–20, 2008.

[7] M. Wasilewska and I. Gosk-Bierska, "Thromboembolism associated with atrial fibrillation as a cause of limb and organ ischemia," *Advances in Clinical and Experimental Medicine*, vol. 22, no. 6, pp. 865–873, 2013.

[8] M. Lichtenberg, F.-W. Stahlhoff, and D. Boese, "Endovascular treatment of acute limb ischemia and proximal deep vein thrombosis using rotational thrombectomy: a review of published literature," *Cardiovascular Revascularization Medicine*, vol. 14, no. 6, pp. 343–348, 2013.

43

High Output Cardiac Failure Resolving after Repair of AV Fistula in a Six-Month-Old

Uygar Teomete,[1] Rubee Anne Gugol,[2] Holly Neville,[3] Ozgur Dandin,[4] and Ming-Lon Young[2]

[1]University of Miami Miller School of Medicine, Department of Radiology, Miami, FL 33136, USA
[2]University of Miami Miller School of Medicine, Department of Pediatrics, Miami, FL 33136, USA
[3]Division of Pediatric Surgery, DeWitt Daughtry Family Department of Surgery, University of Miami Miller School of Medicine, Miami, FL 33136, USA
[4]University of Miami Miller School of Medicine, Department of Surgery, Ryder Trauma Center, Miami, FL 33136, USA

Correspondence should be addressed to Ozgur Dandin; dandinozgur@gmail.com

Academic Editor: Moses Elisaf

Background. Acquired AVF in pediatrics are commonly caused by iatrogenic means, including arterial or venous punctures. These fistulae can cause great hemodynamic stress on the heart as soon as they are created. *Case.* A six-month-old 25-week gestation infant was referred for respiratory distress. Initial exam revealed tachypnea, tachycardia, and hypertension. There was a bruit noted on her left arm. An ultrasound showed an arteriovenous fistula. Its location, however, precluded intervention because of the high risk for limb-loss. An echocardiogram showed evidence of pulmonary hypertension that was treated with sildenafil and furosemide. However, no improvement was seen. On temporary manual occlusion of the fistula, the patient was noted to have increased her blood pressure and decreased her heart rate, suggesting significant hemodynamic effect of the fistula. The fistula was subsequently ligated and the patient clinically and echocardiographically improved. *Conclusion.* A patient in high output cardiac failure or pulmonary artery hypertension, especially premature patients with preexisting lung disease, should be probed for history of multiple punctures, trauma, or surgery and should have prompt evaluation for AVF. If it can be diagnosed and repaired, most of the cases have been shown to decrease the stress on the heart and reverse the pathologic hemodynamics.

1. Introduction

Arteriovenous fistulae (AVF) are anomalous communications between an artery and a vein. These malformations are known to increase cardiac output and have hemodynamic consequences [1]. They can be congenital or acquired. In the pediatric population, the most common cause of an acquired AVF is single or repeated diagnostic or therapeutic arterial or venous punctures. Particularly vulnerable patients include those with multiple medical problems, because of the need for chronic vascular access.

2. Case Presentation

A six-month-old female infant was referred to cardiology due to progressively increasing oxygen requirements and cardiomegaly on chest X-ray. She was born at 25 weeks of gestation and had multiple medical problems in the early neonatal period including retinopathy of prematurity, hyaline membrane disease, gastroesophageal reflux, severe liver dysfunction, and suspected necrotizing enterocolitis. She had a history of ligation of her patent arterial duct on the 16th day of life. On physical exam her respiratory rate was 65, her heart rate was 153, and blood pressure was 130/80 mmHg. Her oxygen saturation was in the low 90s on 30% FiO_2 (fraction of inspired oxygen). Her lung sounds were coarse. Her heart had regular rate and rhythm, with no murmurs. Her abdomen showed a liver edge that was palpable three centimeters below the right subcostal margin. She had a palpable bruit at the left antecubital fossa. Pulses were normal and equal on all extremities, and there were no obvious discrepancies in limb lengths. An echocardiogram showed severe pulmonary

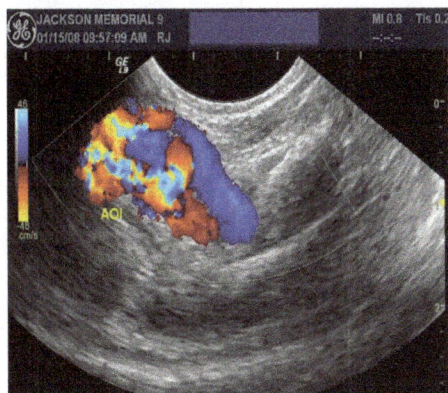

FIGURE 1: The distal left brachial artery to brachial vein fistula.

artery hypertension with mild right ventricular and atrial dilatation, with a patent foramen ovale shunting right to left. Biventricular systolic function was normal, with no evidence of left ventricular hypertrophy or dilatation. A duplex ultrasound of the left upper extremity showed presence of an AVF between the left brachial artery and vein as evidenced by increased flow obtained from the left brachial artery with dilated, tortuous brachial veins demonstrating arterialized flow along the length of the veins. Velocity measurements of up to 692 cm/second were obtained at the level of the AVF (Figures 1 and 2).

The calculated blood flow in the fistula was estimated to be about 450–500 mL/min, which is equivalent to up to twice the estimated total cardiac output for this patient. The fistula was not ligated because its location was high risk for limb-loss. She was managed with diuresis and blood pressure control. One month later, she was reevaluated for recurrent and progressive episodes of desaturations and respiratory distress. On physical exam her vital signs showed a respiratory rate of 60 per minute, and oxygen saturations were between 90–95% on oxygen supplementation by nasal cannula. Her blood pressure was 52/32 mmHg, and the heart rate was 134–148 beats per minute. Cardiac exam demonstrated normal S1 and S2, no murmurs, and an intermittent gallop. Electrocardiogram showed normal sinus rhythm with right atrial enlargement and right axis deviation and T-wave inversion in the lateral leads, suggesting right ventricular strain. The echocardiogram suggested elevated pulmonary artery systolic pressures, which were 2/3 of the systemic pressure. The right ventricle showed mildly depressed systolic function.

The patient was started on sildenafil for management of the pulmonary hypertension, but this did not alter the measured pulmonary pressures upon echocardiographic reevaluation one week later. On careful assessment of the left antecubital fossa, with temporary manual occlusion of the affected area, there was a decrease in the heart rate from 128 bpm to 102 bpm, and an increase in the blood pressure from 76/55 to 92/57 mmHg (positive Nicoladoni-Branham sign [2, 3]). An echocardiogram that was done simultaneously showed a decrease in the flow through the right ventricle. The fistula was subsequently surgically ligated without complications.

Repeat physical exam showed normalization of the patient's blood pressure and heart rate readings. She was quickly weaned to room air. A repeat echocardiogram done thirteen days after the repair showed no evidence of pulmonary artery hypertension.

3. Discussion

Arteriovenous fistulae are among the rare but well-documented causes of congestive heart failure [4–7]. In pediatrics, AVF can be congenital or acquired, the latter, not uncommonly secondary to iatrogenic causes including single or multiple arterial and/or venous punctures. The hemodynamic effects of AVF have been evaluated in many studies on patients in whom AVF are surgically created for hemodialysis [8, 9]. Cardiac output is said to increase greatly and immediately on opening of an AVF. This is secondary to an increase in the sympathetic tone, leading to increased stroke volume and heart rate. In only three days there are altered echocardiographic parameters evident after creation of an AVF. There have been notable increases in left atrial diameter, left ventricular diastolic dimension, shortening fraction, and cardiac output. There also are changes that suggest increased cardiac volume loading and decreased left ventricular compliance (decreased diastolic function).

There can be up to a 6-fold increase in blood flow in a single fistula [10]. "Fistular cardiopathy" is described in a study by Dallo et al. in 1984, when they studied 33 cases of acquired systemic arteriovenous fistulae from 1945 to 1981 and they observed that a syndrome of hyperkinetic hemodynamics resulting in heart failure developed from four days to 31 years after the initial insult and was related to the magnitude of the arteriovenous shunt [11]. The study by Iwashima in 2002 [8] showed that there is alteration in left ventricular diastolic filling pattern, which is suggestive of diastolic dysfunction. There is pseudonormalization of the systolic function as the left ventricular diastolic dimension increases with increased cardiac output. The left atrial systolic dimensions increased significantly within two weeks after creation of the fistula; left ventricular end diastolic dimensions increased significantly within one week. The left ventricular systolic dimension was not noted to change.

The above echocardiographic findings become more prominent as the heart is exposed to continued volume overload. Pulmonary artery hypertension, a less recognized consequence of AVF, has been described in many case reports. Peripheral arteriovenous shunting has been compared to the development of pulmonary hypertension due to congenital heart left-to-right intracardiac shunts [4]. Compensatory mechanisms from sustained volume overload and high cardiac output, over time, can lead to irreversible cardiac hypertrophy and ventricular dilatation. Pulmonary artery remodeling, consisting of endothelial proliferation, vascular smooth muscle hypertrophy, plexiform lesions, and other histopathologic changes, is seen in patients with left-to-right shunts (i.e., atrial septal defects, ventricular septal defects, or patent arterial ducts) which are all secondary to exposure of the pulmonary vascular bed to high volume [4, 6].

Vessel	Velocities within the vessel (cm/sec)				
	Proximal part of vessel ⟵⟶ Area of greatest turbulence ⟵⟶ Distal part of vessel				
L axillary V	96.5				
L brachial A	131.4	176.2	692.1	58.4	112.9
L brachial V	94.2	141.9		127.6	
L ulnar A					80.7
L ulnar V					46.5
L radial A					33.0
L radial V					10.0

FIGURE 2: A representation of findings from the Doppler ultrasound of the left arm (L: left, V: vein, and A: artery).

Pulmonary artery hypertension in our patient was complicated albeit masked by the presence of hyaline membrane disease from her prematurity, and the alterations in the right ventricular dimensions and function may already have begun earlier. The rapid progression of systolic dysfunction, however, shows the impact of the excessive venous return to the heart.

A small fraction of AVF spontaneously regress (<3%) [12]. Most of these lesions, however, need to be repaired. There have been cases wherein prolonged exposure to such a high output state predisposes the patient to even worse pulmonary artery hypertension after repair [13]. This underscores the need for urgent intervention in this lesion. In our patient the immediate effect of manually occluding the AVF showed a significant drop in the heart rate and an increase in the blood pressure, classically described as the Nicoladoni-Branham sign [2, 3].

The diagnosis AVF can be clinically made based on a simple palpable thrill and a machinery murmur over the affected area [14]. Other findings may consist of high cardiac output state, such as the Nicoladoni-Branham sign, peripheral edema distal to the fistula, limb length discrepancy, ulcers, or gangrene, related to insufficiency [15]. Diagnosis can be confirmed with color Doppler ultrasonography, digital subtraction angiography, or magnetic resonance angiography. The gold standard is to demonstrate on contrast angiography direct imaging of the abnormal arteriovenous communication and definition of the adjacent vessels [5, 16]. However systemic and neurologic complications related to contrast angiography occur in patients. Also hemodynamic and cardiac electrophysiologic changes are seen during iv contrast agent injection. MRI has the advantage of avoiding X-ray radiation exposure especially in pediatric patients. But patients with any metallic materials within the body and who have any history of claustrophobia are not suitable for this procedure. Color Doppler ultrasonography has high accuracy rates and can be performed fast and at bedside but usually it has operator dependent results. Additional to these diagnostic procedures, contrast enhanced ultrasound (CEUS) can be another option. AVF has risk of life threatening complications including spontaneous bleeding [17]. Compared to standard US, CEUS may be useful and has high sensitivity for detecting potential bleeding and active bleeding with low complication rates [18, 19]. When heart failure is present, electrocardiograms may show ST-T-wave changes from right and/or left ventricular strain, ventricular hypertrophy, and/or atrial hypertrophy [20]. Echocardiograms may show a hyperdynamic myocardium, volume overload, pulmonary hypertension, atrial and/or ventricular dilatation, and signs of possible diastolic or systolic dysfunction [8, 9].

In conclusion, acquired AVF in pediatrics are commonly caused by iatrogenic means, including arterial or venous punctures. These fistulae can cause great hemodynamic stress on the heart as soon as they are created. A patient in high output cardiac failure or pulmonary artery hypertension, especially in patient who is premature with preexisting lung disease, should be probed for history of multiple punctures, trauma, or surgery and should have prompt evaluation for AVF. If discovered, it should be addressed in a timely manner. If repaired, most of these cases have been shown to decrease the stress on the heart and reverse the pathologic hemodynamics.

Ethical Approval

All procedures performed in this study involving human participants were in accordance with the ethical standards of the institutional research committee and with the 1964 Helsinki Declaration and its later amendments or comparable ethical standards.

References

[1] E. Aitken, D. Kerr, C. Geddes, C. Berry, and D. Kingsmore, "Cardiovascular changes occurring with occlusion of a mature arteriovenous fistula," *The Journal of Vascular Access*, vol. 16, no. 6, pp. 459–466, 2015.

[2] H. H. Branham, "Aneurysmal varix of the femoral artery and vein following a gunshot wound," *International Journal of Surgery*, vol. 3, pp. 250–251, 1890.

[3] S. Velez-Roa, J. Neubauer, M. Wissing et al., "Acute arteriovenous fistula occlusion decreases sympathetic activity and improves baroreflex control in kidney transplanted patients," *Nephrology Dialysis Transplantation*, vol. 19, no. 6, pp. 1606–1612, 2004.

[4] S. Bhatia, J. Morrison, T. Bower, and M. McGoon, "Pulmonary hypertension and arteriovenous fistulas," *Mayo Clinic Proceedings*, vol. 78, pp. 908–912, 2003.

[5] A. Pagel, A. Bass, S. Strauss, E. Peleg, and M. J. Rapoport, "High output cardiac failure due to iatrogenic A-V fistula in scar: a report of a case and review of the literature," *Cardiovascular Surgery*, vol. 11, no. 4, pp. 317–319, 2003.

[6] A. K. Gerke and J. Wilson, "Complete resolution of severe high output heart failure and pulmonary hypertension after repair of longstanding arteriovenous fistula," *CHEST Journal*, vol. 132, no. 4, article 729S, 2007.

[7] S. Singh, M. Elramah, S. S. Allana et al., "A case series of real-time hemodynamic assessment of high output heart failure as a complication of arteriovenous access in dialysis patients," *Seminars in Dialysis*, vol. 27, no. 6, pp. 633–638, 2015.

[8] Y. Iwashima, T. Horio, Y. Takami et al., "Effects of the creation of arteriovenous fistula for hemodialysis on cardiac function and natriuretic peptide levels in CRF," *American Journal of Kidney Diseases*, vol. 40, no. 5, pp. 974–982, 2002.

[9] C. Basile, C. Lomonte, L. Vernaglione, F. Casucci, M. Antonelli, and N. Losurdo, "The relationship between the flow of arteriovenous fistula and cardiac output in haemodialysis patients," *Nephrology Dialysis Transplantation*, vol. 23, no. 1, pp. 282–287, 2008.

[10] G. M. London, A. P. Guerin, and S. J. Marchais, "Hemodynamic overload in end-stage renal disease patients," *Seminars in Dialysis*, vol. 12, no. 2, pp. 77–83, 1999.

[11] L. Dallo, C. Pastrana, G. Rodríguez, O. Medina Mora, R. Barragán, and D. Bialostozky, "Acquired systemic arteriovenous fistulas: experience of 33 cases," *Archivos del Instituto de Cardiologia de Mexico*, vol. 54, no. 2, pp. 159–166, 1984.

[12] H. B. Shumaker and E. E. Wayson, "Spontaneous care of aneurysms and arteriovenous fistulas with some notes on intravascular thrombosis," *The American Journal of Surgery*, vol. 79, article 532, 1950.

[13] T. Nara, D. Yoshikawa, S. Saito, Y. Kadoi, T. Morita, and F. Goto, "Perioperative management of biventricular failure after closure of a long-standing massive arteriovenous fistula," *Canadian Journal of Anesthesia*, vol. 48, no. 6, pp. 588–591, 2001.

[14] B. E. Cil, I. Akmangit, B. Peyniercioglu, M. Karcaaltincaba, and S. Cekirge, "Iatrogenic femoral arteriovenous fistula: endovascular treatment with covered stent implantation and 4-year follow-up," *Diagnostic and Interventional Radiology*, vol. 12, no. 1, pp. 50–52, 2006.

[15] S. D. Megremis, M. A. Christaki, N. K. Mourkoyiannis, G. S. Papadopoulos, and A. M. Tsilimigaki, "Iatrogenic brachial arteriovenous fistula in a child," *Journal of Ultrasound in Medicine*, vol. 25, no. 6, pp. 809–812, 2006.

[16] B. B. Das and J. Sharma, "Acquired brachial arteriovenous fistula in an ex-premature infant," *Clinical Pediatrics*, vol. 41, no. 2, pp. 131–132, 2002.

[17] K. C. Zorn, C. L. Starks, O. N. Gofrit, M. A. Orvieto, and A. L. Shalhav, "Embolization of renal-artery pseudoaneurysm after laparoscopic partial nephrectomy for angiomyolipoma: case report and literature review," *Journal of Endourology*, vol. 21, no. 7, pp. 763–768, 2007.

[18] A. Helck, R. T. Hoffmann, W. H. Sommer et al., "Diagnosis, therapy monitoring and follow up of renal artery pseudoaneurysm with contrast-enhanced ultrasound in three cases," *Clinical Hemorheology and Microcirculation*, vol. 46, no. 2-3, pp. 127–137, 2010.

[19] A. Helck, W. H. Sommer, M. Wessely, M. Notohamiprodjo, M. Reiser, and D. A. Clevert, "Benefit of contrast enhanced ultrasound for detection of ischaemic lesions and arterio venous fistulas in renal transplants—a feasibility study," *Clinical Hemorheology and Microcirculation*, vol. 48, no. 1-3, pp. 149–160, 2011.

[20] J. Ellis, R. Martin, P. Wilde, A. Tometzki, J. Senkungu, and D. Nansera, "Echocardiographic, chest X-ray and electrocardiogram findings in children presenting with heart failure to a Ugandan paediatric ward," *Tropical Doctor*, vol. 37, no. 3, pp. 149–150, 2007.

44

Endovascular Management of Right Subclavian Artery Pseudoaneurysm due to War Injury in Adolescent Patient

Onur Saydam,[1] **Deniz Şerefli,**[1] **Mehmet Atay,**[2] **and Cengiz Sert**[1]

[1]*Tepecik Training and Research Hospital, Department of Cardiovascular Surgery, 35170 İzmir, Turkey*
[2]*Bakirkoy Dr. Sadi Konuk Training and Research Hospital, Department of Cardiovascular Surgery, 34147 İstanbul, Turkey*

Correspondence should be addressed to Onur Saydam; onursaydam@hotmail.com

Academic Editor: Jaw-Wen Chen

Today there is a widespread use of endovascular treatment (EVT) for traumatic vascular injuries in adults, but there is lack of evidence of its use in adolescent patients with vascular injuries. With this case, we present successful EVT of 14-year-old adolescent with a right subclavian artery pseudoaneurysm (SAP) due to war injury. SAP was successfully excluded with deployment of 6×50 mm flexible, self-expanding covered nitinol stent graft (The GORE® VIABAHN® Endoprosthesis (W.L. Gore & Associates, Flagstaff, AZ)). Patient was discharged from hospital 2 days after the procedure with dual antiplatelet therapy (clopidogrel and aspirin). 3 months after discharge control DUS showed patent stent graft without any residual lesions. As a result, EVT is an alternative approach to treatment of SAP. It is safe, effective, and less invasive therapy for SAP in adults as well as in adolescents. We aim to contribute to the literature with this first case report.

1. Introduction

Nowadays war related injuries have begun to appear with increase in frequency in Turkey due to state of war in neighboring countries. The usage of firearms and explosive weapons in these situations can cause vascular injuries [1]. Subclavian artery pseudoaneurysm (SAP) or rupture is not common but can occur due to clavicle fracture, firearms, and other trauma [2]. Because of close relation to vital structure and noncompressibility, SAP remains a challenging problem for surgeons. Currently less invasive techniques rather than open surgery (OS) are being discussed for SAP in adult patients [3, 4]. However, there is lack of evidence of usage of endovascular therapy (EVT) in adolescents suffering SAP. We report a case of an adolescent with traumatic SAP, which was formed secondary to war injury and was successfully treated by EVT.

2. Case Report

A 14-year-old boy was admitted to emergency department with complaint of pain in right upper pectoral area. Physical examination revealed a wound scar with a diameter of 0.5×0.2 mm and a pulsatile mass with a diameter of 6×6 cm in the right upper pectoral area. There was also a scar related to thorax drainage tube in the mid-clavicular line, which was placed 2 months before in a hospital right after the explosion in Syria (Figure 1(a)). The reason of placement of drainage tube remained unknown due to lack of medical records. Anamnesis revealed that the pulsatile mass was growing with each passing day. He was hemodynamically stable. Right upper extremity pulses were palpable and no signs were observed pointing to circulatory disorder. Color Doppler Ultrasonography (DUS) showed a large SAP (5×5 cm) with a yin yang sign. SAP was originating from right subclavian artery (RSA) and it was approximately 2.5 mm wide. Contrast enhanced computed tomography angiography was performed to evaluate the vascular dimensions. Proximal RSA diameter was 5.3 mm and distal RSA was 5.2. We preferred EVT and performed the procedure under general anesthesia. Heparin was administered to maintain activated coagulation time above 250 seconds. Retrograde percutaneous approach from the right femoral artery to RSA with insertion of 5F vascular sheath into common femoral

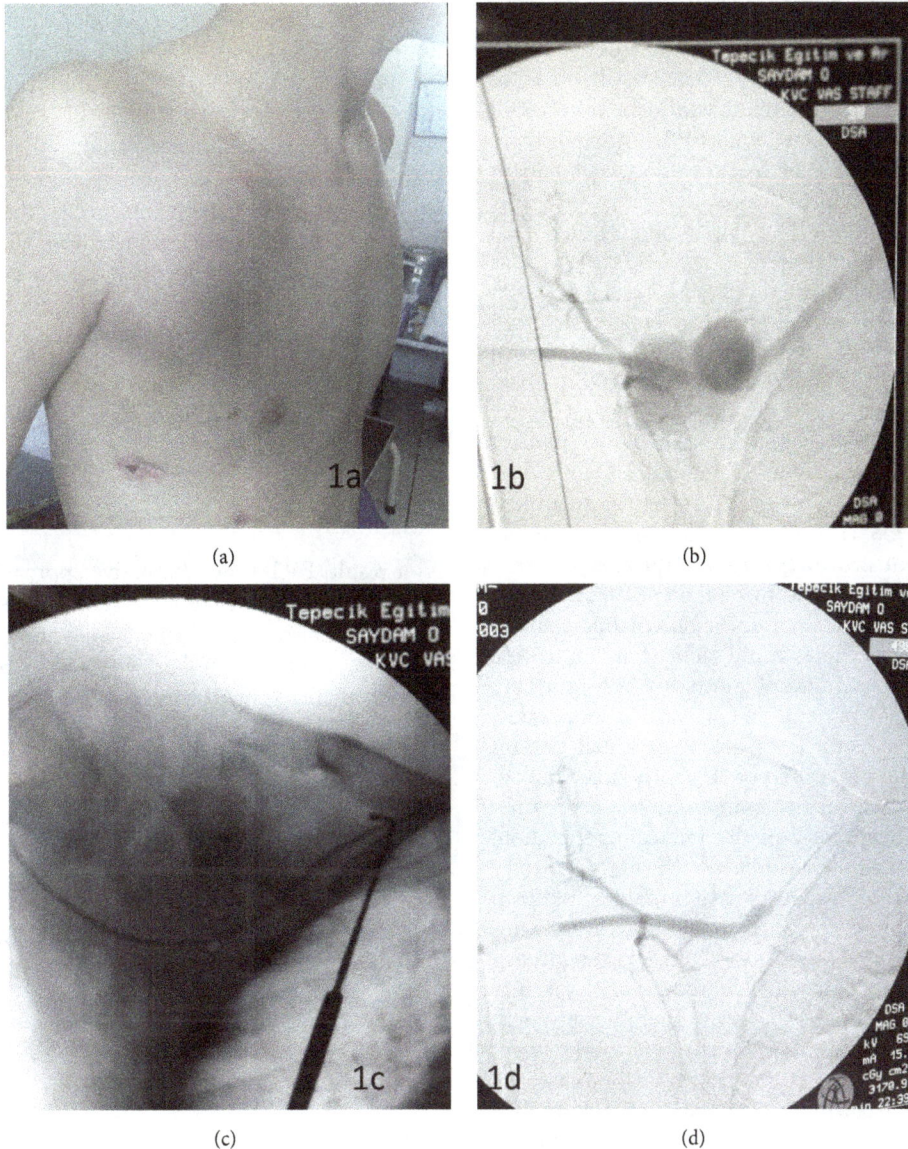

FIGURE 1: (a) Large subclavian pseudoaneurysm pulsatile sac with palpable trill. (b) Angiogram of pseudoaneurysm sac originated from the right subclavian artery. (c) Passing the lesion with 0.035 hydrophilic guide wire with the help of 5F straight selective multipurpose diagnostic catheter. (d) Final selective angiogram of the right subclavian artery with a complete hemostasis and preserved subclavian artery branches.

artery was performed. Selective angiography of the RSA with 5F pigtail catheter via left anterior oblique view with an angle 25° showed an SAP (Figure 1(b)). We passed the lesion with 0.035 hydrophilic guide wire with the help of 5F straight selective multipurpose diagnostic catheter (Figure 1(c)). We removed 5F vascular sheath and exchanged with 7F vascular sheath. SAP was excluded with deployment of 6 × 50 mm flexible, self-expanding covered nitinol stent graft (GORE VIABAHN Endoprosthesis (W.L. Gore & Associates, Flagstaff, AZ)). Postdilation inside of the stent graft with balloon angioplasty was performed. We preserved the RSA branches (Figure 1(d)). Control angiography showed SAP was completely excluded and there was no extravasation. Blood flow of the upper extremity was normal. 7F vascular sheath was removed and manual compression was applied

to vascular access site. He was extubated in the operation room. The total duration of the operation was 20 minutes. No loading dose was given for clopidogrel and aspirin. The treatment was started right after the procedure with 1 mg/kg clopidogrel and 2 mg/kg of aspirin. 0.01 cc/kg enoxaparin was administered 2 hours after the operation. The patient discharged from hospital on postoperative day 2 without any vascular access site related complication. 3 months after discharge control DUS showed patent stent graft without any residual lesions.

3. Discussion

Today there is a widespread use of endovascular treatment for traumatic vascular injuries in adults, but there is lack of evidence of its use in adolescent patients with vascular injuries. With this case report, we aim to contribute to the literature with this first case report, to the best of our knowledge in adolescent patients with penetrating SAP caused by war injury and treated with EVT. Although there is a case report about EVT of SAP in adolescent patient with Ehlers-Danlos syndrome (EDS), before the trauma our patient was totally healthy [5]. EDS is a dominantly inherited connective tissue disorder and EDS type 4 (the vascular type) is mainly caused by a deficit of type 3 fibrillar collagen which is constituent of arterial wall [6]. Differently from EDS patients we accept that our patient has healthy arterial wall and this may lead to difference in results. RSA arises from brachiocephalic artery and extends to the lateral border of the first rib. RSA injuries can be seen 5–10% percent in the population and most of these injuries are caused by penetrating traumas [7]. OS or EVT can be the treatment strategies for SAP. OS is usually safe but because of the injury risk of adjacent structures during surgical exploration complication rates are reported to be up to 24% in OS [8]. According to studies, depending on hemodynamic stability at presentation, mortality rates could range from 5% to 30% [9, 10]. Because of the significant morbidity and mortality rates, we preferred EVT rather than OS. Also, in some cases, thoracotomy may be required to obtain proximal control of the artery and in our case possible adhesions due to tube replacement might further complicate the procedure. There are some handicaps for EVT in adolescent population. Vascular access is one of these problems. The brachial artery is mostly used in adult patients, as it provides a direct, shorter, and less tortuous approach [11]. In our patient after DUS evaluation we have chosen femoral retrograde approach rather than RSA because of the need for the use of 7F vascular sheath in order to introduce stent graft. The other problem for usage of EVT in adolescents is the diameter of the target vessel because of continuing vessel growth. In our case, the diameter of RSA was 5.2 mm and because RSA is mobile and can be exposed to rotational forces during abduction and anteflexion of the arm we preferred to use 6 mm × 50 mm GORE VIABAHN Endoprosthesis (W.L. Gore & Associates, Flagstaff, AZ) rather than bare-metal stent. It is a nitinol supported flexible, self-expanding stent graft made of an expanded polytetrafluoroethylene. Unlike the bare-metal self-expanding stents we did not oversize VIABAHN stent. Because according to studies oversizing the VIABAHN stents by more than 20% of the vessel diameter will end up with significantly lower patency rates [12]. A study revealed that stent sizes of 6 mm and above for RSA would keep the patient asymptomatic in adult population [13]. Patency is an important issue for stent grafts. There are studies on this stent graft which show good patency rates [14, 15]. Postprocedural management is also having positive impact on patency of the graft. The optimal duration of dual antiplatelet therapy with aspirin and clopidogrel after endovascular treatment remains controversial [16, 17]. Dual antiplatelet therapy with aspirin and clopidogrel with loading dose is mostly recommended for 6 months in adults. There are also studies suggesting more aggressive and longer antithrombotic regimens after VIABAHN stent graft placement [18]. Because of lack of

evidence for loading dose of clopidogrel in adolescent we did not use loading dose and because of long life expectancy we planned to give clopidogrel for 6 months and 100 mg aspirin therapy for life long. Although all these were taken into consideration there are some studies that show 16.7%–34% thrombosis rates [19, 20]. Being different than SAP, these studies are mostly made on occlusive disease which is progressing disease and may not have adequate inflow and outflow and this situation can affect the patency rates of the graft. Nevertheless, stent thrombosis does not preclude future revascularization, which, if necessary, can be done under less emergent circumstances after the acute injury has resolved [21].

4. Conclusion

As a result, EVT is an alternative approach to treatment of SAP. It is safe and effective as well as less invasive therapy for SAP. It can also be performed safely in adolescent patients. Periodic patient follow-ups with DUS and postprocedural therapy strategies may have a positive impact on patency. But there is still lack of knowledge for long-term effectiveness and patency.

Authors' Contributions

All authors of this research paper have directly participated in the planning, execution, or analysis of this study; they have read and approved the final version submitted.

References

[1] H. R. Champion, J. B. Holcomb, and L. A. Young, "Injuries from explosions: physics, biophysics, pathology, and required research focus.," *The Journal of trauma*, vol. 66, no. 5, pp. 1468–1477, 2009.

[2] J. A. Serrano, "Acute subclavian artery pseudoaneurysm after closed fracture of the clavicle," *Acta Orthop Belg*, vol. 69, no. 6, p. 555, 2003.

[3] T. Yamagami, R. Yoshimatsu, O. Tanaka et al., "A case of iatrogenic subclavian artery injury successfully treated with endovascular procedures," *Annals of Vascular Diseases*, vol. 4, no. 1, pp. 53–55, 2011.

[4] S. Kuma, K. Morisaki, A. Kodama et al., "Ultrasound-guided percutaneous thrombin injection for post-catheterization pseudoaneurysm," *Circulation Journal*, vol. 79, no. 6, pp. 1277–1281, 2015.

[5] P. I. Rossi, L. A. Scher, S. G. Friedman, M. H. Hall, R. A. Boxer, and M. G. Bialer, "Subclavian artery pseudoaneurysm in type IV Ehlers-Danlos syndrome," *Journal of Vascular Surgery*, vol. 27, no. 3, pp. 549–551, 1998.

[6] D. P. Germain, "Ehlers-Danlos syndrome type IV," *Orphanet Journal of Rare Diseases*, vol. 2, no. 1, article 32, 2007.

[7] C. E. Hyre, D. F. Cikrit, S. G. Lalka, A. P. Sawchuk, M. C. Dalsing, and J. J. Schuler, "Aggressive management of vascular injuries of the thoracic outlet," *Journal of Vascular Surgery*, vol. 27, no. 5, pp. 880–885, 1998.

[8] V. Kalakuntla, "Six-year experience with management of subclavian artery injuries," *Am Surg*, vol. 66, no. 10, pp. 927-30, 2000.

[9] D. Demetriades, S. Chahwan, H. Gomez et al., "Penetrating injuries to the subclavian and axillary vessels," *Journal of the American College of Surgeons*, vol. 188, no. 3, pp. 290–295, 1999.

[10] S. M. George Jr., M. A. Croce, T. C. Fabian et al., "Cervicothoracic arterial injuries: Recommendations for diagnosis and management," *World Journal of Surgery*, vol. 15, no. 1, pp. 134–139, 1991.

[11] P. Leonardou and P. Pappas, "Urgent endovascular treatment of iatrogenic subclavian artery rupture: Report of three cases," *Ulusal Travma ve Acil Cerrahi Dergisi*, vol. 18, no. 6, pp. 527–530, 2012.

[12] K. McQuade, D. Gable, G. Pearl, B. Theune, and S. Black, "Four-year randomized prospective comparison of percutaneous ePTFE/nitinol self-expanding stent graft versus prosthetic femoral-popliteal bypass in the treatment of superficial femoral artery occlusive disease," *Journal of Vascular Surgery*, vol. 52, no. 3, pp. 584–e7, 2010.

[13] K. Kumar, G. Dorros, M. C. Bates, L. Palmer, L. Mathiak, and C. Dufek, "Primary stent deployment in occlusive subclavian artery disease," *Catheterization and Cardiovascular Diagnosis*, vol. 34, no. 4, pp. 281–285, 1995.

[14] J. Lammer, T. Zeller, and K. A. Hausegger, "Heparin-bonded covered stents versus bare-metal stents for complex femoropopliteal artery lesions: the randomized VIASTAR trial (viabahn endoprosthesis with propaten bioactive surface [VIA] versus bare nitinol stent in the treatment of long lesions in superficial femoral artery occlusive disease)," *Journal of the American College of Cardiology*, vol. 62, no. 15, pp. 1320–1327, 2013.

[15] M. Bosiers, K. Deloose, J. Callaert et al., "Superiority of stent-grafts for in-stent restenosis in the superficial femoral artery: Twelve-month results from a multicenter randomized trial," *Journal of Endovascular Therapy*, vol. 22, no. 1, pp. 1–10, 2015.

[16] P. Alonso-Coello, S. Bellmunt, C. McGorrian et al., "Antithrombotic therapy in peripheral artery disease," in *Antithrombotic Therapy and Prevention of Thrombosis*, vol. 141, 2 Supplement, pp. e669S–e690S, 2012.

[17] A. Visona, "Antithrombotic treatment before and after peripheral artery percutaneous angioplasty," *Blood Transfus*, vol. 7, no. 1, pp. 18–23, 2009.

[18] B. W. Ullery, K. Tran, N. Itoga, K. Casey, R. L. Dalman, and J. T. Lee, "Safety and efficacy of antiplatelet/anticoagulation regimens after Viabahn stent graft treatment for femoropopliteal occlusive disease," *Journal of Vascular Surgery*, vol. 61, no. 6, pp. 1479–1488, 2015.

[19] P. C. Johnston, S. M. Vartanian, S. J. Runge et al., "Risk factors for clinical failure after stent graft treatment for femoropopliteal occlusive disease," *Journal of Vascular Surgery*, vol. 56, no. 4, pp. 998–1007.e1, 2012.

[20] M. Fischer, C. Schwabe, and K.-L. Schulte, "Value of the hemobahn/viabahn endoprosthesis in the treatment of long chronic lesions of the superficial femoral artery: 6 Years of experience," *Journal of Endovascular Therapy*, vol. 13, no. 3, pp. 281–290, 2006.

[21] E. S. Xenos, M. Freeman, S. Stevens, D. Cassada, J. Pacanowski, and M. Goldman, "Covered stents for injuries of subclavian and axillary arteries," *Journal of Vascular Surgery*, vol. 38, no. 3, pp. 451–454, 2003.

45

A Case of Superficial Femoral Arteriovenous Fistula and Severe Venous Stasis Ulceration, Managed with an Iliac Extender Prosthesis

Nicole Ilonzo, Selena Goss, Chun Yang, and Michael Dudkiewicz

Mount Sinai St. Luke's-West, New York, NY, USA

Correspondence should be addressed to Nicole Ilonzo; nilonzo@chpnet.org

Academic Editor: Muzaffer Sindel

Most femoral artery arteriovenous fistulas occur as a result of percutaneous interventions. However, arteriovenous fistulas can occur in the setting of trauma, with resultant consequences such as heart failure, steal syndrome, or venous insufficiency. Indications for endovascular repair in this setting are limited to patients who are at too high risk for anesthesia, have a hostile groin, or would not survive significant bleeding. We report the case of a traumatic femoral arteriovenous fistula, causing severe venous insufficiency and arteriomegaly, in a 58-year-old male, with history of traumatic gunshot wound complicated by popliteal DVT. Surgical options for arteriovenous fistula include open and endovascular repair but this patient's fistula was more suitable for endovascular repair for reasons that will be discussed.

1. Introduction

This is a case of an arteriovenous fistula causing severe venous insufficiency with ensuant venous stasis ulceration. Venous insufficiency is a disease that affects anywhere from <1 to 40% of females and <1 to 17% of males [1]. Patients with chronic venous insufficiency can develop complications from this disease, with the most severe being venous stasis ulcerations.

2. Case Presentation

A 58-year-old male presented to the emergency department with right lower extremity swelling and a large ulceration on his right lateral leg for nearly six years (Figure 1). The patient had been treated in Guyana with topical agents and dressing changes, without improvement. In the ED, right lower extremity duplex demonstrated popliteal vein thrombosis as well as traumatic fistula between superficial femoral vein and superficial femoral artery. Duplex ultrasound also showed distal femoral vein to measure 4.36 cm AP, mid femoral vein 1.12 cm, and an enlarged lymph node noted in the groin measuring 4.56 × 1.60 cm. CT angiogram of the abdomen, pelvis, and lower extremities showed right superior femoral

arteriovenous fistula and a tortuous right common iliac artery that may be causing a May Thurner's type compression of the R common iliac vein (Figure 2).

Patient subsequently underwent bilateral extremity angiogram and selective catheterization of the right common iliac artery via retrograde left femoral approach. Angiogram revealed a patent but enlarged right common femoral artery, a patent right profunda artery, and a patent and enlarged right superficial femoral artery (SFA) with a distal arteriovenous (AV) fistula connecting the superficial femoral artery to the femoral vein with venous flow upwards (Figure 3). On pelvic imaging, there also appeared to be very late venous filling possibly of a venous malformation, which was not seen on previous imaging (Figure 4). There was a large venous aneurysm just distal to the fistulous tract. The remainder of the arterial outflow was normal giving rise to a patent popliteal artery and patent tibial trifurcation.

The decision was made to pursue endovascular repair of the patient's fistula. Given concerns that the SFA was so enlarged and at risk for significant hemorrhage, a superficial femoral artery cutdown was performed (Figure 5). The SFA was dissected free from its surrounding structures. The anterior wall of the SFA was punctured in an antegrade

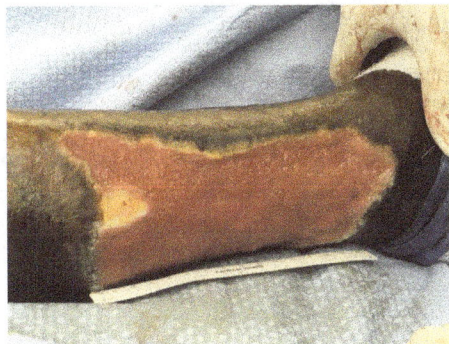

FIGURE 1: Right lateral leg venous stasis ulcer.

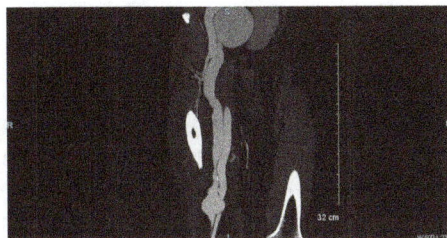

FIGURE 2: CT angiogram showing a superficial femoral arteriovenous fistula with arteriomegaly of the right external iliac artery.

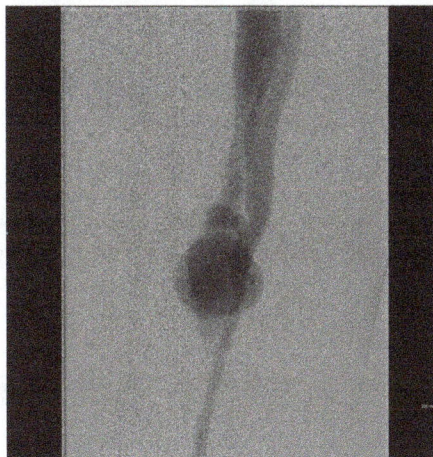

FIGURE 3: Right lower extremity angiogram showing a patent and enlarged right superficial femoral artery with a distal AV fistula connecting the superficial femoral artery to the femoral vein with venous flow upwards.

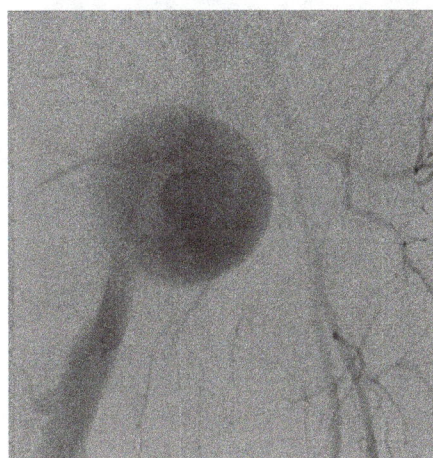

FIGURE 4: Right lower extremity angiogram showing possibility of a venous malformation, which was not seen on previous imaging.

fashion and a 12-French sheath was then placed. There was some bleeding around the 12-French sheath which required clamping of the proximal superficial femoral artery with a vascular clamp. A Gore iliac branch endoprosthesis which measured 10 mm distally 16 mm proximally for a length of 7 cm was opened and deployed in standard fashion across the arteriovenous fistula. It was postdilated using an angioplasty balloon. After postdilation angioplasty there was good apposition against the wall and the fistula filled very slowly via collaterals and not via inline flow (Figure 6). In addition, the patient maintained his outflow via the popliteal artery. Split thickness graft was placed over the ulcer and negative pressure therapy was utilized. The VAC was taken down and there was excellent take of the skin graft. Patient has subsequently undergone Unna booth therapy and the wound has healed completely after 3 months (Figure 7).

3. Discussion

The scoring system used to classify and stage venous insufficiency is called the clinical manifestations, etiological factors, anatomical distribution, and pathophysiological conditions classification (CEAP classification) [2, 3]. This patient, with a CEAP classification of C6 for active venous ulceration, required surgical intervention. The key to treatment of this venous stasis ulceration was to interrupt the fistula [4].

Traumatic arteriovenous fistulae can be repaired by open or endovascular approaches [5, 6]. This patient's fistula was best managed with an endovascular approach but there were limitations given the proximal and distal landing zones were significantly different in size. Using a standard Viabahn stent

would be a suboptimal choice for this reason. Therefore, the decision was made to use a Gore Excluder Iliac branch endoprosthesis, which could adjust for this asymmetry. As described by the manufacturer, the Gore Excluder Iliac branch endoprosthesis is indicated for treatment of infrarenal artery aneurysms. The graft is exclusively designed for the iliac artery [7]. However, it was used with excellent effect in this context.

Of note, there may be an element of residual venous hypertension secondary to compression of the right external iliac vein by the hypertrophied right external iliac artery. We anticipate further healing of his venous stasis ulcer now that the patient's venous insufficiency is largely corrected with the stent. However, if his venous disease did not seem to improve significantly, we would have attempted to treat the external iliac vein compression with a stent in hopes of providing patency to the vein.

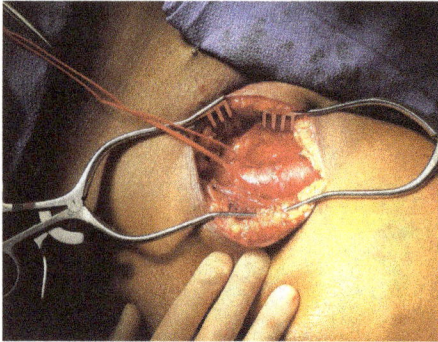

FIGURE 5: A superficial femoral artery cutdown was performed revealing an enlarged SFA.

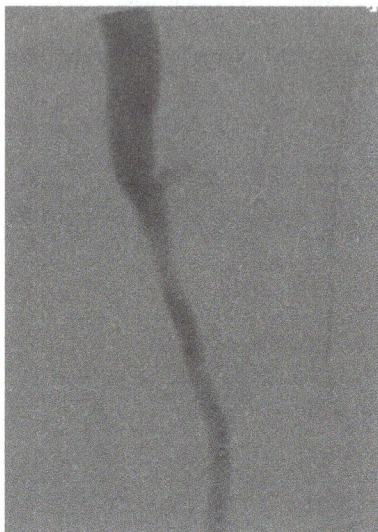

FIGURE 6: Superficial femoral arteriovenous fistula occluded after placement of iliac extender stent.

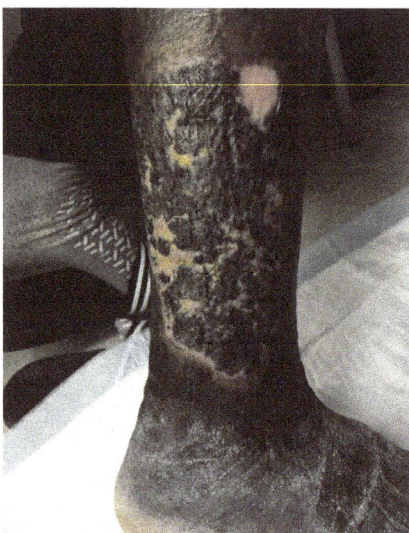

FIGURE 7: Wound healed within 3 months.

References

[1] J. L. Beebe-Dimmer, J. R. Pfeifer, J. S. Engle, and D. Schottenfeld, "The epidemiology of chronic venous insufficiency and varicose veins," *Annals of Epidemiology*, vol. 15, no. 3, pp. 175–184, 2005.

[2] S. Krishnan and S. C. Nicholls, "Chronic venous insufficiency: clinical assessment and patient selection," *Seminars in Interventional Radiology*, vol. 22, no. 3, pp. 169–177, 2005.

[3] B. Vasudevan, "Venous leg ulcers: Pathophysiology and Classification," *Indian Dermatology Online Journal*, vol. 5, no. 3, p. 366, 2014.

[4] R. Chiesa, E. M. Marone, C. Limoni, M. Volontè, and O. Petrini, "Chronic venous disorders: correlation between visible signs, symptoms, and presence of functional disease," *Journal of Vascular Surgery*, vol. 46, no. 2, pp. 322–330, 2007.

[5] E. Aslim, "Traumatic arteriovenous fistulae 25 years after gunshot injury," *European Journal of Vascular and Endovascular Surgery*, vol. 52, no. 3, p. 316, 2016.

[6] P. C. Thompson, B. W. Ullery, D. Fleischmann, and V. Chandra, "Novel approach to a giant external iliac vein aneurysm secondary to posttraumatic femoral arteriovenous fistula," *Vascular and Endovascular Surgery*, vol. 49, no. 5-6, pp. 148–151, 2015.

[7] "Instructions for use for GORE EXCLUDER AAA Endoprosthesis," https://www.goremedical.com/products/excluder—ifu/instructions.

46

Endovascular Management of Middle Aortic Syndrome Presenting with Uncontrolled Hypertension

Owen S. Glotzer ⓘ, Kathryn Bowser, F. Todd Harad, and Sandra Weiss

The Heart and Vascular Center, Christiana Care, Newark, DE 19713, USA

Correspondence should be addressed to Owen S. Glotzer; owen.s.glotzer@christianacare.org

Academic Editor: Nikolaos Papanas

Middle Aortic Syndrome is a rare vascular disorder consisting of narrowing or stenosis of the distal thoracic or abdominal aorta. It is described in the literature in the form of case studies and case series. The authors present an unusual case of Middle Aortic Syndrome attributed to Takayasu's arteritis in a 60-year-old female who presented to the emergency department with uncontrolled hypertension. Traditional intervention involves open surgical bypass. This case study reviews the published literature on this rare syndrome and illustrates a successful alternative to open surgery through an endovascular approach.

1. Introduction

Middle Aortic Syndrome is a rare vascular disorder consisting of narrowing or stenosis of the distal thoracic or abdominal aorta. This constellation of anatomic abnormalities and symptoms is generally attributed to either a developmental/congenital disorder or to inflammatory vasculitis such as Takayasu's arteritis (TAK). Organ and muscle malperfusion distal to the affected aorta can lead most commonly to lower extremity claudication, resistant hypertension, and abdominal pain [1, 2]. It is classically identified during the first three decades of life and has been traditionally treated with open surgery [3–6]. The authors present a unique case of severe abdominal aortic stenosis in a 60-year-old female who presented with uncontrolled hypertension.

2. Case Report

A 60-year-old female presented to the outpatient cardiology clinic for evaluation of worsening chronic hypertension for which she had been on hydrochlorothiazide/Valsartan for 10 years. Her systolic blood pressure exceeded 200 mmHg in the office, and aggressive medical therapy was initiated in the outpatient setting. She returned to the emergency department the following day with headache and malaise and systolic blood pressure above 200 mmHg for which she was treated and discharged.

She returned to the emergency department again 5 days later, this time with complaints of word finding difficulty, blurred vision, and lower extremity tingling. Her blood pressure on presentation was 216/81 mmHg. She was admitted, and workup demonstrated no acute intracranial process or carotid stenosis. Echocardiography revealed mild concentric left ventricular hypertrophy with a preserved ejection fraction. Her blood pressure continued to be refractory to medical therapy despite five antihypertensive agents and eventual initiation of an esmolol infusion. A renal artery ultrasound identified renal artery stenosis with flow at the arterial origin measuring 350 cm/s on the right and 208 cm/s on the left (Table 1); flow velocity in the supraceliac aorta was also noted to be elevated. She had no history of kidney disease and no elevation of her creatinine. Vascular surgery was consulted and a history of lower extremity claudication was elicited. On exam she had weak but palpable femoral pulses and an audible abdominal aortic bruit; ankle-brachial index measurements were deferred and the patient was scheduled for angiogram.

The patient underwent aortography the following day and on selective angiography the renal arteries were found to be widely patent. Significant stenosis was identified at the distal thoracic aorta extending into the abdominal aorta but terminating proximal to the celiac trunk. The degree of stenosis was deemed to be greater than 90% and a pressure gradient between the upper extremity and intra-aortic measurements

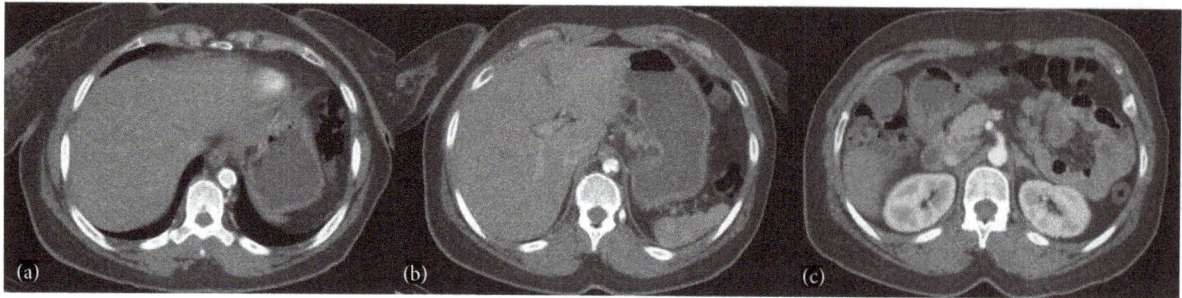

FIGURE 1: (a) Aorta proximal to stenosis with circumferential calcification measuring 9 mm lumen and 14 mm external diameter. (b) Aorta at the level stenosis with a luminal diameter of 5 mm. (c) Aorta distal to stenosis with a 14 mm wall and a patent lumen.

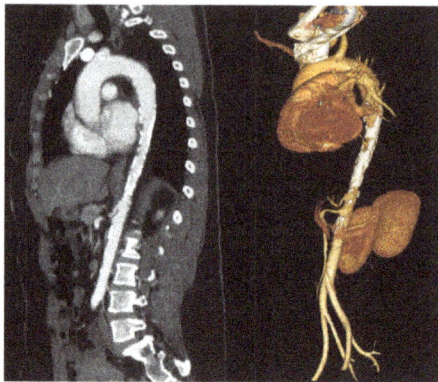

FIGURE 2: CTA of showing the area of stenosis in the supraceliac aorta with 3D reconstruction.

TABLE 1: Renal artery duplex measurements.

Criteria	Right Kidney	Left Kidney
Size (cm)	8.71	10.26
Velocity (cm/s)		
Origin	350	208
Proximal	175	211
Mid	49	112
Distal	41	NR
RI		
Upper	0.64	0.59
Mid	0.69	0.57
Lower	0.71	0.50
RAR	2.69	1.67

RI = resistive indices, RAR = renal to aortic ratio, and NR = not recorded

exceeded 100 mmHg. CTA was subsequently performed to evaluate the extent of the lesion and confirmed a stenosis 1.3 cm proximal to the celiac origin measuring 5 mm at its narrowest point (Figures 1 and 2). The patient underwent arteriogram; the stenosis was successfully navigated and a Protege 14 × 40 x 12 mm nitinol stent (Medtronic Vascular, Santa Rosa CA) was delivered followed by a 10 mm post-dilation balloon. A completion arteriogram demonstrated excellent flow across the stent.

After stenting, the patients' systolic blood pressure was 140-160 mmHg, and she experienced resolution of her lower extremity claudication. She was discharged from the hospital on Aspirin and Plavix and a blood pressure regimen consisting of lisinopril, hydralazine, amlodipine, and carvedilol.

She was lost to follow-up until two years later when she returned to the hospital with a blood pressure of 220/85 mmHg, with complaints of chest discomfort. CTA demonstrated stenosis in the distal portion of the aortic stent. An angiogram was performed, and the stent was ballooned to 12 mm. Pressure gradient measurements taken before and after dilatation decreased from 60 mmHg to 20 mmHg. On follow-up one year later, she continued to experience excellent blood pressure control.

3. Discussion

Middle Aortic Syndrome is a rare clinical presentation with only case studies and case series reported in the literature [4, 5, 7–9]. There is no characteristic presentation, but this syndrome can lead to severe hypertension, diminished or absent femoral pulses, lower extremity claudication, incongruent extremity pressure measurements, and audible arterial bruits. Laboratory analysis can show elevation of inflammatory markers such as erythrocyte sedimentation rate (ESR) and C-reactive protein (CRP). [10]

The classic imaging findings of Middle Aortic Syndrome have been described as an hour glass shaped aorta identified on CT scan or arteriography. Classification of this syndrome is based on the most proximal portion of the aorta affected [5, 6]. Distal lesions are more often associated with renal and/or splanchnic arterial disease, which is consistent with the case presented here as the infraceliac aorta was of normal caliber and there was no associated narrowing in the renal or splanchnic vasculature.

It is difficult to attribute the location and degree of narrowing to atherosclerotic disease alone given her lack of risk factors such as obesity, diabetes mellitus, or smoking history and lack of arterial calcification in other areas. Attributing her stenosis to congenital anomaly seems even more implausible given her age at presentation. Although large vessel arteritis is generally diagnosed in patients before the age of 30, adult onset TAK is well described [3, 11–13]. According to the American College of Rheumatology, three of six criteria are required for the diagnosis of TAK: onset at or before 40 years of age, 10 mmHg difference in brachial pressures, decreased pulsation in a brachial artery, subclavian or aortic bruit, narrowing/occlusions of the aorta, its primary branches or major proximal arteries in the extremities, and claudication of the extremities [14–16]. Although ESR and CRP were never obtained during her workup, according to these criteria the patient meets criteria for TAK.

Another point of interest is the ultrasound demonstrating flow acceleration in the renal arteries, with a lack of renal stenosis present on arteriography or CT. The authors attribute this finding to poststenotic flow acceleration centered at the level of the renal arteries, which is further supported by follow-up duplex study that demonstrates decreased flow velocity through the renal arteries after placement of the aortic stent. The native aorta distal to the stenosed segment measured 14 mm; as such, increased velocity is expected through a 10 mm stent. Placement of a larger stent was thought to pose too high a risk for iatrogenic trauma.

Traditional intervention consists of open surgery with bypass grafting, interposition grafting, or patch aortoplasty [5, 11, 17–20]. However, given the extent and complexity of these procedures, mortality rates have been quoted as high as 13% [21]. More recently, endovascular intervention has been performed with positive results [2, 22–25]. The extent of the lesion, involvement of visceral and/or renal arteries, age, and comorbidities of the patient need to be taken into consideration when selecting the most appropriate therapy [26]. The patient described here achieved blood pressure control and experienced resolution of her associated symptoms; despite the need for reintervention the authors maintain that endovascular therapy was the appropriate approach in this instance. The longevity of aortic stenting for stenotic lesions has yet to be determined, and some patients will require reintervention, as was true in this case. The decreased risk of morbidity and mortality justifies the endovascular approach as the initial intervention in elderly patients or those with significant comorbidities.

4. Conclusion

Middle Aortic Syndrome is a rare entity with an often unclear clinical presentation. The authors of this manuscript add this presentation to the literature regarding hypertension stemming from significant stenosis of the abdominal aorta. This case study demonstrates that the endovascular approach should be viewed as an appropriate early step in the management of hypertension due to aortic stenosis for patients with anatomically amenable lesions, who are at an increased risk of complications from open surgery.

References

[1] T. T. Terramani, A. Salim, D. B. Hood, V. L. Rowe, and F. A. Weaver, "Hypoplasia of the descending thoracic and abdominal aorta: A report of two cases and review of the literature," *Journal of Vascular Surgery*, vol. 36, no. 4, pp. 844–848, 2002.

[2] W. Che, H. Xiong, X. Jiang et al., "Stenting for middle aortic syndrome caused by Takayasu arteritis-immediate and long-term outcomes," *Catheterization and Cardiovascular Interventions*, vol. 91, pp. 623–631, 2018.

[3] J. E. Connolly, S. E. Wilson, P. L. Lawrence, and R. M. Fujitani, "Middle aortic syndrome: Distal thoracic and abdominal coarctation, a disorder with multiple etiologies," *Journal of the American College of Surgeons*, vol. 194, no. 6, pp. 774–781, 2002.

[4] H. D. Kim, M. Kim, S. Kim et al., "Resistant hypertension caused by stenosis of the aorta in elderly women: three case reports," *Clinical Hypertension*, vol. 20, no. 1, 2014.

[5] J. C. Stanley, E. Criado, J. L. Eliason, G. R. Upchurch Jr., R. Berguer, and J. E. Rectenwald, "Abdominal aortic coarctation: Surgical treatment of 53 patients with a thoracoabdominal bypass, patch aortoplasty, or interposition aortoaortic graft," *Journal of Vascular Surgery*, vol. 48, no. 5, pp. 1073–1082, 2008.

[6] L. M. Graham, G. B. Zelenock, E. E. Erlandson, A. G. Coran, S. M. Lindenauer, and J. C. Stanley, "Abdominal aortic coarctation and segmental hypoplasia," *Surgery*, vol. 86, no. 4, pp. 519–529, 1979.

[7] K. Uwabe, O. Okada, and M. Harada, "Ascending to descending aorta bypass for middle aortic syndrome," *Circulation Journal*, vol. 71, no. 7, pp. 1162-1163, 2007.

[8] K. C. A. Cheng and Y. L. Li, "Mid-aortic syndrome secondary to Takayasu's disease," *BMJ Case Reports*, vol. 2017, 2017.

[9] K. Yakut and I. Erdogan, "Case report of a rarely seen long segment middle aortic syndrome," *Turk Kardiyoloji Dernegi Arsivi-Archives of the Turkish Society of Cardiology*, vol. 45, no. 2, pp. 181–183, 2017.

[10] R. Serra, L. Butrico, F. Fugetto et al., "Updates in pathophysiology, diagnosis and management of takayasu arteritis," *Annals of Vascular Surgery*, vol. 35, pp. 210–225, 2016.

[11] B. Segers, M. Derluyn, J.-P. Barroy, and A. P. Brunet, "Isolated supradiaphragmatic descending thoracic aorta stenosis in a Takayasu's disease: Surgical cure," *European Journal of Cardio-Thoracic Surgery*, vol. 20, no. 6, pp. 1243–1245, 2001.

[12] Y. Qi, L. Yang, H. Zhang et al., "The presentation and management of hypertension in a large cohort of Takayasu arteritis," *Clinical Rheumatology*, vol. 37, no. 10, pp. 2781–2788, 2018.

[13] F. A. Aeschlimann, L. Barra, R. Alsolaimani et al., "Presentation and disease course of childhood- versus adult-onset Takayasu Arteritis," *Arthritis & Rheumatology*, 2018.

[14] W. P. Arend, B. A. Michel, D. A. Bloch et al., "The American College of Rheumatology 1990 criteria for the classification of Takayasu arteritis," *Arthritis & Rheumatology*, vol. 33, no. 8, pp. 1129–1134, 1990.

[15] K. L. Huang, Y. C. Lin, and K. L. Oller, "An Unusual Cause of Abdominal Pain in a Young, Hypertensive Female," *Gastroenterology*, vol. 154, no. 3, pp. e10–e11, 2018.

[16] B. Patel, A. Tiwari, S. R. K. Dubey, G. C. Bhatt, P. Tiwari, and B. D. Bhan, "Takayasu arteritis presenting with malignant hypertension; a rare manifestation of a rare disease: a case report and review of the literature," *Tropical Doctor*, vol. 47, no. 1, pp. 60–63, 2017.

[17] C. A. Hinojosa, J. E. Anaya-Ayala, A. Torres-Machorro, R. Lizola, and H. Laparra-Escareno, "Middle aortic syndrome in Takayasu's arteritis: Report of two surgical cases," *Annals of Vascular Surgery*, vol. 34, pp. 270.e13–270.e17, 2016.

[18] A. Chitrakar, K. R. Shrestha, and U. K. Shrestha, "Middle aortic syndrome with renal artery stenosis," *Journal of Surgical Case Reports*, vol. 2017, no. 9, 2017.

[19] K. T. Delis and P. Gloviczki, "Middle Aortic Syndrome: From Presentation to Contemporary Open Surgical and Endovascular Treatment," *Perspectives in Vascular Surgery and Endovascular Therapy*, vol. 17, no. 3, pp. 187–203, 2005.

[20] H. J. Kim, J.-W. Choi, H. Y. Hwang, and H. Ahn, "Extra-anatomic ascending aorta to abdominal aorta bypass in Takayasu arteritis patients with mid-aortic syndrome," *The Korean Journal of Thoracic and Cardiovascular Surgery*, vol. 50, no. 4, pp. 270–274, 2017.

[21] A. V. Pokrovsky, T. A. Sultanaliev, and A. A. Spiridonov, "Surgical treatment of vasorenal hypertension in nonspecific aorto-arteritis (Takayasu's disease)," *Journal of Cardiovascular Surgery*, vol. 24, no. 2, pp. 111–118, 1983.

[22] M. Di Santo, É. V. Stelmaszewski, and A. Villa, "Endovascular intervention in takayasu arteritis. Case report," *Archivos Argentinos de Pediatría*, vol. 114, no. 3, pp. e147–e150, 2016.

[23] Y. P. Diao, Y. X. Chen, S. Yan et al., "Efficacy and safety analysis of surgical bypass and endovascular management in the treatment of 116 Takayasu arteritis," *Zhonghua Yi Xue Za Zhi*, vol. 96, no. 6, pp. 447–450, 2016.

[24] J. Jung, G. Song, S. Choi, Y. Lee, and J. Kim, "Endovascular intervention versus surgery in patients with takayasu arteritis: a meta-analysis," *European Journal of Vascular and Endovascular Surgery*, vol. 55, no. 6, pp. 888–899, 2018.

[25] D. Saadoun, M. Lambert, T. Mirault et al., "Retrospective analysis of surgery versus endovascular intervention in Takayasu arteritis a multicenter experience," *Circulation*, vol. 125, no. 6, pp. 813–819, 2012.

[26] S. M. Kim, I. M. Jung, A. Han et al., "Surgical Treatment of Middle Aortic Syndrome with Takayasu Arteritis or Midaortic Dysplastic Syndrome," *European Journal of Vascular and Endovascular Surgery*, vol. 50, no. 2, pp. 206–212, 2015.

47

Anomalous Right Subclavian Artery-Esophageal Fistulae

Courtney Brooke Shires ⑩[1] **and Michael J. Rohrer**[2]

[1]Department of Otolaryngology, Head and Neck Surgery, University of Tennessee Health Science Center, 910 Madison Ave., Suite 430, Memphis, TN 38163, USA

[2]Department of Surgery, Division of Vascular and Endovascular Surgery, University of Tennessee Health Science Center, 910 Madison Ave., Second Floor, Memphis, TN 38163, USA

Correspondence should be addressed to Courtney Brooke Shires; cshires1@gmail.com

Academic Editor: Muzaffer Sindel

An aberrant right subclavian artery (ARSA) is the most common aortic arch anomaly, but only 19 previous cases of ARSA-esophageal fistula have been reported. Six patients have survived their bleeding episode. We describe the case of a 44-year-old woman who developed massive hemoptysis. Laryngoscopy, bronchoscopy, head and neck angiogram, and median sternotomy did not reveal what was presumed initially to be a tracheoinnominate fistula. Contrasted CT showed an anomalous subclavian artery posterior to the esophagus. Given the technical challenge of approaches for this pathology, the patient was unfit for open surgical repair. Therefore, endovascular covered stent grafts were deployed spanning the segment of the subclavian artery in continuity with the esophagus, via a right brachial artery approach. Unfortunately, the patient died after successful placement of the grafts.

1. Introduction

Artery-esophageal fistulae are rare but can cause massive and life-threatening hemorrhage. Prompt diagnosis and treatment are mandatory if the patient is to be saved, since these fistulae are fatal in a majority of cases. These fistulae most often develop secondary to prior thoracic operations, infection, neoplasm, foreign body, or radiotherapy and typically involve a fistula between the esophagus and the adjacent descending thoracic aorta [1–3]. Fistulae between the subclavian artery and esophagus are extremely rare and anatomically possible in the presence of an anomalous right subclavian artery which arises from the proximal descending thoracic aorta and courses behind the esophagus to supply the right arm.

2. Case Report

A 44-year-old woman with a history of gastroesophageal reflux disease and hypertension presented with worsening shortness of breath. She was found to have pneumonia and required intubation. She developed multiple complications, including sepsis, adult respiratory distress syndrome, acute renal failure, intensive care neuropathy, cardiac arrhythmias, and cardiac arrest. Approximately three weeks after hospitalization, a tracheostomy tube was placed. She then developed intra-abdominal abscesses after a gastrostomy tube became dislodged. She underwent exploratory laparotomy with abscess drainage and closure of the gastrostomy and was maintained on total parenteral nutrition.

Four months after admission to the hospital, a nasogastric tube was placed and enteral nutrition was started. Sixteen days later, she experienced an episode of substantial bleeding, and it was not clear whether this came from the airway or oropharynx. Her hematocrit was 20 percent, platelets were 396,000, and blood urea nitrogen was 13 mg/dL. She was resuscitated with packed red blood cells, platelets, cryoprecipitate, and fresh frozen plasma; selective carotid arteriography of the head and neck, direct laryngoscopy, and bronchoscopy were unremarkable.

Three days later, she again experienced severe bleeding, which was initially felt to have originated from her airway. She was taken to the operating room by the vascular surgery team

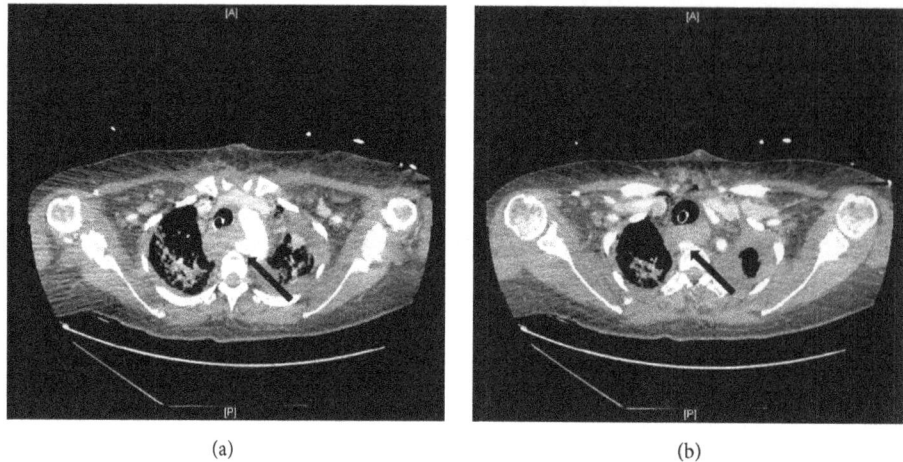

(a) (b)

FIGURE 1: Sequential CT scan images show origin of right subclavian artery from the proximal descending thoracic aorta ((a), black arrow) and coursing posterior to the esophagus ((b), black arrow).

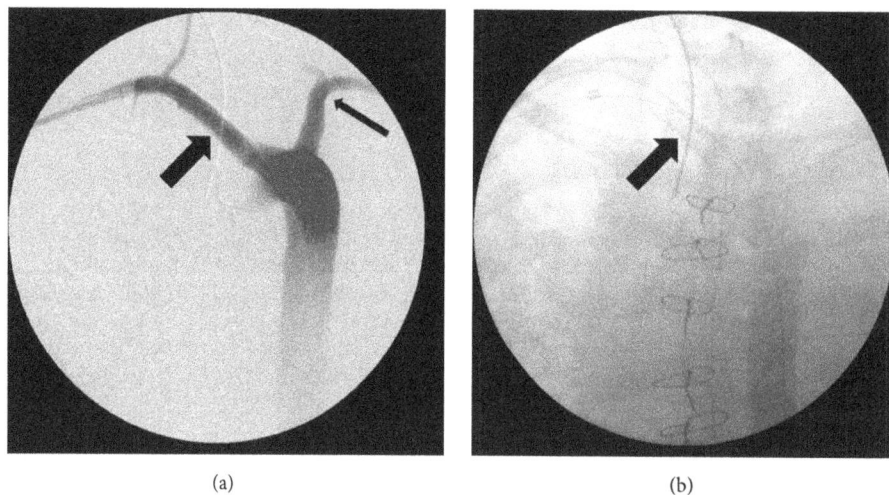

(a) (b)

FIGURE 2: (a) Intraoperative angiogram performed in an AP projection through a sheath positioned in the right axillary artery from a right brachial approach. The right subclavian artery is seen (wide arrow) as is the left subclavian artery (narrow arrow). (b) Intraoperative image in the same projection after deployment of a balloon expandable covered stent at level of esophageal-arterial communication. The arrow indicates the position of the covered stent.

with the preoperative impression that she had a tracheoinnominate fistula. Median sternotomy revealed a right carotid artery arising directly from the aortic arch with no innominate or right subclavian artery in the anterior mediastinum. No artery to trachea fistula was identified and a provisional diagnosis of aberrant right subclavian artery with subclavian to esophageal fistula was made given the observation of the absence of the subclavian and innominate arteries in the usual location. The sternotomy was closed and a CT of the chest was performed, which demonstrated the anomalous right subclavian artery without aneurysmal degeneration (Figures 1(a) and 1(b)). She was taken back to the operating room for endovascular covered stent grafting of the segment of the subclavian artery in continuity with the esophagus. An angiogram was performed (Figure 2(a)) and three covered stents were deployed to span the artery-esophageal fistula via

a right brachial artery approach (Figure 2(b)). Successful control of the bleeding was accomplished, but she experienced a cardiopulmonary arrest and died despite resuscitative efforts.

3. Discussion

The presence of an aberrant right subclavian artery (ARSA) is the most common aortic arch anomaly, present in 0.2–2.5% of the population [4, 5]. The discovery of this variation is usually an incidental finding on imaging studies performed for other reasons, but the anomaly is more prevalent in patients with Down's syndrome and patients with chromosome 22q11 deletions [5–8]. Previous reports have suggested that this anomaly is more common in females (65–72%), but in another study it had equal sex prevalence [6]. When an anomalous subclavian artery is present, it courses posterior to the esophagus in

80% of cases, between the esophagus and trachea in 15%, and anterior to the trachea in 5% [9, 10]. This anomalous artery often becomes aneurysmal, resulting in the development of what is known as "Kommerell's diverticulum."

Despite the relative frequency of ARSA, our case of ARSA-esophageal fistula is only the twentieth reported case of ARSA-esophageal fistula, which has involved both aneurysmal and nonaneurysmal anomalous arteries. None of the patients who developed an ARSA-esophageal fistula associated with an aneurysmal artery have survived, and none of the first ten reported cases of nonaneurysmal ARSA-esophageal fistula survived their bleeding episode. Hemorrhage was fatal in fourteen of these twenty patients, bringing the mortality rate in reported cases to 70%.

Diagnosis of the ARSA-esophageal fistula is challenging. In most cases, esophagoscopy cannot be used to assist in diagnosis of acute hemorrhage because of the extreme volume of hematemesis [3]. Upper endoscopy has been used in six reported cases and was able to identify the source of bleeding in only three patients [11–13]. This is comparable to the sensitivity of EGD in diagnosing artery-esophageal fistulas of 38% [11]. The risk of EGD dislodging a hemostatic clot and inciting recurrent hemorrhage has been recognized, and McFaddin et al. advocated EGD in the operating room with preparation for thoracotomy should this become necessary [3, 14]. In stable patients, cervicothoracic CT scanning with contrast for visualization of ARSA is the modality of choice. CT scanning can provide strong support of the diagnosis of artery-esophageal fistula [3]. Angiography can be performed in the operating room and can definitively define the presence of the anomalous subclavian artery and therefore heighten the index of suspicion for the presence of an anomalous subclavian to esophageal fistula.

Management of patients with bleeding from an anomalous subclavian artery to esophagus fistula is very challenging since bleeding in these patients presents as abrupt, rapidly exsanguinating hematemesis, and the etiology is from an unusual and unexpected source. Sentinel bleeding was reported in four of the twenty patients with ARSA-esophageal fistula, including our patient. In most patients with nonaneurysmal ARSA-esophageal fistula, presentation is abrupt, massive arterial bleeding for several days to weeks after placement of a nasogastric or endotracheal tube [3]. The occurrence of an initially limited episode of bleeding provides an opportunity to make an anatomic diagnosis and treat the problem before the final exsanguinating event.

Initial management can involve the use of a Sengstaken-Blakemore tube, which can be used to temporize the bleeding while the patient is stabilized, as in patients with any artery-esophageal fistula. In actively bleeding patients, right thoracotomy is recommended by most physicians to treat the problem. This results in appropriate exposure of both the anomalous artery and esophagus. In general, infants do not require revascularization of the right arm, because of excellent collateral circulation [2]. Adults, however, typically require revascularization after ligation and division of the aberrant vessel to prevent subclavian steal syndrome [13, 15]. Primary esophageal repair should be performed if limited

mediastinal contamination has occurred [2]. Muscle and fascial flaps are useful to provide a barrier between the esophagus and the involved artery.

In patients who are at high surgical risk and not likely to survive a thoracotomy, or those individuals with a limited life expectancy, arteriography with endovascular stent grafting may be used. Inman et al. advocated placing stents to span the width of the posterior esophagus overlapping anomalous artery on both the distal and proximal ends [4]. Although stent graft placement in a contaminated wound is not recommended as definitive therapy, it may be used as a temporizing measure [16, 17]. However, in 2008, Magagna et al. successfully placed an endovascular prosthesis in a ARSA-esophageal fistula of a 73-year-old woman undergoing chemoradiation therapy after total laryngectomy for laryngeal cancer who made a complete and prolonged recovery [18]. We were able to deploy three stents in the right subclavian artery in our patient. Unfortunately, she experienced a cardiac arrest in spite of successful deployment of covered stents and did not survive.

Associated risk factors for the development of ARSA-esophageal fistulization have varied (Table 1). Three patients had previously undergone grafting of the anomalous artery. Four patients were advanced in age and were found to have aneurysms of the ARSA. Three patients, including our patient, had been receiving long term corticosteroids. A child with Down's syndrome experienced fistulization from an esophageal stent placed after caustic ingestion. The most common associated risk factor, however, has been the prolonged presence of a nasogastric tube, which has been the case in thirteen of the nineteen patients reported in the literature. It is evident that prolonged placement of nasogastric or endotracheal tube or vascular grafts may result in significant compression, pressure, or friction with the ARSA, which is adjacent to the esophagus, resulting in formation of a fistula [3].

It is, therefore, logical to recommend avoiding prolonged nasogastric or endotracheal intubation in patients with known aberrant right subclavian artery. Feugier et al. have suggested screening of intensive care patients before long term placement of nasogastric tubes [3]. Transesophageal ultrasound is usually diagnostic, but this diagnosis can often be made as an incidental finding on a chest CT scan ordered for other reasons. The only chest CT that this patient had undergone was obtained earlier in her care when there was concern about contrast-related nephrotoxicity and therefore no intravenous contrast was given. At the time, she had severe lung consolidation and the anomalous artery was not recognized, even in retrospect.

Nasogastric tubes should be removed and gastrostomy performed in patients with ARSA on imaging [3]. Our patient underwent prolonged nasogastric tube placement for nutritive support secondary to dislodged PEG tube with resulting intraabdominal abscesses. Had we known she had an anomalous artery, perhaps reoperative surgical gastrostomy, jejunostomy placement, or the use of TPN would have been appropriate alternative sources of nutrition.

TABLE 1: Reported cases of anomalous subclavian artery-esophageal fistulae.

Study	Age (years)	Sex	Pathology	Cause	Predisposing factors	Time lag after intubation (days)	Outcome	Treatment	Sentinel bleed
Lynn, 1969	57	M		Aneurysm	Aneurysm		Fatal		
Reynes, 1976	72	F		Aneurysm	Aneurysm		Fatal		Yes
Merchant et al., 1977	17	F	Recovery after cesarian section	NGT		9	Fatal		
Livesay et al., 1982	25	M	Head trauma	ETT/NGT		13	Fatal		
Jungck and Puschel, 1983	6	M	Multiple trauma	ETT/NGT		42	Fatal		
Belkin et al., 1984	27	M	ENT cancer	NGT		60	Fatal		
Edwards et al., 1984	36	F	Subarachnoid hemorrhage	NGT	Corticotherapy	27	Fatal		Yes
Gosset et al., 1985	72	F	Recovery after aortic repair	ETT/NGT	Corticotherapy, infection, surgery	30	Fatal		
Guzzeta et al., 1989	0.4	F	Recovery after heart surgery	NGT			Survived		
Kulling, 1989		M			Aneurysm		Fatal		
Ikeda et al., 1991	9	M	Recovery after heart surgery	ETT/NGT	Surgery		Fatal		
Stone, 1990		M					Fatal		
Hirakata et al., 1991	55	M	Esophageal cancer	NGT	Surgery, irradiation, cancer	44	Survived		
Miller et al., 1996	11	F	Intracerebral hemorrhage	ETT/NGT		17	Survived	Surgery	No
Minyard and Smith, 2000	39	F	Head trauma	NGT			Fatal		
Feugier et al., 2003	24	M	Multiple trauma	ETT/NGT	Deceleration syndrome	31	Survived	Surgery	
Eynden, 2006	9	F		Esophageal stent	Caustic ingestion in Down syndrome patient with subsequent esophageal fissures and mediastinitis		Survived	Surgery	Yes
Inman et al., 2008	63	M		Salivary bypass tube	Chemotherapy and radiation, then salvage total laryngectomy and pharyngectomy		Fatal	Endovascular stent	Yes
Magagna et al., 2008	73	F			Laryngectomy, then chemotherapy and radiation therapy		Survived	Stent	Yes
Current study	41	F		NGT, tracheostomy tube	Corticotherapy, sepsis		Fatal	Stent	Yes

4. Conclusion

The course of an anomalous subclavian artery usually brings it posterior and contiguous with the esophagus. Although usually asymptomatic, the presence of prolonged nasogastric intubation may predispose an erosion of the esophagus into the adjacent artery leading to an arterial-esophageal fistula. Subclavian esophageal fistulae do not always present with sentinel bleeding. In stable patients, CT with contrast, angiography, and endoscopy may be useful in diagnosis and may reveal an otherwise unsuspected source. Once a diagnosis is made, bleeding from an ARSA-esophageal fistula may be temporized with a Sengstaken-Blakemore tube. Open surgical repair remains the gold standard of treatment, although endovascular stent grafts may be important to control life-threatening bleeding. The presence of a nasogastric tube is associated with development of these fistulae; therefore, prolonged NG tube placement should be carefully considered in patients with known anomalous right subclavian arteries.

Disclosure

This work was presented as a poster at the American Bronchoesophagological Association, Combined Otolaryngologic Spring Meeting in Chicago, IL, in April 2011.

References

[1] O. Dicle, M. Secil, A. Y. Goktay, and H. Akbaylar, "Subclavian artery aneurysm with oesophagoarterial fistula," *British Journal of Radiology*, vol. 72, pp. 1208–1210, 1999.

[2] R. G. Miller, D. K. Robie, S. L. Davis et al., "Survival after aberrant right subclavian artery-esophageal fistula: Case report and literature review," *Journal of Vascular Surgery*, vol. 24, no. 2, pp. 271–275, 1996.

[3] P. Feugier, L. Lemoine, L. Gruner, M. Bertin-Maghit, B. Rousselet, and J.-M. Chevalier, "Arterioesophageal fistula: a rare complication of retroesophageal subclavian arteries," *Annals of Vascular Surgery*, vol. 17, no. 3, pp. 302–305, 2003.

[4] J. C. Inman, P. Kim, and R. McHugh, "Retroesophageal subclavian artery - esophageal fistula: A rare complication of a salivary bypass tube," *Head & Neck*, vol. 30, no. 8, pp. 1120–1123, 2008.

[5] T. Nakatani, S. Tanaka, and S. Mizukami, "Anomalous triad of a left-sided inferior vena cava, a retroesophageal right subclavian artery, and bilateral superficial brachial arteries in one individual," *Clinical Anatomy*, vol. 11, no. 2, pp. 112–117, 1998.

[6] J. S. Easterbrook, "Identification of aberrant right subclavian artery on MR images of the cervical spine," *Journal of Magnetic Resonance Imaging*, vol. 2, no. 5, pp. 507–509, 1992.

[7] W. B. Goldstein, "Aberrant subclavian artery in mongolism," *The American Journal of Roentgenology Radium Therapy and Nuclear Medicine*, vol. 93, pp. 131–134, 1965.

[8] K. Momma, R. Matsuoka, and A. Takao, "Aortic arch anomalies associated with chromosome 22q11 deletion (CATCH 22)," *Pediatric Cardiology*, vol. 20, no. 2, pp. 97–102, 1999.

[9] A. Arkin, "Double aortic arch with total persistence of the right and isthmus stenosis of the left arch: A new clinical and X-ray picture. Report of six cases in adults," *American Heart Journal*, vol. 11, no. 4, pp. 444–474, 1936.

[10] M. M. Gomes, P. E. Bernatz, and R. J. Forth, "Arteriosclerotic aneurysm of an aberrant right subclavian artery.," *British Journal of Diseases of the Chest*, vol. 54, no. 6, pp. 549–552, 1968.

[11] G. D. Perdue Jr., R. B. Smith III, J. D. Ansley, and M. J. Costantino, "Impending aortoenteric hemorrhage. The effect of early recognition on improved outcome," *Annals of Surgery*, vol. 192, no. 3, pp. 237–243, 1980.

[12] D. Sosnowik, R. Greenberg, S. Bank, and L. M. Graver, "Aortoesophageal fistula: early and late endoscopic features," *American Journal of Gastroenterology*, vol. 83, no. 12, pp. 1401–1404, 1988.

[13] D. L. Akers Jr., R. J. Fowl, J. Plettner, and R. F. Kempczinski, "Complications of anomalous origin of the right subclavian artery: case report and review of the literature," *The Annals of Thoracic Surgery*, vol. 44, pp. 86–89, 1987.

[14] D. M. McFaddin and C. Dang, "Management of aortoesophageal fistula. a case report," *The American Surgeon*, vol. 51, no. 9, pp. 548–550, 1985.

[15] J. M. Smith, G. J. Reul, and D. C. Wukasch, "Retroesophageal subclavian arteries: surgical management of symptomatic children. cardiovascular diseases," *Bulletin of the Texas Heart Institute*, vol. 6, no. 3, pp. 331–334, 1979.

[16] F. M. Warren, J. I. Cohen, G. M. Nesbit, S. L. Barnwell, M. K. Wax, and P. E. Andersen, "Management of carotid 'blowout' with endovascular stent grafts," *The Laryngoscope*, vol. 112, no. 3, pp. 428–433, 2002.

[17] H. W. Pyun, D. H. Lee, H. M. Yoo et al., "Placement of covered stents for carotid blowout in patients with head and neck cancer: follow-up results after rescue treatments," *American Journal of Neuroradiology*, vol. 28, no. 8, pp. 1594–1598, 2007.

[18] P. Magagna, N. Abbiate, G. Mansi et al., "Endovascular treatment of aberrant right subclavian (lusorian) artery to oesophagus fistula: A case report," *Vascular and Endovascular Surgery*, vol. 42, no. 4, pp. 394–396, 2008.

48

Recurrent Upper Extremity Thrombosis Associated with Overactivity: A Case of Delayed Diagnosis of Paget-Schroetter Syndrome

Himani Sharma and Abhinav Tiwari

Department of Internal Medicine, University of Toledo Medical Center, Toledo, OH, USA

Correspondence should be addressed to Himani Sharma; himani007@gmail.com

Academic Editor: Halvor Naess

Paget-Schroetter syndrome is thrombosis of the axillary-subclavian vein that is associated with strenuous and repetitive activity of the upper extremities. Overuse of the arm coupled with external compression results in microtrauma in the intima of the subclavian vein, resulting in the activation of the coagulation cascade. Diagnosis is usually made by Doppler ultrasound and the treatment involves thrombolysis, while routine surgical decompression of the thoracic outlet is controversial. In this report, we present a case of a patient who presented with a second episode of spontaneous right upper extremity deep venous thrombosis. The first episode was inadequately treated with oral anticoagulation alone. During the second episode, Paget-Schroetter syndrome was diagnosed, after careful review of his occupational history. He subsequently underwent angioplasty and decompression of thoracic outlet with no recurrence of thrombosis in a 12-month follow-up period.

1. Introduction

Paget-Schroetter syndrome (PSS) or "effort" thrombosis of the axillary-subclavian vein is an uncommon cause of deep vein thrombosis (DVT) seen in physically active and otherwise healthy individuals. It was first described by Paget in 1875 and Von Schroetter in 1884 and was named the "Paget-Schroetter syndrome" by Hughes in 1949 [1]. PSS accounts for 30–40% of spontaneous axillary-subclavian vein thrombosis (ASVT) and for 10–20% of all upper extremity deep venous thrombosis (UEDVT) [2]. Despite being a known cause of UEDVT, this entity is usually undiagnosed or misdiagnosed, mainly due to lack of awareness of the syndrome. Pathogenesis involves microtrauma to the intima of vasculature leading to intraluminal clot formation [3]. Diagnosis is usually made by Doppler ultrasound, computed tomography, and magnetic resonance venography. Oral anticoagulation alone is insufficient and catheter-directed thrombolysis (CDT) is usually performed [4]. Doing routine thoracic outlet decompression surgery following pharmacomechanical intervention is a topic of debate. In this report, we describe a case of a 38-year-old male patient who presented with second episode of right UEDVT in one year. Due to rigorous use of his right arm, PSS was suspected and he received pharmacochemical thrombolysis followed by first rib resection (FRR).

2. Case Report

A 38-year-old male patient was admitted with a two-week history of painful swelling of the right upper extremity. He denied any history of fever, rash, joint pain, or insect bite. He gave a history of a right UEDVT, diagnosed one year ago, treated with six months of oral rivaroxaban with no subsequent follow-up visits. On examination, he had a temperature of 37.5°C, a blood pressure of 128/78 mmHg, a pulse rate of 76 beats/minute, a respiratory rate of 18 breaths/minute, and an oxygen saturation of 98% on room air. On inspection, he had noticeable swelling and redness extending from his right wrist to the shoulder, and there was no superficially engorged vein on the arm or the chest. On palpation, he had mild tenderness of the affected area. All peripheral pulses were palpable and capillary refill time at right thumbnail was

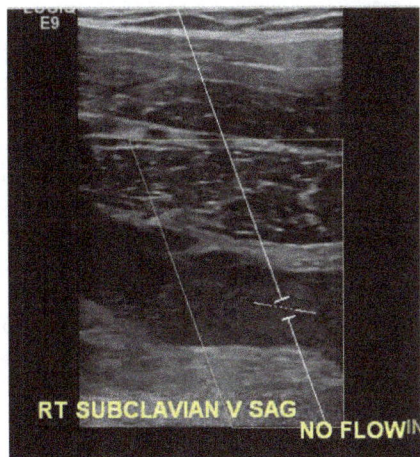

FIGURE 1: Doppler ultrasound showing absence of blood flow in the subclavian vein.

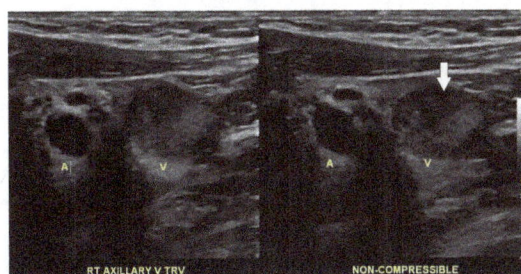

FIGURE 2: Doppler ultrasound showing noncompressibility of the axillary vein (arrow) due to thrombus.

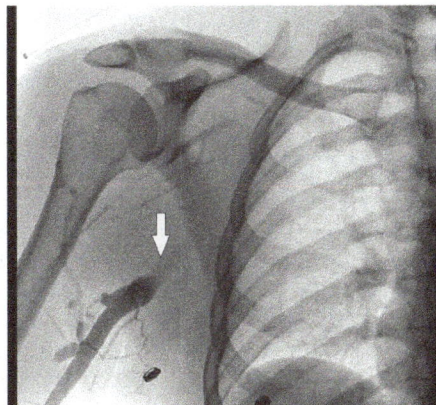

FIGURE 3: Angiogram showing abrupt cut-off in the contrast flow in the axillary vein (arrow) indicating obstruction.

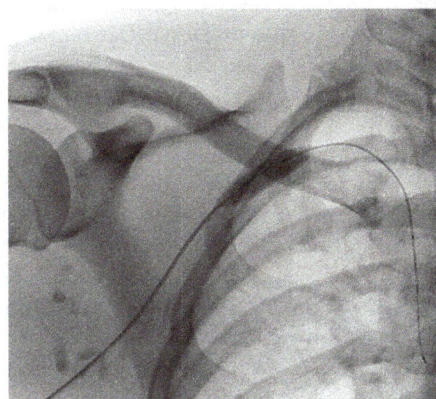

FIGURE 4: Fluoroscopic image showing balloon angioplasty being performed.

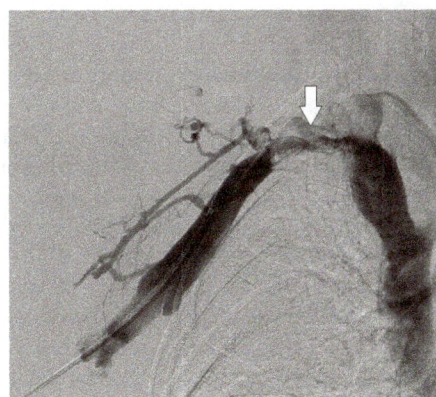

FIGURE 5: Peripheral angiogram showing residual stenosis at the level of clavicle (arrow) after performing thrombectomy and angioplasty.

<2 sec. There was no palpable lymphadenopathy. All of his laboratory workup, including the complete blood count and coagulation profile, was unremarkable. A Doppler ultrasound of the right upper limb showed thrombosis of the right axillary, subclavian vein, and brachial veins (Figures 1 and 2), following which he was started on intravenous (IV) unfractionated heparin. The patient had no history of trauma and no personal history of malignancy or intravenous (IV) drug abuse. The etiology of the recurrent spontaneous DVT was initially unclear; however, on further questioning, the patient mentioned that he was a construction worker and his job involved a rigorous use of right arm with repetitive overhead labor. This additional information about his occupation led to the realization that PSS or effort thrombosis could be an etiology of ASVT in the context of arm activity. Urgent cardiology consult was obtained, and it was decided that the patient should undergo pharmacomechanical thrombolysis. Angiography revealed an abrupt cut-off in the contrast flow in the axillary vein (Figure 3). The AngioJet device was used for an initial run of thrombectomy followed by power pulse spray of tissue plasminogen activator (tPA) throughout the length of the thrombotic segment. Subsequently, thrombectomy was performed in multiple runs along the entire length of the thrombosed vein and repeat images showed a markedly improved contrast flow through the vein. However, there was some residual stenosis in the subclavian vein at the level of the

first rib. Balloon venoplasty was then performed, using a 10 × 20 mm and subsequently using a 10 × 40 mm Charger balloon (Figure 4). Repeat venography revealed the presence of mild residual stenosis at the level of the first rib (Figure 5). Due to this residual stenosis, it was decided to surgically resect the first rib. During the surgical procedure, the subclavian vein was found to be thickened and had few collaterals, some of which were taken down. Intraoperatively, it was also noticed that the space between the first rib and the clavicle was extremely narrow and hypertrophied subclavius muscle was compressing the vein. Careful dissection of the subclavius muscle was performed following which the scalenus anterior and scalenus medius muscles were identified and removed in piecemeal. Lastly, the middle part of the first rib was transected. The patient tolerated the procedure well and was discharged on the second postoperative day on rivaroxaban for 6 months. The patient, at 6- and 12-month follow-up had no recurrence of symptoms while he continued his job as a construction worker.

3. Discussion

Upper extremity DVT can have a primary etiology, which accounts for about 20% of cases and includes either acquired or congenital anatomical anomalies. The remainder, 80% cases, are caused by secondary factors including the use of central venous or dialysis catheter, pacemaker insertion, and parenteral nutrition. Other secondary causes are the use of oral contraceptive pills, hypercoagulable state, and surgery on the upper arm [3]. Upper extremity DVT caused by secondary factors is usually treated with removal of the offending agent combined with anticoagulation use. Primary effort thrombosis or PSS is a rare entity with incidence between 1 and 2 per 100,000 population per year [3] and accounts for 1–4% of all venous thrombosis [4, 5]. About 60% to 80% of patients report repetitive and rigorous upper extremity activity, such as pitching, swimming, weight lifting, or even manual labor, at the onset of symptoms [6–8]. Therefore, it is more commonly seen in the dominant arm [9]. PSS is a sequela of thoracic outlet syndrome (TOS), as it involves compression of the subclavian vein, as it courses over the first rib, posterior to the clavicle in the anterior-most part of the thoracic outlet. Numerous factors can lead to its extrinsic compression, including anomalous subclavius or scalenus anterior, a long transverse process of the cervical spine, cervical rib, abnormal insertion of the first rib, congenital fibromuscular bands, or narrowing of the costoclavicular space from the depression of the shoulder [3, 10]. Subclavian vein is also subjected to intrinsic trauma due to repetitive shoulder-arm motion causing microscopic intimal tears in the vessel wall. It is postulated that chronic compression and microintimal trauma cause inflammation, which eventually leads to intimal hyperplasia and fibrosis of connective tissue surrounding the vein [11]. Fibrosis and scarring of tissue surrounding the vein decrease the mobility, thus making it susceptible to injury. Patients with effort thrombosis have an acute or subacute presentation and typically presents with a painful swollen and erythematous arm. On palpation, the arm is cold and tender with palpable venous cords [9, 12]. A duplex ultrasound scan is diagnostic with 56% to 100% sensitivity and 94% to 100% specificity for detecting DVT [8]. Once the diagnosis of PSS is established, a venography is recommended for both confirmation and therapeutics. A clot is usually visualized in the subclavian vein at the costoclavicular area or sometimes even more distally. The

presence of collaterals also supports the diagnosis of PSS [3]. It is recommended to initiate treatment with parenteral anticoagulation when the diagnosis of PSS is confirmed [13]. Thrombolytic therapy is of most benefit to patients who have moderate-to-severe symptoms related to sudden axillosubclavian thrombosis. Catheter-directed pharmacological thrombolysis restores vein patency in 64 to 84% cases, with improved patency rates associated with earlier initiation of therapy [14]. Despite limited data on utility, mechanical thrombolysis (EKOS catheter, AngioJet) is often used in combination with pharmacologic thrombolysis [15]. Occasionally, percutaneous transluminal angioplasty (PTA) is performed to keep the vein open following thrombolysis if thoracic outlet decompression is contemplated [3]. There is conflicting data regarding routine resection of the first rib at the time of diagnosis of PSS. Some studies have shown that both nonsurgical and surgical groups show decent outcomes if the first rib is left alone [16–18]. However, many other observational studies suggest that there is a lower rate of recurrent thrombosis with reduced long-term morbidity with surgical decompression of the thoracic outlet, as compared to a more conservative approach [3, 19]. A meta-analysis showed that the symptom relief (95%) and vein patency rate (98%) were significantly more in the surgical group as compared to the group in which the rib is not removed (54% and 48%, resp.) [20]. In a retrospective study involving 22 patients with PSS, it was shown that pharmacomechanical thrombolysis followed by FRR had successful vein patency rate of 86% and all except 1 of the 22 patients were asymptomatic. The mean follow-up time was 25 ± 17 months [21]. In our case, the inciting events were repetitive endovascular trauma and external compression, which were not addressed during the first episode of DVT with anticoagulation alone; hence he presented with a second episode. In conclusion, occupational or recreational history plays a pivotal role in diagnosing PSS and failure to perform thrombectomy and surgical decompression may result in recurrent episodes of upper extremity DVT in such cases.

Disclosure

All the authors of this paper have reviewed the document in its entirety and agree with the structure and content.

References

[1] E. S. R. Hughes, "Venous obstruction in the upper extremity; Paget-Schroetter's syndrome; a review of 320 cases," *Surgery, gynecology & obstetrics*, vol. 88, no. 2, pp. 89–127, 1949.

[2] E. Bernardi, R. Pesavento, and P. Prandoni, "Upper extremity deep venous thrombosis," in *Seminars in Thrombosis and Hemostasis*, vol. 32, no. 07, pp. 729–736, Thieme Medical Publishers, Inc., New York, NY, USA, October 2006.

[3] K. A. Illig and A. J. Doyle, "A comprehensive review of Paget-Schroetter syndrome," *Journal of Vascular Surgery*, vol. 51, no. 6, pp. 1538–1547, 2010.

[4] V. Vijaysadan, A. M. Zimmerman, and R. E. Pajaro, "Paget-Schroetter syndrome in the young and active," *The Journal of the American Board of Family Practice*, vol. 18, no. 4, pp. 314–319, 2005.

[5] P. Prandoni, "Upper extremity deep vein thrombosis," *Current Opinion in Pulmonary Medicine*, vol. 5, no. 4, pp. 222–226, 1999.

[6] Y. Sternbach and R. M. Green, "Endovascular and surgical management of acute axillary-subclavian venous thrombosis," in *Handbook of Venous Disease*, Hodder Arnold, London, UK, 2nd edition, 2001.

[7] H. V. Joffe, N. Kucher, V. F. Tapson, and S. Z. Goldhaber, "Upper-extremity deep vein thrombosis: a prospective registry of 592 patients," *Circulation*, vol. 110, no. 12, pp. 1605–1611, 2004.

[8] B. O. Mustafa, S. W. Rathbun, T. L. Whitsett, and G. E. Raskob, "Sensitivity and specificity of ultrasonography in the diagnosis of upper extremity deep vein thrombosis: A systematic review," *Archives of Internal Medicine*, vol. 162, no. 4, pp. 401–404, 2002.

[9] B. Lindblad, L. Tengborn, and D. Bergqvist, "Deep vein thrombosis of the axillary-subclavian veins: epidemiologic data, effects of different types of treatment and late sequele," *European Journal of Vascular Surgery*, vol. 2, no. 3, pp. 161–165, 1988.

[10] N. A. Mall, G. S. Van Thiel, W. M. Heard, G. A. Paletta, C. Bush-Joseph, and B. R. Bach Jr., "Paget-Schroetter Syndrome: a review of effort thrombosis of the upper extremity from a sports medicine perspective," *Sports Health*, vol. 5, no. 4, pp. 353–356, 2013.

[11] S. Aziz, C. J. Straehley, and T. J. Whelan Jr., "Effort-related axillo-subclavian vein thrombosis. A new theory of pathogenesis and a plea for direct surgical intervention," *The American Journal of Surgery*, vol. 152, no. 1, pp. 57–61, 1986.

[12] J. T. Adams and J. A. DeWeese, "Effort thrombosis of the axillary and subclavian veins," *Journal of Trauma and Acute Care Surgery*, vol. 11, no. 11, pp. 923–930, 1971.

[13] C. Kearon, E. A. Akl, A. J. Comerota et al., "Antithrombotic therapy for VTE disease: antithrombotic therapy and prevention of thrombosis, 9th ed: American College of Chest Physicians evidence-based clinical practice guidelines," *Chest*, vol. 141, no. 2, pp. e419S–e494S, 2012.

[14] A. Vik, P. A. Holme, K. Singh et al., "Catheter-directed thrombolysis for treatment of deep venous thrombosis in the upper extremities," *CardioVascular and Interventional Radiology*, vol. 32, no. 5, pp. 980–987, 2009.

[15] H. S. Kim, A. Patra, B. E. Paxton, J. Khan, and M. B. Streiff, "Catheter-directed thrombolysis with percutaneous rheolytic thrombectomy versus thrombolysis alone in upper and lower extremity deep vein thrombosis," *CardioVascular and Interventional Radiology*, vol. 29, no. 6, pp. 1003–1007, 2006.

[16] I. Martinelli, T. Battaglioli, P. Bucciarelli, S. M. Passamonti, and P. Mannuccio Mannucci, "Risk factors and recurrence rate of primary deep vein thrombosis of the upper extremities," *Circulation*, vol. 110, no. 5, pp. 566–570, 2004.

[17] D. Lechner, C. Wiener, A. Weltermann, L. Eischer, S. Eichinger, and P. A. Kyrle, "Comparison between idiopathic deep vein thrombosis of the upper and lower extremity regarding risk factors and recurrence," *Journal of Thrombosis and Haemostasis*, vol. 6, no. 8, pp. 1269–1274, 2008.

[18] A. Hingorani, E. Ascher, E. Lorenson et al., "Upper extremity deep venous thrombosis and its impact on morbidity and mortality rates in a hospital-based population," *Journal of Vascular Surgery*, vol. 26, no. 5, pp. 853–860, 1997.

[19] H. C. Urschel Jr. and A. N. Patel, "Surgery remains the most effective treatment for Paget-Schroetter syndrome: 50 years' experience," *The Annals of Thoracic Surgery*, vol. 86, no. 1, pp. 254–260, 2008.

[20] J. Lugo, A. Tanious, P. Armstrong et al., "Acute paget-schroetter syndrome: Does the first rib routinely need to be removed after thrombolysis? Presented at the second annual International Society for Vascular Surgery Meeting, Miami, FL, 2013.," *Annals of Vascular Surgery*, vol. 29, no. 6, pp. 1073–1077, 2015.

[21] J. M. Kärkkäinen, H. Nuutinen, T. Riekkinen et al., "Pharmacomechanical Thrombectomy in Paget–Schroetter Syndrome," *CardioVascular and Interventional Radiology*, vol. 39, no. 9, pp. 1272–1279, 2016.

49

Left Brachiocephalic Vein Stenosis due to the Insertion of a Temporal Right Subclavian Hemodialysis Catheter

Eleni I. Skandalou,[1] **Fani D. Apostolidou-Kiouti,**[2]
Ilias D. Minasidis,[1] **and Ioannis K. Skandalos**[2]

[1]*Renal Unit "Therapeutiki", Thessaloniki, Greece*
[2]*Surgical Department, General Hospital "Agios Pavlos", Thessaloniki, Greece*

Correspondence should be addressed to Eleni I. Skandalou; skandaloueleni@gmail.com

Academic Editor: Nikolaos Papanas

Central vein stenosis/occlusion is a common well-described sequel to the placement of hemodialysis catheters in the central venous system. The precise mechanisms by which central vein stenosis occurs are not well known. Current concepts in central vein stenosis pathophysiology focus on the response to vessel injury model, emphasizing the process of trauma. A case of left brachiocephalic vein stenosis due to the insertion and function of a temporary right subclavian hemodialysis catheter is presented. The purpose of the manuscript is to emphasize that, with the introduction of a temporary subclavian hemodialysis catheter via the right subclavian vein apart from causing concurrent stenosis/infarction of the right subclavian and right brachiocephalic vein, it is also possible to cause stenosis of the left brachiocephalic vein (close to its contribution to the superior vena cava) although the catheter tip is placed in the correct anatomical position in the superior vena cava.

1. Introduction

Central vein stenosis/occlusion is a common well-described sequel to the placement of hemodialysis catheters in the central venous system [1, 2]. This situation, in the dialysis patients, is a serious problem and it has a greater impact on the blood inflow compared with stenosis of a peripheral vein, because the central veins represent the final common pathway for blood flow from the periphery to the heart. Central vein stenosis obviates the possibility of creating a new arteriovenous hemodialysis vascular access on the affected side, as the hemodialysis vascular access is frequently lost with the stenosis progression [3]. A consequence of a central vein stenosis is diminished long-term patency of an ipsilateral arteriovenous vascular access. A case of left brachiocephalic vein stenosis due to the insertion and function of a temporary right subclavian hemodialysis catheter is presented.

2. Case Presentation

A 53-year-old man with end stage renal disease, due to renovascular hypertension, started dialysis with right subclavian temporal dialysis catheter four years ago. The introduction of the temporary right subclavian hemodialysis catheter, in the first hospital where the patient was managed, took place with chest X-ray confirmation of the correct catheter tip position in the superior vena cava. A natural radial-cephalic arteriovenous vascular access was created 3 months after that. The performed vascular access needed 6 weeks for its maturation, so the temporal hemodialysis catheter was removed 4.5 months after its insertion. The arteriovenous vascular access was in function for 7 months. The vascular access thrombosis was managed by another ipsilateral proximally brachiocephalic arteriovenous anastomosis which was used directly, due to already maturation of the cephalic vein. In the laboratory investigation, the patient was found to be in procoagulant state with heterozygous factor V (Leiden). A gradually aggravated left upper arm swelling followed by left chest wall swelling and collateral veins dilatation was manifested (Figure 1).

The vascular access angiography showed a large stenosis of the left brachiocephalic vein close to its contribution to the superior vena cava (Figure 2), obviously at the contact

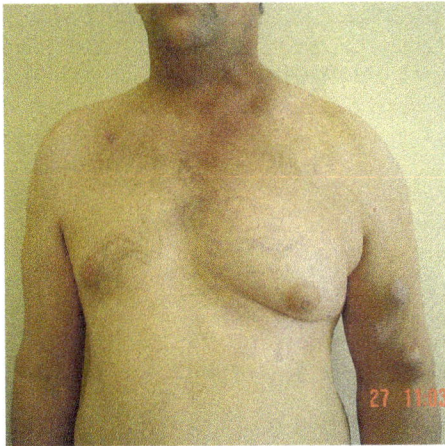

FIGURE 1: Swelling of the left upper arm and left chest wall. Right subclavian scar.

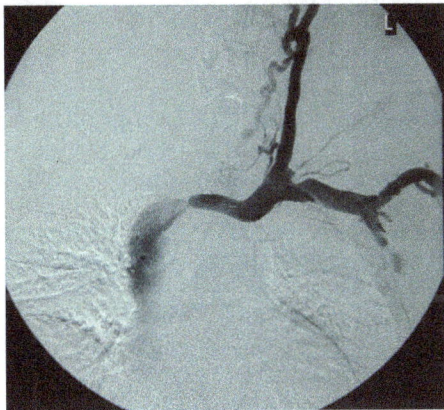

FIGURE 2: Vascular access angiography: stenosis of the left brachiocephalic vein close to the superior vena cava.

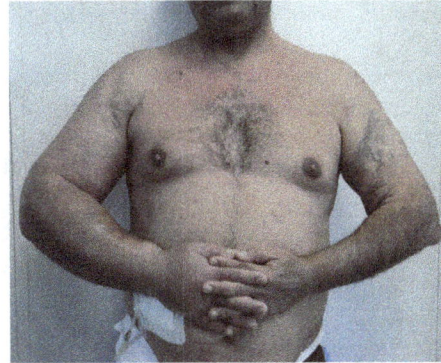

FIGURE 3: Excessive edema of the right upper arm. Inserted peritoneal dialysis catheter.

point with the tip of the initially introduced temporary right subclavian catheter. Because of the patient's thrombophilic status, a percutaneous angioplasty (PTA) and stenting of the venous stenosis were not attempted.

After that, a right natural radial-cephalic arteriovenous anastomosis was performed and after its maturation the left arm vascular access was ligated. The new vascular access was in use for 16 months, with incidents of venous thrombotic events, progressive right upper arm edema, and venous hypertension (right subclavian vein stenosis). Patient did not show any signs or symptoms related to cerebral oedema and/or brain disorders.

We moved on peritoneal dialysis to manage our patient (Figure 3).

3. Discussion

The precise mechanisms by which central vein stenosis occurs are not well known. Current concepts in central vein stenosis pathophysiology focus on the response to vessel injury model, emphasizing the process of trauma [4], catheter's material and catheter's contact to venous intima, uremic environment, inflammation, intimal hyperplasia, and a fibrotic response. Regardless of the predominant underlying cause, the final result is the same. There is an upregulation of proinflammatory transcription factors and profibrotic genes, which in turn causes smooth muscle proliferation and thickening of the venous intima [2, 5]. The resulting venous stenosis/obstruction causes venous hypertension. This condition is related to oedema of the arm, difficulty using the vascular access or its loss, and arm dysfunction [2].

The use of silicone catheters for subclavian cannulation is safe and effective to provide temporary vascular access for acute hemodialysis. The incidence of subclavian vein stenosis due to the use of silicone catheters is lower compared to polytetrafluoroethylene and polyurethane catheters. In a comparative study, the polyurethane catheters were also found to be less traumatic than the polytetrafluoroethylene catheters for the venous intima [6].

The initial stenosis is located at the point of the venous wall trauma caused by the insertion of a venous catheter. Furthermore, the direct contact of the catheter with the venous endothelium into the venous lumen and the venous intima trauma caused by the constant venous movement associated with the procedures of breathing and heart function are causes of venous stenosis. The above causes may lead to generation of thrombin, platelet activation, expression of P-selectin, and an inflammatory reaction with increased inflammatory markers [7]. In an autopsy study, there was found that even temporary catheters were associated with focal and local endothelial damage, endothelial denudation and attached organized thrombus, endothelial cells, and collagen [5]. Histological examination of samples of subclavian vein stenosis confirmed endothelial hyperplasia, indicating the presence of fibrous tissue.

Inflammation has an important role in central venous stenosis. The pathology associated with this lesion is characterized by neointimal hyperplasia, which is a common response closely related to vessel injury and inflammation [5, 8]. In our case, the right subclavian catheter tip, lead in a straight route through the right brachiocephalic vein, could be in contact and cause injury to the left brachiocephalic vein endothelium at the point near to its junction to the superior vena cava.

Another mechanism of vascular wall damage is the blood flow turbulence at the catheter's insertion site due to constriction of the vein lumen as well as the turbulence of the blood inflow to the venous blood system from the catheter's tip during the hemodialysis [9]. In our case, the mechanism of intima damage from the blood flow turbulence obviously contributed to the stenosis, due to the proximity or contact of the tip of the right subclavian catheter to the left brachiocephalic vein endothelium at the point near to its junction to the superior vena cava.

Moreover, the hypothesis of uremic environment effect has been supported by recent findings of intimal changes in the cephalic vein of renal failure patients, even prior to arteriovenous fistula (AVF) creation [10]. Intravascular thrombosis can be caused by the release of profibrotic cytokines that are associated with platelet aggregation.

In the 1980s the subclavian venous access was already in a wide use, and a link between subclavian venous catheterization and central venous stenosis was identified back then. In the early 1990s, a removal of the subclavian to the jugular vein catheterization was observed and this option withstood time. Unfortunately, even nowadays, more than 30 years after, the subclavian catheterization continues to be used, even for temporal hemodialysis catheter insertion. Regarding the right subclavian vein catheterization, the venous anatomy should be taken into consideration, as there are two angles in the catheter route: the subclavian to internal jugular junction and the contribution of two brachiocephalic veins to form the superior vena cava. The particularity of this anatomy resulted, in our case, in the left brachiocephalic vein stenosis by a temporal right subclavian hemodialysis catheter. We must note that the initial right subclavian vein catheterization was the cause of all problems that occurred and of such a short time (less than 3 years) of possibility for the patient's therapy by hemodialysis.

4. Conclusion

A temporal right subclavian hemodialysis catheter can cause stenosis, not only to the ipsilateral, but also to the heterolateral brachiocephalic vein, with devastating consequences for the creation and function of a hemodialysis arteriovenous vascular access in both arms, as well as for the arm function.

References

[1] V. N. Krishna, J. B. Eason, and M. Allon, "Central Venous Occlusion in the Hemodialysis Patient," *American Journal of Kidney Diseases*, vol. 68, no. 5, pp. 803–807, 2016.

[2] A. S. Yevzlin, "Hemodialysis catheter-associated central venous stenosis," *Seminars in Dialysis*, vol. 21, no. 6, pp. 522–527, 2008.

[3] K. A. Illig, "Management of central vein stenoses and occlusions: The critical importance of the costoclavicular junction," *Seminars in Vascular Surgery*, vol. 24, no. 2, pp. 113–118, 2011.

[4] A. K. Agarwal, "Central Vein Stenosis: Current Concepts," *Advances in Chronic Kidney Disease*, vol. 16, no. 5, pp. 360–370, 2009.

[5] A. R. Forauer and C. Theoharis, "Histologic changes in the human vein wall adjacent to indwelling central venous catheters," *Journal of Vascular and Interventional Radiology*, vol. 14, no. 9 I, pp. 1163–1168, 2003.

[6] H. Tanabe, R. Murayama, K. Yabunaka et al., "Low-angled peripheral intravenous catheter tip placement decreases phlebitis," *Journal of Vascular Access*, vol. 17, no. 6, pp. 542–547, 2016.

[7] T. Palabrica, R. Lobb, B. C. Furie et al., "Leukocyte accumulation promoting fibrin deposition is mediated in vivo by P-selectin on adherent platelets," *Nature*, vol. 359, no. 6398, pp. 848–851, 1992.

[8] A. Torres, D. Hernández, S. Suria et al., "Subclavian catheter-related infection is a major risk factor for the late development of subclavian vein stenosis," *Nephrology Dialysis Transplantation*, vol. 8, no. 3, pp. 227–230, 1993.

[9] S. Unnikrishnan, T. N. Huynh, B. C. Brott et al., "Turbulent flow evaluation of the venous needle during hemodialysis," *Journal of Biomechanical Engineering*, vol. 127, no. 7, pp. 1141–1146, 2005.

[10] M. A. Wali, R. A. Eid, M. Dewan, and M. A. Al-Homrany, "Intimal Changes in the Cephalic Vein of Renal Failure Patients before Arterio-Venous Fistula (AVF) Construction," *Journal of Smooth Muscle Research*, vol. 39, no. 4, pp. 95–105, 2003.

50

A Case of Unusual Vascularization of Upper Abdominal Cavity Organs

Natalia Mazuruc,[1] **Serghei Covantev**(iD),[2] **and Olga Belic**[1]

[1]*Department of Human Anatomy, State University of Medicine and Pharmacy «Nicolae Testemitanu», Chisinau, Moldova*
[2]*Laboratory of Allergology and Clinical Immunology, State University of Medicine and Pharmacy «Nicolae Testemitanu», Chisinau, Moldova*

Correspondence should be addressed to Serghei Covantev; kovantsev.s.d@gmail.com

Academic Editor: Muzaffer Sindel

We describe a case report of multiple arterial variations of internal organs of upper abdominal cavity in a cadaver of 63-year-old female. There were several developmental variations of the vascular supply of the stomach, pancreas, spleen, and liver. There were several accessory arteries: left gastric, left hepatic, and posterior gastric artery as well as several arteries that had abnormal origin. The variations were discovered during macroscopical dissection at the department of human anatomy. It should be noted that multiple developmental variation can be common in clinical practice and clinicians should be aware of them during diagnostic and interventional procedures.

1. Introduction

The upper part of abdominal cavity is limited by the diaphragm from the top, from the sides by lateral abdominal walls and from the inferior part by the transverse colon and its mesentery. This anatomical region is particularly important for hepatopancreatobiliary, vascular, and transplant surgeons as it is rich in anatomical variations that can compromise the procedure. The vascularization of upper abdominal cavity' organs has been studied abundantly [1].

The celiac trunk provides the vascular supply of the upper abdominal organs. Uflacker classified the celiac trunk into 8 types: classic coeliac trunk, hepatosplenic trunk, hepato-gastric trunk, hepatosplenicmesenteric trunk, gastrosplenic trunk, coeliac-mesenteric trunk, and no coeliac trunk [2]. Michel classified the vascular supply of the liver in 10 types and later Hiatt modified this classification [3, 4]. The splenic artery may have two, three, four, and five terminal branches or enter the splenic tissue without branching. A more complex classification is provided by Vandamme and Bonte who describe bifurcation of the splenic artery into two rami lienalis where the gastroepiploic artery is a collateral of the splenic stem; trifurcation of the splenic artery; truncus lienogastroepiploicus [5].

Detailed knowledge of topographical and morphological as well as the functional possibilities of the anatomical regional and its surrounding structures including collateral paths of vascularization is essential for surgical procedures [6]. It is important to limit the risk of vascular injury, particularly in the presence of anatomical variations for a variety of procedures and especially in transplant surgery [7].

2. Anatomical Case

During the macroscopical dissection of a 63-year-old female cadaver we determined several anomalies of the vascularization of upper abdominal cavity organs.

The celiac trunk branched into two vessels: the left gastric artery and a hepatosplenic trunk, which further divided into splenic and common hepatic arteries (Figure 1).

The splenic artery in its proximal part had a sinuous trajectory. In the medium part of the vessel the artery had a curve with the base situated superiorly which then continued in a straight manner in the prehilar area. In the hilar region the splenic artery branches into three branches of the first order, two of which were terminal and entered directly into splenic parenchyma.

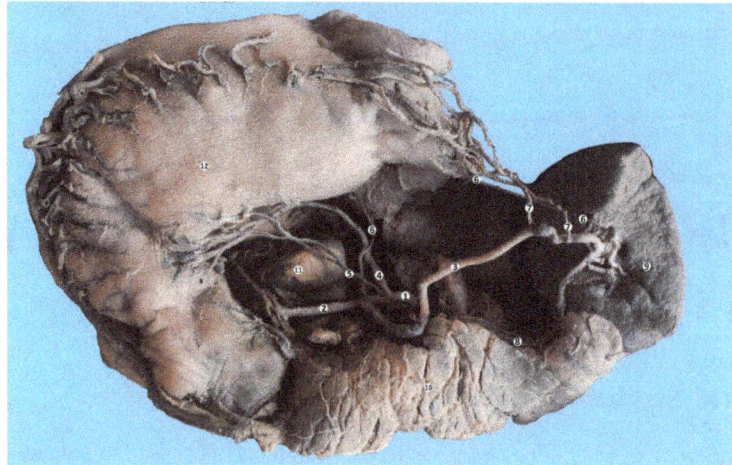

FIGURE 1: The branches of the celiac trunk. Macrospecimen (female, 63 years old). 1: celiac trunk, 2: common hepatic artery, 3: splenic artery, 4: left gastric artery, 5: accessory left gastric artery, 6: posterior gastric artery, 7: left gastroepiploic artery 8: splenic vein, 9: spleen, 10: pancreas, 11: caudate lobe of the liver, and 12: stomach.

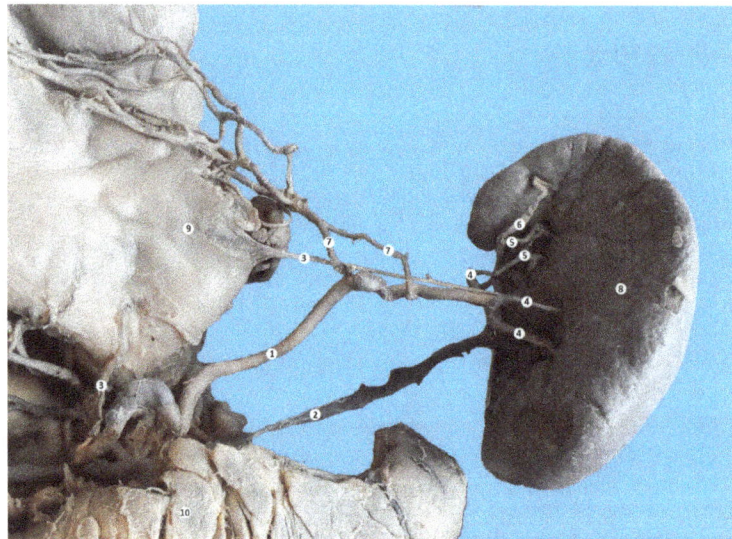

FIGURE 2: The branches of splenic artery. Macrospecimen (female, 63 years old). 1: splenic artery, 2: splenic vein, 3: posterior gastric artery, 4: splenic arteries of the first order 5: splenic arteries of the second order, 6: superior polar artery 7: left gastroepiploic artery 8: spleen, 9: stomach, and 10: pancreas.

The superior splenic branch of the first order divided into two second order branches. From the superior second order branch a superior polar branch took origin (Figure 2). From the distal third of the splenic artery took origin two left gastroepiploic arteries (at 8 and 10 cm, respectively) which participated in the vascularization of the posterior stomach wall and the great omentum.

We should also mention the presence of two posterior gastric arteries, which also branched from the splenic artery. The first posterior gastric artery took origin from the site, where the splenic artery branched from the hepatosplenic trunk and passed to the fundus of the stomach. The second posterior gastric artery is a more common variant that took origin from the second branch of the first order (Figures 1 and 2). The lesser curve of the stomach was vascularized by two

left gastric arteries and right gastric artery. The accessory left gastric artery branched from the proximal third of the splenic artery (2,7 cm from its origin).

The common hepatic artery passed near the right side of the caudate lobe of the liver and at the level of the pancreas head (after giving a gastroduodenal branch) continued into proper hepatic artery which branched into left hepatic arteries and a larger right hepatic artery (Figure 3).

A rare variation is also the presence of an accessory left hepatic artery, which began from the proper hepatic artery and supplied the left and the caudate lobes of the liver. From the proper hepatic artery took origin the superior duodenal artery that passed to the bulb of the duodenum. The proper hepatic artery then gave off its terminal branches: the right and left hepatic arteries. The intermediate hepatic artery

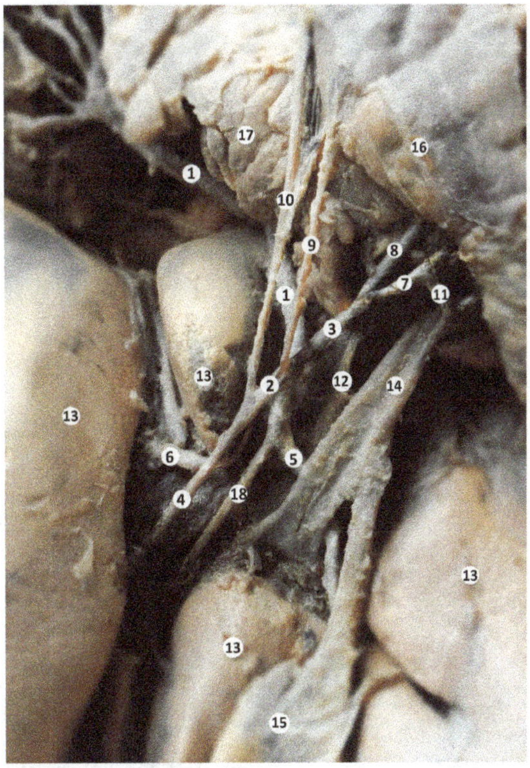

FIGURE 3: Liver blood supply. Macrospecimen (female, 63-year-old). 1 – common hepatic artery, 2 – proper hepatic artery, 3 – gastroduodenal artery, 4 – left hepatic artery, 5 – right hepatic artery, 6 – accessory left hepatic artery, 7 – right gastroepiploic artery, 8 – superior posterior pancreaticoduodenal artery, 9 – superior duodenal artery, 10 – right gastric artery, 11 – the branch of the superior anterior pancreaticoduodenal artery, 12 – portal vein, 13 – liver, 14 – common bile duct, 15 – gall bladder, 16 – duodenum, 17 – pancreas, 18 – intermediate hepatic artery.

branched from the right hepatic artery and passed to the quadrate lobe of the liver (Figure 3).

The cystic artery was situated behind the cystic duct, outside the Calot triangle, and had only a posterior branch that entered and vascularized the posterior wall of the gallbladder (Figure 4).

The gastroduodenal artery gave two branches: the posterior superior pancreaticoduodenal artery and the right gastroepiploic artery. From the right gastroepiploic artery branched the superior anterior pancreaticoduodenal artery and a short branch to the common bile duct (Figures 3, 4, and 5). A graphical representation of all of the anatomical variations is present in Figure 6.

3. Discussions

Based on the current data from the literature there are multiple types of liver and gallbladder vascularization. Watson and Harper (2015) report that the hepatic artery can have variable origin (10 types based on Michels classification, 1955). There are often accessory left and right hepatic arteries (10-20% of cases) [8].

The trifurcation of the hepatic artery can be encountered in approximately 3.3% of cases [9]. The gastroduodenal artery can have the accessory branches or, in rare cases, be absent. In 11% of cases, patients may have an arterial pattern, which is not described in Michel's classification

[10]. Although, the presence of accessory hepatic arteries is not uncommon the combination of accessory hepatic arteries and extrahepatic arteries (duodenum and pancreas) is rare. Therefore, the present case demonstrates an even more complicated vascular anatomy at the level of hepatogastric and hepatoduodenal ligament. A vessel is named "additions" or "accessory" typically when the second vessel is smaller in diameter or has an abnormal origin.

De Martino RR and coworkers consider that the anomalies of the splenic artery can be part of the celiac trunk anomalies. The vessel may start from the aorta with one or two branches. It also may take origin from left gastric, middle colic, or left hepatic artery [11]. The present case is an example of hepatosplenic trunk (type II variation by Uflacker). A type II celiac trunk anatomy is found in 7.1-8% of cases [12, 13].

The vascularization of the stomach is also highly variable. The left gastric artery can take origin from aorta, celiac trunk, or accessory left hepatic artery (1-16%) and left hepatic artery (10%) [11] or may have a common trunk with the hepatic artery (1.7%) [9].

Accessory gastric arteries are often present and most commonly originates from hepatic vessels (21.2%) [14]. The right gastric artery more often originates from proper hepatic artery (53%), from the area where the common hepatic artery bifurcates (20%), from left hepatic artery (15%), and less common from gastroduodenal artery (8%) or common hepatic artery (4%) [15]. The present case is uncommon since

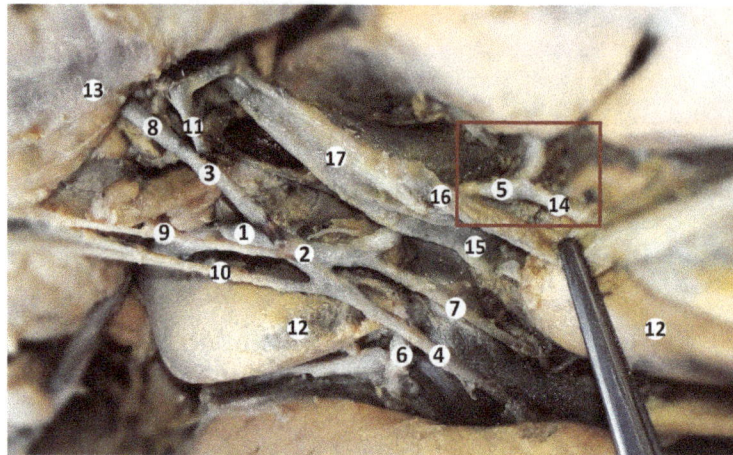

Figure 4: Cystic artery. Macrospecimen (female, 63 years old). 1: common hepatic artery, 2: proper hepatic artery, 3: gastroduodenal artery, 4: left hepatic artery, 5: right hepatic artery, 6: accessory left hepatic artery, 7: intermediate hepatic artery, 8: superior posterior pancreaticoduodenal artery, 9: superior duodenal artery, 10: right gastric artery, 11: right gastroepiploic artery, 12: liver, 13: duodenum, 14: cystic artery, 15: hepatic duct, 16: cystic duct, and 17: common bile duct.

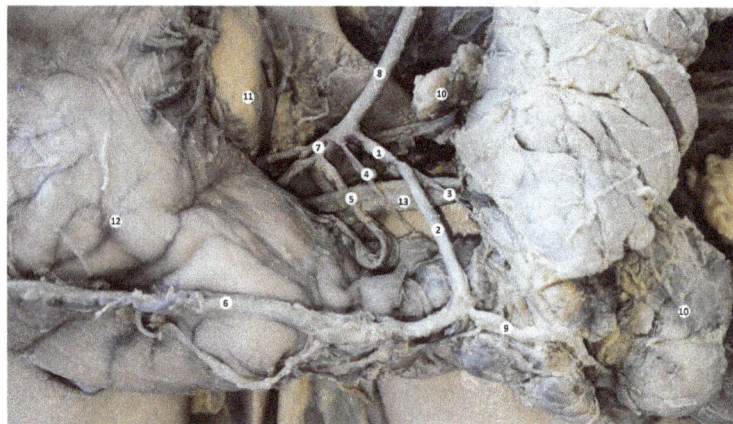

Figure 5: The branches of pancreaticoduodenal artery. Macrospecimen (female, 63 years old). 1: gastroduodenal artery, 2: right gastroepiploic artery, 3: superior posterior pancreaticoduodenal artery, 4: superior duodenal artery, 5: right gastric artery, 6: right gastroepiploic artery, 7: proper hepatic artery, 8: common hepatic artery, 9: superior anterior pancreaticoduodenal artery, 10: pancreas, 11: liver, 12: stomach, and 13: common bile duct.

the lesser curve of the stomach was vascularized by two left gastric arteries and right gastric artery. The accessory left gastric artery branched from the proximal third of the splenic artery. This is a rare case and to our knowledge not previously reported in the literature.

The posterior gastric artery is a branch of the splenic artery and supplies the posterior stomach wall. For the first time it was mentioned by Walther in 1729 and after that rediscovered by Suzuki and coworkers in 1978. This artery can be found in 4 to 100%. Nevertheless, the authors report that it is present in 37.5-48% of cases [16, 17]. Okabayashi and coworkers report that computer tomography detects the posterior gastric artery in 98% and it usually begins from the splenic artery and rarely from the celiac trunk [18]. Two posterior gastric arteries to our knowledge were not previously reported in the literature.

Finally, there are incidental findings that developmental variations of vascular supply are linked to anomalies of the organs shape [19, 20]. Although case reports do not count as evidence-based medicine, they still represent valuable material for evaluation. Therefore, arterial variations should be studied in more detail taking into account organ morphology.

4. Conclusion

During the macroscopical dissection, we determined the accessory arteries of the upper abdominal cavity: left gastric, left hepatic, and two posterior gastric arteries, which have clinical importance in surgery. Textbook anatomy gives an overview of the most common type of developmental variation. Nevertheless, during interventional procedures one may encounter cases that are more complex. The presence

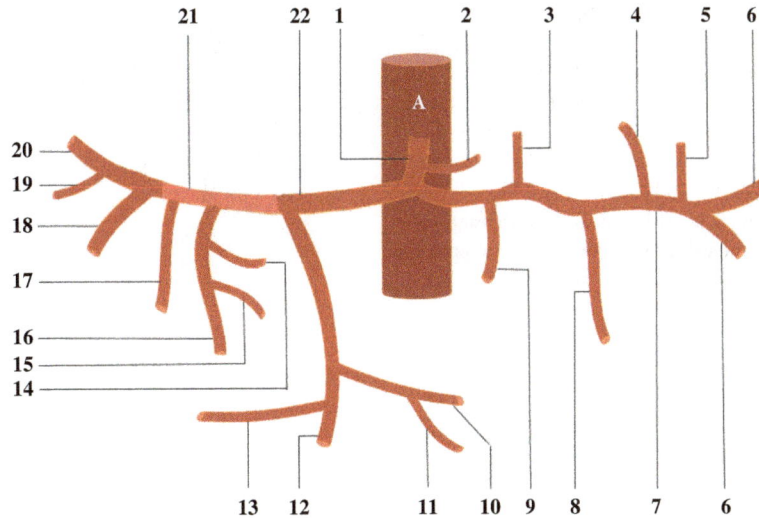

FIGURE 6: A: abdominal aorta; 1: celiac trunk, 2: left gastric artery, 3: accessory left gastric artery, 4: second left gastroepiploic artery, 5: second posterior gastric artery, 6: terminal branches of the splenic arteries, 7: splenic arteries, 8: left gastroepiploic artery, 9: posterior gastric artery, 10: right gastroepiploic artery, 11: superior anterior pancreaticoduodenal artery, 12: gastroduodenal artery, 13: posterior superior pancreaticoduodenal artery, 14: right gastric artery, 15: superior duodenal artery, 16: left hepatic artery, 17: accessory left hepatic artery, 18: intermediate hepatic artery, 19: cystic artery, 20: right hepatic artery, 21: proper hepatic artery, and 22: common hepatic artery.

of accessory gastric arteries may complicate gastric resections. Hepatic vascular anatomy is important during hepatic transplant and resections in case of pathological processes (for example, tumors). Finally, lesions to the posterior gastric arteries can lead to the necrosis of the posterior part of the stomach with drastic complications. Modern procedures in hepatopancreatobiliary and vascular surgery still depend on the knowledge of the regional anatomy and this case demonstrates there is much that can be learned from cadaver dissections.

References

[1] R. S. Tubbs, M. M. Shoja, and M. Loukas, *Bergman's Comprehensive Encyclopedia of Human Anatomic Variation*, John Wiley & Sons, Inc., Hoboken, NJ, USA, 2016.

[2] R. Uflacker, *Atlas of Vascular Anatomy: An Angiographic Approach*, Williams and Wilkins, Baltimore, 1997.

[3] N. A. Michels, "Newer anatomy of the liver and its variant blood supply and collateral circulation," *The American Journal of Surgery*, vol. 112, no. 3, pp. 337–347, 1966.

[4] J. R. Hiatt, J. Gabbay, and R. W. Busuttil, "Surgical anatomy of the hepatic arteries in 1000 cases," *Annals of Surgery*, vol. 220, no. 1, pp. 50–52, 1994.

[5] J. P. J. Vandamme and J. Bonte, "Systematisation of the arteries in the splenic hilus," *Cells Tissues Organs*, vol. 125, no. 4, pp. 217–224, 1986.

[6] O. Belic, N. Mazuruc, and S. Covantev, "Anatomical variations of the splenic artery," *Online J Health Allied Scs*, vol. 16, no. 2, 2017.

[7] R. Dalle Valle, E. Capocasale, MP. Mazzoni, N. Busi, and M. Sianesi, "Pancreas procurement technique. Lessons learned from an initial experience," *Acta bio-medica : Atenei Parmensis*, vol. 77, no. 3, pp. 152–156, 2006.

[8] C. J. E. Watson and S. J. F. Harper, "Anatomical variation and its management in transplantation," *American Journal of Transplantation*, vol. 15, no. 6, pp. 1459–1471, 2015.

[9] S. A. Araujo Neto, H. A. Franca, C. F. de Mello Júnior et al., "Anatomical variations of the celiac trunk and hepatic arterial system: An analysis using multidetector computed tomography angiography," *Radiologia Brasileira*, vol. 48, no. 6, pp. 358–362, 2015.

[10] C. Duran, S. Uraz, M. Kantarci et al., "Hepatic arterial mapping by multidetector computed tomographic angiography in living donor liver transplantation," *Journal of Computer Assisted Tomography*, vol. 33, no. 4, pp. 618–625, 2009.

[11] R. R. De Martino, "Normal and variant mesenteric anatomy," in *Mesenteric Vascular Disease: Current Therapy*, S. G. Oderich, Ed., pp. 9–23, Springer, New York, NY, USA, 2015.

[12] D. F. Pinal-Garcia, C. M. Nuno-Guzman, M. E. Gonzalez-Gonzalez, and T. R. Ibarra-Hurtado, "The celiac trunk and its anatomical variations: A cadaveric study," *Journal of Clinical Medicine Research*, vol. 10, no. 4, pp. 321–329, 2018.

[13] L. Selvaraj, "Study of normal branching pattern of the coeliac trunk and its variations using CT angiography," *Journal of Clinical and Diagnostic Research*, vol. 9, no. 9, pp. AC01–AC4, 2015.

[14] K. Ishigami, K. Yoshimitsu, H. Irie et al., "Accessory left gastric artery from left hepatic artery shown on MDCT and conventional angiography: Correlation with CT hepatic arteriography," *American Journal of Roentgenology*, vol. 187, no. 4, pp. 1002–1009, 2006.

[15] I. Eckmann and V. Krahn, "Frequency of different sites of origin of the right gastric artery," *Anatomischer Anzeiger*, vol. 155, no. 1-5, pp. 65–70, 1984.

[16] W. Trubel, E. Turkof, A. Rokitansky, and W. Firbas, "Incidence, anatomy and territories supplied by the posterior gastric artery," *Cells Tissues Organs*, vol. 124, no. 1-2, pp. 26–30, 1985.

[17] A. S. Berens, F. V. Aluisio, G. L. Colborn, S. W. Gray, and J. E. Skandalakis, "The incidence and significance of the posterior gastric artery in human anatomy," *Journal of the Medical Association of Georgia*, vol. 80, no. 8, pp. 425–428, 1991.

[18] T. Okabayashi, M. Kobayashi, S. Morishita et al., "Confirmation of the posterior gastric artery using multi-detector row computed tomography," *Gastric Cancer*, vol. 8, no. 4, pp. 209–213, 2005.

[19] S. Covantev, N. Mazuruc, and O. Belic, "Bifid pancreas tail and superior horizontal pancreatic artery of Popova: an unusual duet," *Russian Open Medical Journal*, vol. 7, no. 2, p. e0203, 2018.

[20] V. Rakesh, S. Nayak, B. K. Potu, V. R. Vollala, and T. Pulakunta, "Twisted renal vessels producing an abnormal shape of the right kidney," *Singapore Medical Journal*, vol. 49, no. 9, pp. e252–e253, 2008.

51

A Case of Atrioventricular Block Potentially Associated with Right Coronary Artery Lesion and Ticagrelor Therapy Mediated by the Increasing Adenosine Plasma Concentration

Xiaoye Li,[1] **Ying Xue,**[1] **and Hongyi Wu** ⓘ[2]

[1]*Department of Pharmacy, Zhongshan Hospital, Fudan University, Shanghai, China*
[2]*Department of Cardiology, Zhongshan Hospital, Fudan University, Shanghai, China*

Correspondence should be addressed to Hongyi Wu; wu.hongyi@zs-hospital.sh.cn

Academic Editor: Atila Iyisoy

Purpose. To report a case of atrioventricular block (AVB) which might be associated with the right coronary artery lesion and the novel oral antithrombotic drug ticagrelor mediated by the increasing adenosine plasma concentration (APC). *Case Report.* A 65-year-old man was given loading dose of ticagrelor (180 mg) before coronary angiography with total thrombotic occlusion of right coronary artery and one stent was implanted. On second day after successful percutaneous coronary intervention, ECG monitoring showed second-degree (Mobitz type I) AVB with prolonged PR interval (299 ms). Hypothesis was drawn that elevated APC levels caused by ticagrelor would be the reason for AVB after excluding combination drugs or underlying disease. APC might be an indicator of this side effect caused by the P2Y12 receptor inhibitors. On fourth day after shifting to clopidogrel, the ECG showed normal sinus rhythm and PR interval depressed to 190 ms and APC dropped from 1.62 umol/L to 0.92 umol/L. The bradycardia and AVB did not occur in the three-month follow-up. *Conclusion.* It was important to take the ticagrelor induced bradycardia into account particularly with the myocardial infarction of right coronary artery, treated with atrioventricular block drugs after initiating ticagrelor. Also, we should shift ticagrelor to clopidogrel if AVB occurred.

1. Introduction

Ticagrelor produced faster and stronger inhibition of platelet aggregation than clopidogrel [1]. Most patients can tolerate it well, but some severe adverse drug reaction may occur including dyspnea and asymptomatic bradycardia after medication with ticagrelor [2]. In the PLATO trial, a high proportion of asymptomatic bradycardia symptoms (2.2%) occurred with ticagrelor therapy. But this transient and asymptomatic side effect did not need pacemaker [3].

Many animal and cell experiments disclosed that ticagrelor could inhibit the cellular uptake of adenosine through equilibrative nucleoside transporter 1 leading to the increase of adenosine plasma concentration (APC) [4]. These findings led to the hypothesis that this side effect of ticagrelor was mediated with adenosine which might slow down the conduction of atrioventricular nodes.

Here we reported a case about atrioventricular block (AVB) associated with ticagrelor therapy for acute coronary syndrome (ACS) patient who had a high level of APC which might be the mechanism of this adverse drug reaction. The patient was diagnosed with acute inferior wall ST-elevation myocardial infarction (STEMI).

2. Case Presentation

A 61-year-old male patient suffered a sudden chest pain lasting for 5 minutes accompanied with sweating, dizziness, amaurosis, nausea, and vomiting. The chest pain and tightness had no significant relief after two sublingual tablets of nitroglycerin. He had a history of hypertension of 10 years with the medication of metoprolol sustained release tablets (23.75 mg) and ramipril (2.5 mg). His admission electrocardiogram (ECG) showed normal sinus rhythm and 1 mm ST-segment elevation in lead II, lead III, and lead aVF. The repeated troponin T test was positive at 0.148 ng/mL and the patient was diagnosed with acute inferior wall STEMI. With initial diagnosis of STEMI, he

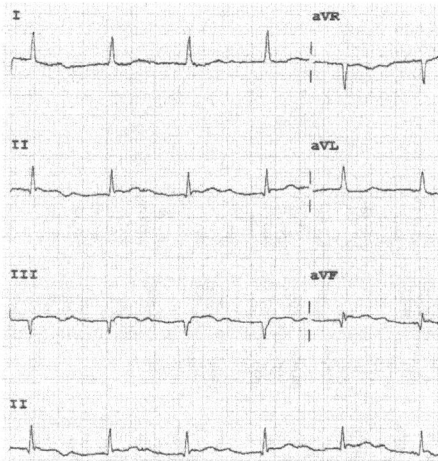

FIGURE 1: Second-degree (Mobitz type I) AVB.

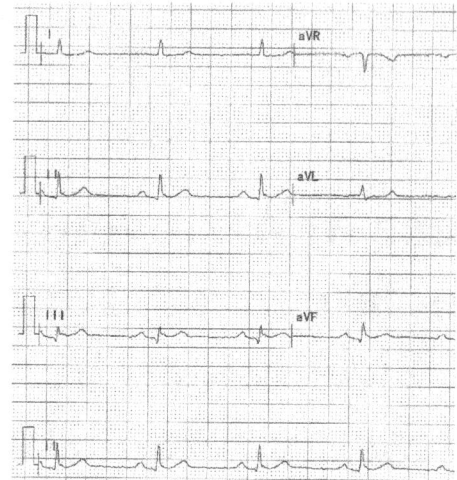

FIGURE 2: Normal sinus rhythm.

had an emergency coronary angiography intervention after receiving a loading dose of ticagrelor (180 mg) and aspirin (300 mg). He was treated with metoprolol sustained release tablets (23.75 mg), rosuvastatin (5 mg), ramipril (2.5 mg), low molecular weight heparin (4000 IU Q12 h), and isosorbide mononitrate sustained release tablets (40 mg) for improving myocardial ischemia. The emergency coronary angiography revealed total thrombotic occlusion of right coronary artery (RCA) and one stent (2.4 mm × 18 mm sirolimus-eluting stent, EXCEL, China) was implanted in the RCA. The blood pressure (BP) was 125/72 mmHg and heart rate (HR) was 76 bpm after percutaneous coronary intervention (PCI) operation without prolonged PR interval (192 ms) and ST segment depressed to baseline. The patient was prescribed the maintenance dose of ticagrelor (90 mg bid) and the symptoms were asymptomatic and hemodynamically stable. On the second day after operation, the ECG monitoring showed second-degree (Mobitz type I) AVB with prolonged PR interval (299 ms) (Figure 1). The BP was 90/50 mmHg and HR was 45 bpm. Although beta-block might cause AVB, the patient was medicated with metoprolol sustained release tablets for many years and maintained the regular dose after onset. This side effect might be induced by ticagrelor which increased the APC. We switched the P2Y12 inhibitor from ticagrelor to clopidogrel. The APC detected by fluorescent probe adenosine assay kit (Bio Vision, Milpitas, CA 95035, USA) was 1.62 umol/L on the second day after operation. On the fourth day after shifting to clopidogrel, the ECG showed normal sinus rhythm and PR interval depressed to 190 ms (Figure 2). The BP was 104/64 mmHg and HR was 59 bpm. The APC was 0.92 umol/L. The bradycardia and AVB did not occur in the three-month follow-up.

3. Discussion

Ticagrelor bound directly, changed the conformation of the P2Y12 receptor, and resulted in a reversible inhibition of the receptor [5]. It can produce much faster and more efficacious P2Y12 effect than clopidogrel for the ACS patients [6]. In the PLATO trial ticagrelor was linked to increase the incidence of

ventricular pauses which were predominantly asymptomatic. The incidence of acute intermittent ventricle in ticagrelor group was 6% and the incidence of intermittent ventricle was 2.2% in one-month follow-up and ticagrelor-related intermittent ventricle was self-limiting and had no impact on efficacy or safety outcomes in acute coronary syndrome (ACS) patients [3].

AVB could be caused by the delay or block conduction in any area of the atrioventricular system. AVB might be transient where the underlying etiology was reversible such as in myocarditis, in myocardial ischemia, or after cardiovascular surgery. The coronary blood flow supply of sinoatrial (SA) and AV nodes was produced by the SA and AV nodal branches most commonly originating from the RCA [7]. Therefore the reduced RCA blood flow was associated with a variety of conduction disturbances. The patient had a total thrombotic occlusion of RCA, with one stent implanted. So the RCA lesion might be responsible for this conduction disturbance in our case.

AVB could occur during the drug therapy including β-blockers and digoxin, or non-DHP CCBs might cause AV block, primarily in the AV nodal area. In our case, the patient was medicated with metoprolol sustained release tablets for over 10 years. So it was not logical to think this newly occurring conduction disturbance was associated with metoprolol.

Another important point related to this conduction disturbance might be the medication of ticagrelor. After medication with the loading dose of ticagrelor (180 mg), the BP was 90/50 mmHg and HR was 45 bpm. Pharmacology screening showed the inhibition of adenosine uptake into human erythrocytes as one of the most potent off-target activities of ticagrelor [4]. However this mechanism of ticagrelor was shown to have specific side effects such as bradycardia and dyspnea, which could also be triggered by APC increase. The APC that was detected by fluorescent probe adenosine assay kit decreased significantly after switching the P2Y12 inhibitor from ticagrelor to clopidogrel. The latest research discovered that the ticagrelor could inhibit the adenosine uptake by red blood cells in ACS patients, leading to the increase in APC similar to what was observed for dipyridamole [4].

Adenosine exerted cardiac electrophysiological effects through activation of A_1R. It had a negative chronotropic effect through suppression of the automaticity of cardiac pacemakers and a negative dromotropic effect on the inhibition of AVB [8]. Adenosine was rapidly taken up by cells through sodium-independent equilibrative nucleoside transporters and sodium-dependent concentrative nucleoside transporters compared with placebo in in vitro experiment [9]. The effect of ticagrelor influencing adenosine concentrations may convey unique properties of the drug not shared by other P2Y12 antagonists such as clopidogrel, prasugrel, and cangrelor.

4. Conclusion

In our case, the right coronary artery lesion and medication with ticagrelor might be the main reasons for the AVB. Extreme caution and close ECG monitoring after initiation of the antiplatelet drug ticagrelor were needed in terms of development of the myocardial infarction with right coronary artery.

Authors' Contributions

All authors had access to the data, participated in the preparation of the manuscript, and approved this manuscript.

References

[1] D. J. Angiolillo, F. Franchi, R. Waksman et al., "Effects of ticagrelor versus clopidogrel in troponin-negative patients with low-risk ACS undergoing ad hoc PCI," *Journal of the American College of Cardiology*, vol. 67, no. 6, pp. 603–613, 2016.

[2] M. A. Velders, J. Abtan, D. J. Angiolillo et al., "Safety and efficacy of ticagrelor and clopidogrel in primary percutaneous coronary intervention," *Heart*, vol. 102, no. 8, pp. 617–625, 2016.

[3] L. Wallentin, R. C. Becker, and A. Budaj, "Ticagrelor versus clopidogrel in patients with acute coronary syndromes," *New England Journal of Medicine*, vol. 361, no. 11, pp. 1045–1057, 2009.

[4] M. Cattaneo, R. Schulz, and S. Nylander, "Adenosine-mediated effects of ticagrelor: Evidence and potential clinical relevance," *Journal of the American College of Cardiology*, vol. 63, no. 23, pp. 2503–2509, 2014.

[5] N. Ferri, A. Corsini, and S. Bellosta, "Pharmacology of the new P2Y12 receptor inhibitors: insights on pharmacokinetic and pharmacodynamic properties," *Drugs*, vol. 73, no. 15, pp. 1681–1709, 2013.

[6] F. Franchi, F. Rollini, J. R. Cho et al., "Impact of escalating loading dose regimens of ticagrelor in patients with st-segment elevation myocardial infarction undergoing primary percutaneous coronary intervention: results of a prospective randomized pharmacokinetic and pharmacodynamic investigation," *JACC: Cardiovascular Interventions*, vol. 8, no. 11, article no. 2124, pp. 1457–1467, 2015.

[7] S. D. Pokorney, C. Radder, P. J. Schulte et al., "High-degree atrioventricular block, asystole, and electro-mechanical dissociation complicating non-ST-segment elevation myocardial infarction," *American Heart Journal*, vol. 171, no. 1, pp. 25–32, 2016.

[8] L. Bonello, M. Laine, N. Kipson et al., "Ticagrelor increases adenosine plasma concentration in patients with an acute coronary syndrome," *Journal of the American College of Cardiology*, vol. 63, no. 9, pp. 872–877, 2014.

[9] J. J. J. Van Giezen, J. Sidaway, P. Glaves, I. Kirk, and J.-A. Björkman, "Ticagrelor inhibits adenosine uptake in vitro and enhances adenosine-mediated hyperemia responses in a canine model," *Journal of Cardiovascular Pharmacology and Therapeutics*, vol. 17, no. 2, pp. 164–172, 2012.

52

Haematochezia from a Splenic Artery Pseudoaneurysm Communicating with Transverse Colon

James O'Brien, Francesca Muscara, Aser Farghal, and Irshad Shaikh

Department of General Surgery, Norfolk and Norwich University Hospital, Colney Lane, Norwich, Norfolk NR4 7UY, UK

Correspondence should be addressed to James O'Brien; james.obrien1@nhs.net

Academic Editor: Nikolaos Papanas

Splenic artery aneurysms (SAA) are the third most common intra-abdominal aneurysm. Complications include invasion into surrounding structures often in association with preexisting pancreatic disease. We describe an 88-year-old female, with no history of pancreatic disease, referred with lower gastrointestinal bleeding. CT angiography showed a splenic artery pseudoaneurysm with associated collection and fistula to the transverse colon at the level of the splenic flexure. The pseudoaneurysm was embolised endovascularly with metallic microcoils. Rectal bleeding ceased. The patient recovered well and follow-up angiography revealed no persistence of the splenic artery pseudoaneurysm. SAA rupture results in 29%–50% mortality. Experienced centres report success with the endovascular approach in haemodynamically unstable patients, as a bridge to surgery, and even on a background of pancreatic disease. This case highlights the importance of prompt CT angiography, if endoscopy fails to identify a cause of gastrointestinal bleeding. Endovascular embolisation provides a safe and effective alternative to surgery, where anatomical considerations and local expertise permit.

1. Introduction

Splenic artery aneurysms (SAA) are defined as a ≥1 cm dilatation of the artery diameter and are the third most common intra-abdominal aneurysm [1]. The majority of SAA are detected as incidental findings, but if they present with rupture, a high mortality rate results [2]. Complications include invasion into and communication with surrounding structures, often in association with preexisting pancreatic disease [1, 3]. Traditionally, treatment of SAA was through surgery, but endovascular therapy is now established with minimal morbidity and mortality [4]. We describe successful endovascular management of a splenic artery pseudoaneurysm, with a fistula between the pseudoaneurysm and the transverse colon, in a patient without coexisting pancreatic disease.

2. Case Report

An 88-year-old Caucasian female was referred from the emergency department with lower gastrointestinal bleeding. She gave a history of five episodes of fresh rectal bleeding with blood separate from the stools, of one day's duration. This was preceded by one day of loose stools and a constant low grade central abdominal pain. There were no other associated upper or lower gastrointestinal symptoms and no systemic disturbance. Past medical history included atrial fibrillation for which she was prescribed warfarin. She was a nonsmoker with minimal alcohol intake.

On examination, body mass index was 23 and blood pressure 140/70 with an irregular heart rate of 80 bpm, a respiratory rate of 18, and oxygen saturation 100% on room air. Examination of the abdomen elicited tenderness in the periumbilical region with no peritonism. On digital rectal examination the rectum was empty with no masses and no perianal disease. Dark blood was noted on the glove with no clots. Haematological and biochemical investigation revealed haemoglobin was 103 g/L (normal range 115–160 g/L), C-reactive protein 210 mg/L (<10 mg/L), and international normalised ratio 4.47 (target 2.5). Urea and electrolytes, liver function, and serum amylase were normal. Electrocardiogram confirmed atrial fibrillation.

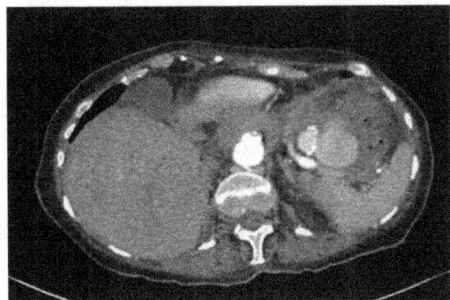

FIGURE 1: CT angiography axial plane demonstrating splenic artery pseudoaneurysm.

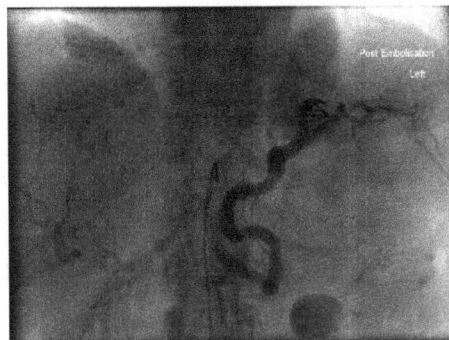

FIGURE 2: Coeliac arteriography coronal plane demonstrating embolisation of the splenic artery pseudoaneurysm.

The patient was managed with intravenous fluid replacement and 10 mg vitamin K. Warfarin was stopped. A flexible sigmoidoscopy was performed with no polyps or masses identified and fresh blood and clots seen throughout the sigmoid colon. The patient continued to report bleeding and repeat haemoglobin had decreased to 81 g/L. Two units of packed red cells were transfused and an oesophagogastroduodenoscopy revealed atrophic gastritis and a prepyloric erosion unlikely to be the source of bleeding. Following this computed tomography (CT) angiography showed a splenic artery pseudoaneurysm with associated collection and fistula to the transverse colon at the level of the splenic flexure (Figure 1).

Radiology consult was obtained and the pseudoaneurysm embolised via catheter directed metallic microcoils. Upon completion no further contrast extravasation was seen, with cessation of flow through the fistula (Figure 2). Rectal bleeding ceased and there were no complications. The patient recovered well and was discharged. A follow-up CT angiography at 6 weeks after embolisation revealed no persistence of the splenic artery pseudoaneurysm.

3. Discussion

Visceral artery aneurysms are rare and reported prevalence in the population varies from 0.1 to 10.4% [5–8]. SAA are the most common type, accounting for 30%–60% [5]. SAA account for up to 60% of all splanchnic artery aneurysms, followed by aneurysms of the hepatic (20%), superior mesenteric (5.9%), and celiac (4%) arteries [9]. Following the aorta and iliac arteries, SAA are the third most common abdominal aneurysm [1, 7].

SAA is a ≥1 cm dilatation of the artery diameter and can be classified as a true or pseudoaneurysm, with the majority (72%) true aneurysms [10]. Most SAA are reported in the main body of the artery, with a majority (74–87%) at the distal third and the mean size 2.1 cm [11–13]. Aneurysm size is not a predictor of rupture [5]. Aetiology is hypothesised as wall degeneration or dilatation of an artery through increased pressure and weakness in the wall [8, 14, 15]. There is increased female : male incidence reported for all SAA [1, 2, 5, 7] and increased male : female incidence reported for giant SAA (defined as a SAA ≥ 5 cm) [2]. Pregnancy, portal hypertension, liver transplant, and pancreatitis are described as particular risk factors, with the latter more closely associated with pseudoaneurysms and the first two factors with true aneurysms [2, 16, 17]. Multiparity has long been associated with increased risk of rupture [1, 7, 18, 19].

20% of SAA are symptomatic and 80% incidental findings [2, 8, 16]. Intervention is recommended for SAA that are symptomatic, increasing in size, found during pregnancy (or in child bearing years), of diameter ≥2 cm (or any size in case of a pseudoaneurysm), as these factors have been described as increasing the risk of rupture [20].

Traditionally 10% of SSA presented with rupture but due to increasing incidental diagnosis this has reduced to 3% [1, 21]. Mortality following rupture was 25% in the 1970s, with little improvement since, and is as high as 100% for pseudoaneurysms [1, 22]. In pregnancy 75% maternal and 95% fetal mortality rates are described. Most aneurysms rupture in this group (95%), with two-thirds during the third trimester [23, 24]. Pathogenesis is hypothesised to be due to the hormonal (oestrogen, progesterone, and relaxin [21, 25, 26]) and physiological changes of pregnancy on the arterial wall and the presence of antenatal comorbidity such as portal hypertension, which is itself a risk factor for SAA [27, 28]. There is an incidence of 7.1–13.0% in this group of patients. Rupture has been described via containment in the lesser sac followed by a second rupture into the greater sac or through a single rupture into the abdomen [26, 29–31]. The symptoms associated with unruptured SAA are usually nonspecific whereas a ruptured SAA almost always presents with hemodynamic instability and severe sudden abdominal pain [1].

Invasion into the stomach, duodenum, pancreatic duct, and colon can result in gastrointestinal bleeding and up to 13% of ruptured SAA have been described as fistulate with these structures [1, 16]. Fistulation to vascular structures such as the splenic and portal veins can cause arteriovenous fistulae resulting in mesenteric steal and small bowel ischaemia [32]. External mass effect on the portal vein can cause portal hypertension and venous congestion [33]. SAA can rupture into pancreatic pseudocysts [20, 34]. 60% of pseudoaneurysms occurring in chronic pancreatitis are SAA [35]. Haemorrhage is described as presenting with a sentinel bleed before major haemorrhage and bleeding as a result of SAA can present with haematemesis, haematochezia, intra-abdominal bleeding, or melaena [1].

This patient presented with rectal bleeding due to fistulation with the transverse colon. Direct colonic involvement presenting with haematochezia without pancreatic involvement is extremely rare in the literature. The first two nonfatal cases of SAA with colonic involvement were reported in 1984 and 2003. In both the SAA communicated with the splenic flexure and required open surgery for definitive treatment [19, 36]. Other authors describe haematochezia from SAA rupturing into a pancreatic pseudocyst with fistula to the colon and in two patients with pancreatitis, a giant pseudoaneurysm communicating with the splenic flexure, and a saccular SAA with a collection extending to the descending colon [3, 37, 38]. Haematochezia from a splenic artery pseudoaneurysm in a patient with a pancreatic pseudocystocolic fistula was successfully treated after the pseudoaneurysm was embolised via catheter directed coils [39]. A patient with chronic pancreatitis underwent successful embolisation of a splenic artery pseudoaneurysm that ruptured into the colon, following a negative laparotomy [40, 41]. The Mayo clinic published an 18-year case series that included a single patient with splenic artery pseudoaneurysm fistulate to the descending colon, without pancreatitis. This patient was treated with surgery. The authors combined their case series with literature review and found 26.2% of splenic pseudoaneurysms present with haematochezia or melaena and in 42% of the 59 patients included, the bleeding originated from the pancreatic duct [20].

Digital subtraction angiography is the preferred modality for delineating SAA and computed tomography for monitoring during conservative management [1]. Endovascular management is now recommended for management of unruptured SAA, including pseudoaneurysms, not involving the splenic hilum [42], through transcatheter embolisation or less commonly stent grafts, with splenic preservation possible [4]. For ruptured SAA or pseudocyst involvement, surgery is recommended [1, 3]. The failure rate of transcatheter embolisation is higher when pseudocyst is present [20]. When a pancreatic pseudocyst is the underlying cause, splenic and pancreatic conserving approaches are described but surgery can be as extensive as aneurysmal resection, splenectomy, and colonic resection with distal pancreatectomy [1]. Ruptured SAA results in high mortality (29%–50%) [20, 43, 44] even following operative management and recent publications advocate endovascular intervention for SAA even on a background of pancreatic disease [45–47]. Experienced centres report success with the endovascular approach even in haemodynamically unstable patients or as a bridge to surgery [44, 48]. Elective laparoscopic approaches have been advocated where loss of splenic function or repeated imaging is contraindicated and where anatomy presents difficulty for embolisation [24, 49]. Zero morbidity or mortality is reported from laparoscopic resection of unruptured SAA [50].

Interventional endovascular treatment for all visceral artery aneurysms is reported with zero mortality for unruptured aneurysms [5, 51]. Although case series for SAA are small, several authors describe zero mortality following endovascular treatment for unruptured SAA since 1987 [43, 44, 52]. Anatomical variation is suggested as the main factor determining successful nonoperative treatment [53]. Aneurysms of the distal artery are more likely to develop complications following endovascular therapy [44]. Recanalisation rates for SAA were quoted as 12.5% in the in 1990s [54]. A large case series in 2015 reports a 93% success rate for all visceral artery aneurysms treated with interventional techniques [5]. Complications of interventional techniques include thrombosis or embolism resulting in organ abscesses and infarction, coil migration, aneurysm recurrence, and local arterial access complications [42]. There is little consensus on follow-up [44].

4. Conclusions

Splenic artery aneurysms and pseudoaneurysms are rarely encountered in routine practice but will increasingly be identified as incidental findings. Patients presenting with haematochezia on a background of pancreatic disease should immediately alert the physician to the possibility of splenic artery aneurysm or pseudoaneurysm, complicated by gastrointestinal involvement. Without this history, cases of rectal bleeding caused by SAA or pseudoaneurysm communicating with the colon present a diagnostic challenge. This highlights the importance of prompt CT angiography, especially if upper and lower gastrointestinal endoscopy fail to identify a cause of bleeding. This case describes a splenic artery pseudoaneurysm with direct colonic involvement, in a patient without a background of pancreatic disease, managed successfully without open surgery. Advances in endovascular embolisation techniques provide a safe and effective alternative to surgery, where anatomical considerations and local expertise permit.

Competing Interests

The authors declare that there are no competing interests regarding the publication of this paper.

References

[1] Y. Al-Habbal, C. Christophi, and V. Muralidharan, "Aneurysms of the splenic artery—a review," *Surgeon*, vol. 8, no. 4, pp. 223–231, 2010.

[2] S. Akbulut and E. Otan, "Management of giant splenic artery aneurysm: comprehensive literature review," *Medicine*, vol. 94, no. 27, Article ID e1016, 2015.

[3] J. Zhao, X. Kong, D. Cao, and L. Jiang, "Hematochezia from splenic arterial pseudoaneurysm ruptured into pancreatic pseudocyst coexisting with fistula to the colon: a case report and literature review," *Gastroenterology Research*, vol. 7, no. 2, pp. 73–77, 2014.

[4] R. Guillon, J. M. Garcier, A. Abergel et al., "Management of splenic artery aneurysms and false aneurysms with endovascular treatment in 12 patients," *CardioVascular and Interventional Radiology*, vol. 26, no. 3, pp. 256–260, 2003.

[5] M. B. Pitton, E. Dappa, F. Jungmann et al., "Visceral artery aneurysms: incidence, management, and outcome analysis in a tertiary care center over one decade," *European Radiology*, vol. 25, no. 7, pp. 2004–2014, 2015.

[6] A. Hossain, E. D. Reis, S. P. Dave, M. D. Kerstein, and L. H. Hollier, "Visceral artery aneurysms: experience in a tertiary-care center," *The American Surgeon*, vol. 67, no. 5, pp. 432–437, 2001.

[7] Y. P. Panayiotopoulos, R. Assadourian, and P. R. Taylor, "Aneurysms of the visceral and renal arteries," *Annals of the Royal College of Surgeons of England*, vol. 78, no. 5, pp. 412–419, 1996.

[8] P. D. Bedford and B. Lodge, "Aneurysm of the splenic artery," *Gut*, vol. 1, pp. 312–320, 1960.

[9] R. Arabia, S. Pellicanò, R. Siciliani, O. L. Dattola, S. Giusti, and L. Terra, "Splenic artery aneurysm and portal hypertension. Report of a case," *Minerva Medica*, vol. 90, no. 4, pp. 143–145, 1999.

[10] S. F. Pasha, P. Gloviczki, A. W. Stanson, and P. S. Kamath, "Splanchnic artery aneurysms," *Mayo Clinic Proceedings*, vol. 82, no. 4, pp. 472–479, 2007.

[11] R. Yadav, M. K. Tiwari, R. M. Mathur, and A. K. Verma, "Unusually giant splenic artery and vein aneurysm with arteriovenous fistula with hypersplenism in a nulliparous woman," *Interactive Cardiovascular and Thoracic Surgery*, vol. 8, no. 3, pp. 384–386, 2009.

[12] T. Karsidag, G. Soybir, S. Tuzun, and C. Makine, "Splenic artery aneurysm rupture," *Chirurgia*, vol. 104, no. 4, pp. 487–490, 2009.

[13] K. Karaman, L. Onat, M. Şirvancı, and R. Olga, "Endovascular stent graft treatment in a patient with splenic artery aneurysm," *Diagnostic and Interventional Radiology*, vol. 11, no. 2, pp. 119–121, 2005.

[14] U. Sadat, O. Dar, S. Walsh, and K. Varty, "Splenic artery aneurysms in pregnancy—a systematic review," *International Journal of Surgery*, vol. 6, no. 3, pp. 261–265, 2008.

[15] M. Chadha and C. Ahuja, "Visceral artery aneurysms: diagnosis and percutaneous management," *Seminars in Interventional Radiology*, vol. 26, no. 3, pp. 196–206, 2009.

[16] Y.-D. Miao and B. Ye, "Intragastric rupture of splenic artery aneurysms: three case reports and literature review," *Pakistan Journal of Medical Sciences*, vol. 29, no. 2, pp. 656–659, 2013.

[17] G. Garbagna, G. Cornalba, and L. Rota, "Splenic artery aneurysms in patients with portal hypertension," *Radiologia Medica*, vol. 66, no. 4, pp. 239–242, 1980.

[18] R. J. Holdsworth and A. Gunn, "Ruptured splenic artery aneurysm in pregnancy. A review," *British Journal of Obstetrics and Gynaecology*, vol. 99, pp. 595–597, 1992.

[19] N. L. Bishop, "Splenic artery aneurysm rupture into the colon diagnosed by angiography," *British Journal of Radiology*, vol. 57, no. 684, pp. 1149–1150, 1984.

[20] D. J. Tessier, W. M. Stone, R. J. Fowl et al., "Clinical features and management of splenic artery pseudoaneurysm: case series and cumulative review of literature," *Journal of Vascular Surgery*, vol. 38, no. 5, pp. 969–974, 2003.

[21] S. G. Mattar and A. B. Lumsden, "The management of splenic artery aneurysms: experience with 23 cases," *The American Journal of Surgery*, vol. 169, no. 6, pp. 580–584, 1995.

[22] J. C. Stanley, N. W. Thompson, and W. J. Fry, "Splanchnic artery aneurysms," *Archives of Surgery*, vol. 101, no. 6, pp. 689–697, 1970.

[23] C. E. Sam, M. Rabl, and E. A. Joura, "Aneurysm of the splenic artery: rupture in pregnancy," *Wiener Klinische Wochenschrift*, vol. 112, no. 20, pp. 896–898, 2000.

[24] J. de Csepel, T. Quinn, and M. Gagner, "Laparoscopic exclusion of a splenic artery aneurysm using a lateral approach permits preservation of the spleen," *Surgical Laparoscopy, Endoscopy and Percutaneous Techniques*, vol. 11, no. 3, pp. 221–224, 2001.

[25] D. O. Selo-Ojeme and C. C. Welch, "Review: spontaneous rupture of splenic artery aneurysm in pregnancy," *European Journal of Obstetrics & Gynecology and Reproductive Biology*, vol. 109, no. 2, pp. 124–127, 2003.

[26] J. E. de Vries, M. E. Schattenkerk, and R. A. Malt, "Complications of splenic artery aneurysm other than intraperitoneal rupture," *Surgery*, vol. 91, no. 2, pp. 200–204, 1982.

[27] M. Puttini, P. Aseni, G. Brambilla, and L. Belli, "Splenic artery aneurysms in portal hypertension," *Journal of Cardiovascular Surgery*, vol. 23, no. 6, pp. 490–493, 1982.

[28] D. Siablis, Z. G. Papathanassiou, D. Karnabatidis, N. Christeas, K. Katsanos, and C. Vagianos, "Splenic arteriovenous fistula and sudden onset of portal hypertension as complications of a ruptured splenic artery aneurysm: successful treatment with transcatheter arterial embolization. A case study and review of the literature," *World Journal of Gastroenterology*, vol. 12, no. 26, pp. 4264–4266, 2006.

[29] J. P. O'Grady, E. J. Day, A. L. Toole, and J. C. Paust, "Splenic artery aneurysm rupture in pregnancy: a review and case report," *Obstetrics & Gynecology*, vol. 50, no. 5, pp. 627–630, 1977.

[30] V. F. Trastek, P. C. Pairolero, J. W. Joyce, L. H. Hollier, and P. E. Bernatz, "Splenic artery aneurysms," *Surgery*, vol. 91, no. 6, pp. 694–699, 1982.

[31] R. S. L. Brockman, "Aneurysm of the splenic artery," *British Journal of Surgery*, vol. 17, no. 68, pp. 692–693, 1930.

[32] F. Sendra, D. B. Safran, and G. McGee, "A rare complication of splenic artery aneurysm: mesenteric steal syndrome," *Archives of Surgery*, vol. 130, no. 6, pp. 669–672, 1995.

[33] M. Vlychou, C. Kokkinis, S. Stathopoulou et al., "Imaging investigation of a giant splenic artery aneurysm," *Angiology*, vol. 59, no. 4, pp. 503–506, 2008.

[34] G. Flati, Å. Andrén-Sandberg, M. La Pinta, B. Porowska, and M. Carboni, "Potentially fatal bleeding in acute pancreatitis: pathophysiology, prevention, and treatment," *Pancreas*, vol. 26, no. 1, pp. 8–14, 2003.

[35] D. K. Bhasin, S. S. Rana, V. Sharma et al., "Non-surgical management of pancreatic pseudocysts associated with arterial pseudoaneurysm," *Pancreatology*, vol. 13, no. 3, pp. 250–253, 2013.

[36] E. T. Ek, C.-A. Moulton, and S. Mackay, "Catastrophic rectal bleeding from a ruptured splenic artery aneurysm," *ANZ Journal of Surgery*, vol. 73, no. 5, pp. 361–364, 2003.

[37] B. Tirpude, H. Bhanarkar, S. Dakhore, and D. Surgule, "Giant splenic artery pseudo aneurysm masquerading as bleeding per rectum—a rare case," *Journal of Evolution of Medical and Dental Sciences*, vol. 2, no. 44, pp. 8569–8573, 2013.

[38] S. Rao, M. Sivina, I. Willis, T. Sher, and S. Habibnejad, "Massive lower gastrointestinal tract bleeding due to splenic artery aneurysm: a case report," *Annals of Vascular Surgery*, vol. 21, no. 3, pp. 388–391, 2007.

[39] B. Taslakian, M. Khalife, W. Faraj, D. Mukherji, and A. Haydar, "Pancreatitis-associated pseudoaneurysm of the splenic artery presenting as lower gastrointestinal bleeding: treatment with transcatheter embolisation," *BMJ Case Reports*, vol. 2012, 2012.

[40] A. Kukliński, K. Batycki, W. Matuszewski, A. Ostrach, Z. Kupis, and T. Łęgowik, "Embolization of a large, symptomatic splenic artery pseudoaneurysm," *Polish Journal of Radiology*, vol. 79, pp. 194–198, 2014.

[41] J. F. Bretagne, D. Heresbach, I. Le Jean-Colin et al., "Splenic pseudoaneurysm rupture into the colon: colonoscopy before and after successful arterial embolization," *Surgical Endoscopy*, vol. 1, no. 4, pp. 229–231, 1987.

[42] J. F. Reidy, P. H. Rowe, and F. G. Ellis, "Technical report: splenic artery aneurysm embolisation—the preferred technique to surgery," *Clinical Radiology*, vol. 41, no. 4, pp. 281–282, 1990.

[43] S. R. Mandel, P. F. Jaques, S. Sanofsky, and M. A. Mauro, "Non-operative management of peripancreatic arterial aneurysms. A 10-year experience," *Annals of Surgery*, vol. 205, no. 2, pp. 126–128, 1987.

[44] R. O. Lakin, J. F. Bena, T. P. Sarac et al., "The contemporary management of splenic artery aneurysms," *Journal of Vascular Surgery*, vol. 53, no. 4, pp. 958–965, 2011.

[45] M. S. Woods, L. W. Traverso, R. A. Kozarek, J. Brandabur, and E. Hauptmann, "Successful treatment of bleeding pseudoaneurysms of chronic pancreatitis," *Pancreas*, vol. 10, no. 1, pp. 22–30, 1995.

[46] A. El Hamel, R. Parc, G. Adda, P. Y. Bouteloup, C. Huguet, and M. Malafosse, "Bleeding pseudocysts and pseudoaneurysms in chronic pancreatitis," *British Journal of Surgery*, vol. 78, no. 9, pp. 1059–1063, 1991.

[47] S. A. Berceli, "Hepatic and splenic artery aneurysms," *Seminars in Vascular Surgery*, vol. 18, no. 4, pp. 196–201, 2005.

[48] I. Vujic, B. L. Andersen, J. H. Stanley, and R. P. Gobien, "Pancreatic and peripancreatic vessels: embolization for control of bleeding in pancreatitis," *Radiology*, vol. 150, no. 1, pp. 51–55, 1984.

[49] A. Pietrabissa, M. Ferrari, R. Berchiolli et al., "Laparoscopic treatment of splenic artery aneurysms," *Journal of Vascular Surgery*, vol. 50, no. 2, pp. 275–279, 2009.

[50] M. J. Arca, M. Gagner, B. T. Heniford, T. Sullivan, and E. G. Beven, "Splenic artery aneurysms: methods of laparoscopic repair," *Journal of Vascular Surgery*, vol. 30, no. 1, pp. 184–188, 1999.

[51] M. Orsi, M. Venturini, F. Morelli et al., "Single-center experience in endovascular treatment of visceral artery aneurysms and pseudoaneurysms with Viabahn covered stent: technical aspects, success rate, complications and MDCT follow-up," in *Proceedings of the Annual Meeting of the European Society of Radiology*, Vienna, Austria, March 2014.

[52] A. Patel, J. L. Weintraub, F. S. Nowakowski et al., "Single-center experience with elective transcatheter coil embolization of splenic artery aneurysms: technique and midterm follow-up," *Journal of Vascular and Interventional Radiology*, vol. 23, no. 7, pp. 893–899, 2012.

[53] S. S. Saltzberg, T. S. Maldonado, P. J. Lamparello et al., "Is endovascular therapy the preferred treatment for all visceral artery aneurysms?" *Annals of Vascular Surgery*, vol. 19, no. 4, pp. 507–515, 2005.

[54] S. C. Carr, W. H. Pearce, R. L. Vogelzang, W. J. McCarthy, A. A. Nemcek Jr., and J. S. T. Yao, "Current management of visceral artery aneurysms," *Surgery*, vol. 120, no. 4, pp. 627–634, 1996.

53

Upper Extremity Deep Vein Thromboses: The Bowler and the Barista

Seth Stake,[1] Anne L. du Breuil,[2] and Jeremy Close[2]

[1]Sidney Kimmel Medical College, Thomas Jefferson University, Philadelphia, PA 19107, USA
[2]Department of Family and Community Medicine, Sidney Kimmel Medical College, Thomas Jefferson University, 833 East Chestnut Street, Suite 301, Philadelphia, PA 19107, USA

Correspondence should be addressed to Seth Stake; sns003@jefferson.edu

Academic Editor: Matthias Reinhard

Effort thrombosis of the upper extremity refers to a deep venous thrombosis of the upper extremity resulting from repetitive activity of the upper limb. Most cases of effort thrombosis occur in young elite athletes with strenuous upper extremity activity. This article reports two cases who both developed upper extremity deep vein thromboses, the first being a 67-year-old bowler and the second a 25-year-old barista, and illustrates that effort thrombosis should be included in the differential diagnosis in any patient with symptoms concerning DVT associated with repetitive activity. A literature review explores the recommended therapies for upper extremity deep vein thromboses.

1. Introduction

Effort thrombosis of the upper extremity refers to a deep venous thrombosis of the upper extremity resulting from repetitive activity of the upper limb [1]. While most cases of effort thrombosis occur in young elite athletes with strenuous upper extremity activity, any repetitive activity capable of damaging vascular endothelium can cause it. This article reports two cases: the first is of a 67-year-old patient who developed upper extremity deep venous thrombosis (UEDVT) after bowling and the second case is of a 25-year-old barista, whose job involved lifting 30-pound bags of coffee over her head, who developed thrombosis of the right central subclavian and axillary vein. These cases illustrate that effort thrombosis should be included in the differential diagnosis in any patient with symptoms concerning deep vein thrombosis (DVT) associated with repetitive activity.

2. Case #1

A 67-year-old man experienced swelling in his proximal right upper extremity the morning after a prolonged game of bowling. He was an avid bowler and part of a competitive league. Over the next three days, the swelling became more prominent and was beginning to cause moderate-to-severe pain and so he was seen in our office. He denied any shortness of breath, chest pain, or history of trauma to his right arm. His past medical history was significant for a heart transplant 11 years earlier due to severe dilated cardiomyopathy that was complicated by thrombosis in his right internal jugular vein and right common femoral vein. He had not been diagnosed with a DVT since that hospital admission and denied any personal or family history of hematologic disease. On physical examination, he had an ill-defined 3 cm mobile, tender mass located deep to the subcutaneous space near the medial aspect of his right bicep. Ultrasound of the right upper extremity revealed acute deep venous thrombosis in the right brachial vein and peripheral axillary vein and acute superficial thrombosis in the right basilic vein (Figure 1).

The patient, who is on tacrolimus secondary to his heart transplant, was treated urgently with enoxaparin and then bridged to warfarin as an outpatient. After completing five weeks of outpatient anticoagulation therapy with warfarin, the patient denied any swelling or discomfort of the right

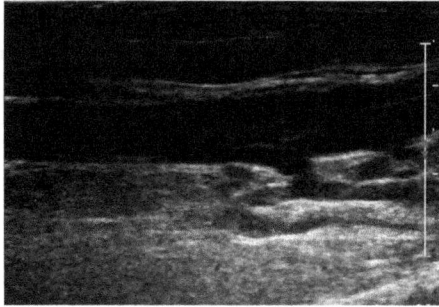

FIGURE 1: Right upper extremity ultrasound of a 67-year-old man revealing acute venous thrombosis in the brachial vein and peripheral axillary vein with acute superficial thrombosis in the right basilica vein.

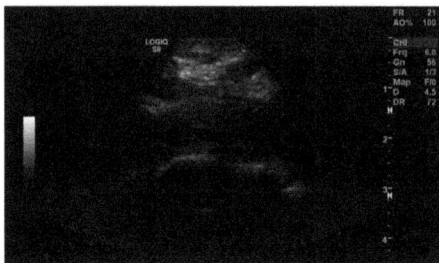

FIGURE 2: Right upper extremity ultrasound of a 25-year-old barista revealing acute thrombosis of the right central subclavian and axillary veins with compression by the first rib.

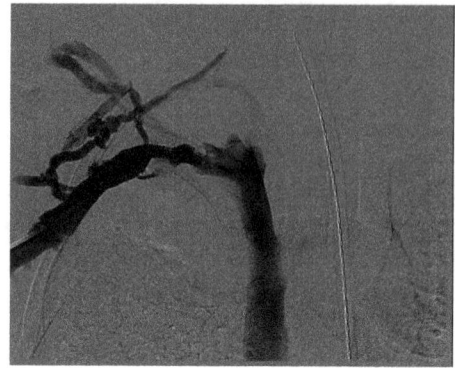

FIGURE 3: Preoperative angiogram of the right upper extremity revealing attenuation of contrast flow at the level of the subclavian vein secondary to thrombosis.

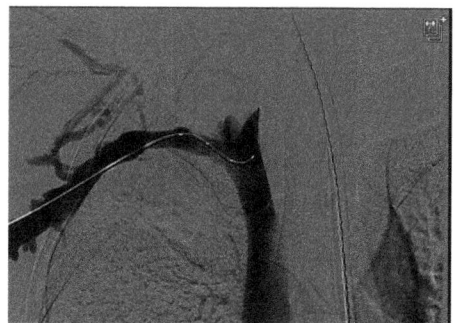

FIGURE 4: Angiogram revealing contrast flow through the subclavian vein status after catheter-directed thrombolysis and balloon angioplasty of the subclavian and axillary veins.

upper extremity. Ultrasound evaluation showed that the thrombi had completely resolved. A sequential musculoskeletal ultrasound did not show any occlusion of blood vessels due to muscle hypertrophy. He was continued on anticoagulation and was approved to continue bowling as tolerated.

3. Case #2

A 25-year-old otherwise healthy woman presented with a four-day history of right arm pain, swelling, heaviness, and redness. She was seen in an urgent care center and then sent to the emergency room for an ultrasound which showed acute thrombosis of the right central subclavian and axillary vein with compression by the first rib (Figure 2). She was discharged by the emergency room on rivaroxaban and advised to follow up at our office. On reviewing her history prior to her visit her physicians were concerned for possible thoracic outlet syndrome and obtained an emergency appointment with the vascular center. The patient had no prior history of DVT or pulmonary embolism (PE). Her job is that of a coffee roaster, and she lifts 30 pounds of coffee over her head all day. She denied any injuries, chest pain, shortness of breath, or lower leg pain or swelling. She also denied any history of any upper extremity catheters.

Patient was admitted and placed on a heparin drip. The next day she underwent catheter-directed thrombolysis, 24 hours of lysis, and then balloon angioplasty of the right subclavian and axillary veins. After thrombolysis a venogram

was performed with the arm abducted, and it showed that the contrast was still not flowing through the subclavian vein (Figures 3 and 4). Then another venogram was done with the arm adducted and it showed that the junction between the first rib and the clavicle was opened and there was flow through the subclavian vein. At that point there was not an obvious filling defect in the subclavian and axillary vein. Two days later she underwent resection of her first rib. After stabilization the patient was discharged on rivaroxaban 15 mg bid for 21 days and then switched to rivaroxaban 20 mg daily. She was seen three weeks later and denied right upper extremity pain, paresthesias, or numbness. She denied any bleeding or bruising, shortness of breath, fever, or chills. She was advised to follow up at 3 months for a follow-up venogram and anticoagulation management.

4. Discussion

Compared to lower extremity DVT, upper extremity DVT (UEDVT) is quite rare, accounting for less than 3% of all venous thromboses [2, 3]. UEDVT is typically classified as being either primary (spontaneous) or secondary in origin. Primary UEDVT is a much rarer disorder (2 per 100,000 persons per year) that refers to either effort thrombosis or idiopathic UEDVT [2, 4, 5]. Secondary UEDVT occurs in patients with known risk factors such as central venous catheters, pacemakers, cancer, or other thrombophilic states. Pulmonary embolism is present in up to one-third of patients with UEDVT and other associated complications such as loss of vascular access, superior vena cava syndrome, and persistent pain and swelling can be devastating [4, 6].

Effort thrombosis is the phenomenon of a deep venous thrombosis in the upper extremity secondary to repetitive upper limb activity. The condition, first described in 1949, classically refers to axillary-subclavian vein thrombosis and is also known as Paget-Schroetter syndrome (PSS). Paget-Schroetter syndrome is a form of thoracic outlet obstruction, which refers to the compression of the neurovascular bundle (brachial plexus, subclavian artery, and subclavian vein) as it exits the thoracic inlet. Effort thrombosis usually follows high-intensity sporting activities such as baseball, wrestling, and swimming. This syndrome occurs in young athletes with hypertrophied muscles or in patients with anatomic abnormalities that constrict the thoracic outlet (cervical rib, hypertrophy of anterior and medial scalene muscles, and abnormal insertion of the costoclavicular ligament) [7]. This leads to compression of the vein, damage to the endothelium, and activation of the coagulation cascade. The repeated trauma to the vessel can result in fibrous tissue formation that persistently compresses the vein and can lead to a cycle of endothelial trauma, thrombosis, and recanalization. Progressive fibrosis of the vascular endothelium may result in extensive collateral formation [3].

Clinically, PSS typically involves the dominant arm. It usually presents in the asymptomatic healthy athlete. When symptomatic, it most frequently presents with swelling and pain [6]. Patients frequently are unable to pinpoint a discrete precipitating event but usually have some form of repetitive upper limb activity. Diagnostic ultrasound is the initial imaging test of choice for diagnosing UEDVT. It is inexpensive, noninvasive, reproducible modality, but it may fail to detect central thrombus if located directly below the clavicle due to acoustic shadowing [6, 8]. Conservative treatment of UEDVT with anticoagulation alone can lead to pulmonary embolism in 6–15% and has a high incidence of recurrent thrombosis and residual venous obstruction in up to 75% of the cases [7].

More aggressive treatment modalities, such as systemic fibrinolysis, are superior to anticoagulation in terms of achieving vein patency but are associated with higher risks of catastrophic bleeding [9]. However, catheter-directed thrombolysis has been reported to be successful in between 62% and 84% of cases provided the symptoms have persisted for less than 10–14 days [10]. Other modes of therapy have been directed at thoracic outlet decompression with resection of the first rib and division of the scalene muscles and the costoclavicular ligament [7, 8, 10, 11]. While some investigators see this treatment as first line, others only recommend it in resistant cases following failed treatment with anticoagulation or fibrinolysis [10]. Research is currently aiming to delineate the factors predicting the need for more aggressive treatments, such as thoracic outlet decompression and catheter-directed thrombolysis [10]. All patients are anticoagulated for 3–6 months after canalization and decompression.

Effort thrombosis has been studied for many years in patients with high-intensity upper arm movement and support that the recognition and urgent treatment of effort thrombosis are important to return these athletes to the field at an equal level of play. In a study done at Washington University four cases of effort thrombosis in major league baseball players diagnosed using contrast venography were all treated with catheter-directed thrombolysis, first-rib resection, and systemic anticoagulation. All four players returned to play at their previous level of competition [12]. Other studies support the recognition of effort thrombosis to prevent catastrophic injury such as the case of a 25-year-old major league pitcher who presented with dizziness and shortness of breath without upper extremity symptoms. He was diagnosed with effort thrombosis and secondary pulmonary embolus and treated successfully with mechanical thrombectomy and catheter-directed venolysis—a lifesaving intervention [1].

These cases represent classic clinical presentations of UEDVT (pain and swelling of the upper extremity). However, while the barista presents with classic PSS, the bowler's three UEDVT start in the middle of his biceps. While the patient had undergone repetitive movements of the upper extremity a few days before, bowling is not typically thought of as being highly intense. A literature review reveals other patients diagnosed with effort thrombosis following mild activity. UEDVT has been diagnosed in patients following games of pool [13], stretching [14], and "Shake Weight" exercises [15]. The case of the pool player involved a 22-year-old pool player who developed UEDVT after a prolonged game of pool. This study suggested that any activity that extends and internally rotates the shoulder can stretch and possibly compress the subclavian vein against the first rib [13].

The bowler's case of effort thrombosis is particularly unusual not only due to mechanism but also due to location. Classically, the damage to the subclavian and axillary veins in PSS is located at the junction of the first rib, clavicle, and the anterior and middle scalene muscles. In the bowler, the axillary vein thrombus was located distal to this point, near the medial border of the biceps muscle. The bowler additionally had a DVT in the brachial vein and a superficial thrombosis in the axillary vein. While the axillary and subclavian veins are classically associated with effort thrombosis, brachial vein thrombosis is not typical [16]. UEDVT involving thrombi in all three of these veins is exceedingly rare. As part of his hypercoagulability workup, our patient needs monitoring for occult malignancy and other secondary causes of UEDVT. Up to one-fourth of patients with idiopathic UEDVT were later diagnosed with malignancy [17], and up to one-third of patients with UEDVT develop PE [18]. As his thrombosis was not located in the thoracic outlet surgical decompression was not an option for him. Therefore, it will be crucial to educate our patient not to hesitate to follow up with any recurrent swelling of the upper extremity or symptoms of pulmonary embolus.

In contrast, the barista is a case of classic PSS caused by thoracic outlet syndrome. As seen on her intraoperative venogram her vein was occluded when her arm was abducted even though the vein was clearly open when her arm was adducted. This case shows the urgent need to refer such patients to vascular surgery for thrombolysis and then resection of the first rib.

In conclusion, these cases illustrate two cases of UEDVT presenting in two patients with histories of repetitive use of their arms, one as a bowler and the other as a barista. Clinical awareness of UEDVT in a patient with recent repetitive upper extremity movement is vital to avoid potentially disastrous complications. In the case of the bowler, treatment with anticoagulation and strict follow-up for the development of hypercoagulable disorders or malignancy have allowed the patient to return to the bowling alley. In the second case urgent awareness of the need to obtain surgical intervention was needed. Even once the thrombosis in her subclavian vein had been removed, she still did not have circulation in her subclavian vein when her arm was abducted. That a surgical intervention almost did not occur was seen when the patient was sent home from the emergency ward on anticoagulation alone. Fortunately, she was seen and referred the next day and operated on expeditiously.

Competing Interests

The authors declare that they have no competing interests.

References

[1] B. D. Bushnell, A. W. Anz, K. Dugger, G. A. Sakryd, and T. J. Noonan, "Effort thrombosis presenting as pulmonary embolism in a professional baseball pitcher," *Sports Health*, vol. 1, no. 6, pp. 493–499, 2009.

[2] E. E. Elman and S. R. Kahn, "The post-thrombotic syndrome after upper extremity deep venous thrombosis in adults: a systematic review," *Thrombosis Research*, vol. 117, no. 6, pp. 609–614, 2006.

[3] L. Zell, W. Kindermann, F. Marschall, P. Scheffler, J. Gross, and A. Buchter, "Paget-Schroetter syndrome in sports activities: case study and literature review," *Angiology*, vol. 52, no. 5, pp. 337–342, 2001.

[4] H. V. Joffe and S. Z. Goldhaber, "Upper-extremity deep vein thrombosis," *Circulation*, vol. 106, no. 14, pp. 1874–1880, 2002.

[5] B. Lindblad, L. Tengborn, and D. Bergqvist, "Deep vein thrombosis of the axillary-subclavian veins: epidemiologic data, effects of different types of treatment and late sequele," *European Journal of Vascular Surgery*, vol. 2, no. 3, pp. 161–165, 1988.

[6] H. V. Joffe, N. Kucher, V. F. Tapson, and S. Z. Goldhaber, "Upper-extremity deep vein thrombosis: a prospective registry of 592 patients," *Circulation*, vol. 110, no. 12, pp. 1605–1611, 2004.

[7] N. A. Mall, G. S. Van Thiel, W. M. Heard, G. A. Paletta, C. Bush-Joseph, and B. R. Bach Jr., "Paget-Schroetter Syndrome: a review of effort thrombosis of the upper extremity from a sports medicine perspective," *Sports Health*, vol. 5, no. 4, pp. 353–356, 2013.

[8] S. J. Melby, S. Vedantham, V. R. Narra et al., "Comprehensive surgical management of the competitive athlete with effort thrombosis of the subclavian vein (Paget-Schroetter syndrome)," *Journal of Vascular Surgery*, vol. 47, no. 4, pp. 809–820.e3, 2008.

[9] S. Sabeti, M. Schillinger, W. Mlekusch, M. Haumer, R. Ahmadi, and E. Minar, "Treatment of subclavian-axillary vein thrombosis: long-term outcome of anticoagulation versus systemic thrombolysis," *Thrombosis Research*, vol. 108, no. 5-6, pp. 279–285, 2002.

[10] K. A. Illig and A. J. Doyle, "A comprehensive review of Paget-Schroetter syndrome," *Journal of Vascular Surgery*, vol. 51, no. 6, pp. 1538–1547, 2010.

[11] H. C. Urschel Jr. and A. N. Patel, "Surgery remains the most effective treatment for Paget-Schroetter Syndrome: 50 years' experience," *The Annals of Thoracic Surgery*, vol. 86, no. 1, pp. 254–260, 2008.

[12] G. S. DiFelice, G. A. Paletta Jr., B. B. Phillips, and R. W. Wright, "Effort thrombosis in the elite throwing athlete," *The American Journal of Sports Medicine*, vol. 30, no. 5, pp. 708–712, 2002.

[13] D. G. Hughes and P. M. Dixon, "Pool players' thrombosis," *The British Medical Journal*, vol. 295, no. 6613, p. 1652, 1987.

[14] H.-W. Liang, T.-C. Su, B.-S. Hwang, and M.-H. Hung, "Effort thrombosis of the upper extremities related to an arm stretching exercise," *Journal of the Formosan Medical Association*, vol. 105, no. 2, pp. 182–186, 2006.

[15] H. Shennib, K. Hickle, and B. Bowles, "Axillary vein thrombosis induced by an increasingly popular oscillating dumbbell exercise device: a case report," *Journal of Cardiothoracic Surgery*, vol. 10, article 1, 2015.

[16] A. Hingorani, E. Ascher, N. Marks et al., "Morbidity and mortality associated with brachial vein thrombosis," *Annals of Vascular Surgery*, vol. 20, no. 3, pp. 297–300, 2006.

[17] R. Sadeghi and M. Safi, "Systemic thrombolysis in the upper extremity deep vein thrombosis," *ARYA Atherosclerosis*, vol. 7, no. 1, pp. 40–46, 2011.

[18] P. Prandoni, P. Polistena, E. Bernardi et al., "Upper-extremity deep vein thrombosis," *Archives of Internal Medicine*, vol. 157, no. 1, pp. 57–62, 1997.

54

A Rare Case of Intermittent Claudication Associated with Impaired Arterial Vasodilation

J. J. Posthuma,[1] K. D. Reesink,[2] M. Schütten,[3] C. Ghossein,[4] M. E. Spaanderman,[4] H. ten Cate,[1] and G. Schep[5]

[1]Laboratory for Clinical Thrombosis and Haemostasis, Department of Internal Medicine, Cardiovascular Research Institute Maastricht, Maastricht University Medical Centre, Maastricht, Netherlands
[2]Department of Biomedical Engineering, Maastricht University Medical Centre, Maastricht, Netherlands
[3]Department of Internal Medicine, Cardiovascular Research Institute Maastricht, Maastricht University Medical Centre, Maastricht, Netherlands
[4]Department of Obstetrics and Gynecology, Maastricht University Medical Centre, Maastricht, Netherlands
[5]Department of Sports Medicine, Máxima Medical Centre, Veldhoven, Netherlands

Correspondence should be addressed to J. J. Posthuma; j.posthuma@maastrichtuniversity.nl

Academic Editor: Antonio Silvestro

Exercise-related intermittent claudication is marked by reduced blood flow to extremities caused by either stenosis or impaired vascular function. Although intermittent claudication is common in the elderly, it rarely occurs in the young and middle-aged individuals. Here, we report a case of exercise-related claudication in a 41-year-old woman, in the absence of overt vascular pathology. Using a series of imaging and functional tests, we established that her complaints were due to impaired arterial vasodilation, possibly due to a defect in nitrous oxide-mediated dilation. The symptoms were reversible upon administration of a calcium antagonist, showing reversibility of the vascular impairment. Identification of reversible vascular "stiffness" merits consideration in young and otherwise healthy subjects with claudication of unknown origin.

1. Introduction

Intermittent claudication is characterized by cramp-like pain in the leg upon exertion, due to insufficient blood flow. Typically, intermittent claudication affects the elderly, most often due to intraluminal stenosis in the peripheral arteries, resulting from atherosclerosis. Intermittent claudication is the commonest presentation of peripheral arterial disease in the elderly [1] but is rare in the young. In younger subjects (<45 years), intermittent claudication may be associated with specific forms of exercise, for example, cycling [2]. Such exercise-related claudication is often due to anatomical malformations such as popliteal artery entrapment or endofibrosis. Here, we present a case of exercise-related claudication in a young woman, apparently associated with reduced arterial vasodilation, in the absence of overt vascular pathology.

2. Case Description

A 41-year-old white European woman presented to our clinic with a 7-year history of unexplained progressive unilateral left thigh pain during cycling, starting at moderate intensity and increasing upon maximal exertion. She had been a spinning instructor for 13 years, with an average of 5 hours per week, before onset of symptoms. In addition, she worked as a firefighter, where she experienced identical complaints during rapid actions, like climbing the stairs. The patient reported a sensation of unilateral muscle fatigue and pain in the left thigh, starting at the vastus medialis and spreading all over the quadriceps, adductors, and biceps femoris, without symptoms in the gluteal region or calf. Complaints vanished within 3 minutes after cessation of exercise and were highly reproducible. There was no history of trauma, while her medical history included right-sided congenital hip dysplasia,

TABLE 1: Laboratory evaluation.

Parameter	Value	Reference range
Hemoglobin (g/dL)	14.18	12–18
Hematocrit (L/L)	0.41	0.36–0.47
Mean corpuscular volume (fL)	96	82–98
Thrombocytes ($\times 10^9$/L)	244	150–400
Leukocytes ($\times 10^9$/L)	5.9	4.5–11
MDRD-eGFR (mL/min/1.73 m)	>60	>60
Creatinine (μmol/L)	80	45–80
C-reactive protein (mg/L)	<1	<10
Erythrocyte sedimentation rate (mm)	2	<30
Total cholesterol (mmol/L)	4.2	1.5–6.5
LDL-cholesterol (mmol/L)	2.3	2.0–4.5
HDL-cholesterol (mmol/L)	1.5	0.9–1.7
Triglyceride (mmol/L)	0.95	0.6–2.2
Cholesterol/HDL ratio	2.8	<8
Total calcium (mmol/L)	2.27	2.10–2.55
Homocysteine (μmol/L)	9.5	<12.2

TABLE 2: Cardiac examination.

Parameter	Results	Reference value
Transthoracic sonography		
Left ventricular ejection fraction (%)	70	>55
End-diastolic volume (ml)	103	56–104
End-systolic volume (ml)	31	19–49
Total peripheral vascular resistance (dyne·s/cm^5)	1621	1200–1600

primary Raynaud's phenomenon, and attention deficit hyperactivity disorder (ADHD), for which she used clomipramine for 10 years. She was on no other drug therapy at time of presentation and had no history of smoking, diabetes, hypertension, hypercholesterolemia, peripheral artery disease, or coronary heart disease. Family history was positive for familial hyperhomocysteinemia, but this was never diagnosed in her.

2.1. Clinical Examination. The woman presented with a height of 172 cm and body weight of 65 kg (body mass index of 22 kg/m^2). Her resting blood pressure was 120/75 mmHg with a heart rate of 61 beats per minute (bpm). Musculoskeletal investigation showed normal back mobility and a full range of motion of hips and knees with normal muscular strength of both legs. In addition, neurological examination was normal in our patient.

2.2. Laboratory Evaluation. Admission laboratory findings included complete blood count, which was unremarkable (Table 1). In addition, haemostatic tests, including activated partial thromboplastin time (aPTT), prothrombin time (PT), INR, fibrinogen, D-dimer, DNA testing for Factor V Leiden and prothrombin G20210A carriership, protein C activity, activated protein C resistance, and free protein S level, were all normal, while no lupus anticoagulants or anti-cardiolipin antibodies were detectable.

2.3. Cardiac Examination. Transthoracic echocardiography showed normal anatomy with normal left ventricular ejection fraction (LVEF) and systolic and diastolic volumes but suggested a slight increase in total peripheral vascular resistance (Table 2).

2.4. Exercise Test. Since symptoms appeared during exercise, a maximal treadmill exercise test was obtained with increasing resistance, starting at 100 Watt and elevating 15 Watt every minute, until exhaustion. Complaints started at 130 Watt and the test was ceased at 260 Watt due to unilateral thigh pain and muscular fatigue. The exercise electrocardiogram (ECG) showed no abnormalities and systolic pressures were obtained before and after exercise from the left brachial and bilateral calf for ankle-brachial index (ABI) calculation. The ABI before exercise was 1.1 on both sides, whereas directly after exercise ABI was reduced for both legs (right: 0.75; left: 0.59), where no alterations upon exercise were expected in a healthy young woman [3] (Table 3).

2.5. Vascular Examination. Prompted by bilateral reduced ABI after exercise and the suggested increased vascular resistance, further vascular examinations were performed. Normal lower limb pulses without audible murmurs and a normal capillary refill (<2 sec) were found in both legs. To investigate whether this patient suffered from endofibrosis, resting arterial duplex ultrasonography was done, which revealed no

TABLE 3: Vascular diameter and intima-media thickness.

Parameter	Results		Reference value
	Left	Right	
Duplex ultrasonography			
Diameter of distal aorta (mm)	14.5		
Diameter of common iliac artery (mm)	9.8	9.9	7.9–11.7
Diameter of external iliac artery (mm)	7.9	7.8	6.7–9.2
Diameter of femoral artery (mm)	10.5	9.2	7.6–8.9
Carotid intima-media thickness (mm)	0.69	0.61	<0.9
Femoral intima-media thickness (mm)	0.78	0.80	<0.9

TABLE 4: Vascular function.

Parameter	Results		Reference value
	Left	Right	
Ankle-brachial index at rest	1.1	1.1	>0.8
Ankle-brachial index after exercise	0.59	0.75	>0.8
Capillary refill at rest (sec)	<2	<2	<2
Vascular function			
Carotid-femoral pulse wave velocity (m/s)	6.74		<10
Peak systolic velocity external iliac artery during hip extension (m/s)	1.41	1.37	0.89–1.41
Peak systolic velocity external iliac artery during hip flexion (m/s)	1.54	1.48	n/a
Carotid distensibility ($\times 10^{-3}/kPa^{-1}$)	16.1		20–30
Brachial flow mediated dilation (%)	1		2.4–8.4
Brachial nitroglycerine mediated dilation (%)	8		20–30
Cutaneous microcirculation			
Capillary density before venous congestion (/mm^2)	74		50.4–85.6
Capillary density after venous congestion (/mm^2)	109		69.5–117.1
Cutaneous blood flow response to warmth (%)	1356		324–1762

stenosis and normal diameters of the external iliac artery and common iliac artery, where femoral arteries appeared to be relatively wide, as might be expected in well-trained individuals [4] (Table 4). In addition, femoral intima-media thickness was within normal range (0.78 mm, reference cut off: <0.9 mm), accompanied by normal peak systolic velocity during hip extension (1.41 m/sec) and flexion (1.54 m/sec) [5]. At the venous level, no signs of (previous) deep vein thrombosis were observed.

Additionally, obstructive vascular pathologies were investigated by multiphase computer tomography angiography (CTA), showing no signs of intraluminal pathologies or aberrant morphology, thereby corroborating the duplex examinations and excluding endofibrosis, popliteal entrapment syndrome, arterial-venous shunts, and venous malformations.

Next, we evaluated arterial function by ultrasonic examination of carotid and brachial artery and tonometric measurement of carotid-femoral pulse wave velocity (cfPWV). Carotid intima-media thickness (0.68 mm, reference cut off: <0.9 mm [6]) and cfPWV (6.74 m/s, reference cut off: <10 m/s [7]) were unremarkable. However, carotid distensibility coefficient was lower than expected (16 × 10^{-3}/kPa, reference value: 20–30 × 10^{-3}/kPa) [8].

Brachial flow-mediated dilation (FMD, was 1%, reference value: 3.0–8.4% [9] and nitroglycerine-mediated dilation, 8%, (reference value: 9.6–18.0% [10]) were markedly reduced. Microcirculatory studies showed normal capillary density before (74/mm^2, reference value: 40.4–85.6/mm^2) and after (109 mm^2, reference value: 69.5–117.1/mm^2) venous congestion [11]. Furthermore, heat-induced cutaneous microvascular dilatation was within normal limits (+1356%, reference value: 324–1762%).

2.6. Therapeutic Strategy. Based on the symptoms and test results, we postulated impaired arterial vasodilation and therapy with isosorbide mononitrate 30 mg twice daily was started, without any effects on the symptoms. This appeared to exclude a lack of nitrous oxide as major underlying defect. In another approach, we prescribed a vasodilating agent, the long-acting calcium antagonist diltiazem 200 mg once daily, through which claudication symptoms were well controlled and blood pressure remained within normal range (24 h measurement: average 110/80 mmHg) without any symptoms of orthostasis. During 2-year follow-up, she experienced no side effects and was able to continue her work as a fire fighter and spinning instructor.

3. Discussion

We described the case of a 41-year-old woman who presented with exercise-related intermittent claudication. Although the patient experienced unilateral symptoms, a bilateral diminished blood flow was found after exercise, as shown by reduced ankle-brachial index, with tendency towards worse flow at the symptomatic side. This pointed towards a vascular origin of the symptoms. First of all, clomipramine-induced vasospasm was considered as a potential cause of symptoms. However, this was deemed unlikely, since the patient had been on clomipramine therapy for 3 years before the onset of symptoms. In addition to this, stopping clomipramine for several months had no effects on symptoms. Therefore, the differential diagnosis of vascular-related claudication during exertion included endofibrosis, atherosclerosis, May-Turner syndrome, Williams syndrome, endothelial dysfunction, eNOS deficiency, scleroderma, Leriche's syndrome, exercise-induced vasospasm, popliteal entrapment syndrome, and Takayasu's disease. Most of these diagnoses could be excluded, due to absence of intraluminal stenosis or aberrant morphology on multiphase CTA and unremarkable laboratory results. In addition, our patient lacked symptoms of skin lesions that were characteristic for scleroderma, thereby unlikely the cause of symptoms in our patient. Since the symptoms were suggestive for endofibrosis, a full work-up according to the latest consensus study was performed [12], including duplex ultrasound with extended leg and in provoked position and multiphase CTA imaging, neither of which showed signs of endofibrosis, thereby basically ruling out the probability that endofibrosis was the cause of symptoms in our patient. This was further supported by increased total peripheral vascular resistance and reduced dilatory response of brachial artery to endothelial-dependent and -independent stimuli, which is very unlikely in endofibrosis. In addition, in the absence of other intraluminal pathologies and aberrant morphology on multiphase CTA, the cause of symptoms in this patient appears to be (subclinically) impaired vascular function rather than intraluminal obstruction or anatomical malformation.

Exercise-induced vasospasm was considered as diagnosis but appears unlikely in the presence of normal arterial diameter and normal peak flow velocities [13]. Reduced vascular function is supported by impaired ABI after exercise, increased total peripheral resistance, and increased systemic arterial stiffness as shown by relatively low carotid distensibility coefficient. Additionally, we consider the decreases in brachial artery flow-mediated dilation (FMD) and nitroglycerin-mediated dilation (NMD) to be important. FMD-induced changes in arterial diameter are caused by shear-stress-induced endothelial release of nitric oxide [14]. Nitric oxide is the major substance, mediating vasodilatation by inducing smooth muscle cell relaxation in the arterial media. Therefore, FMD provides insight in the peripheral artery endothelial function (NO release), as well as the responsiveness to NO smooth muscle in the arterial wall. During NMD assessment, NO is supplemented independent of the endothelium. Therefore, the observed reductions in FMD and NMD of the brachial artery suggest functional impairment of smooth muscle in the arterial wall rather than endothelium-related disease such as endothelial dysfunction and eNOS deficiency. Together with the lack of relief of symptoms with isosorbide mononitrate in this patient, the above seems to indicate that the symptoms may be caused by reduced sensitivity of smooth muscle cells for NO or by NO diffusion impairment. This was supported by relief of symptoms upon addition of a calcium antagonist, since calcium can regulate the vascular contractility in an NO-independent way.

4. Conclusions

This case report illustrates a rare case of symptomatic claudication, most likely due to reduced arterial vasodilation, most likely due to a reduced sensitivity for nitric oxide. While further study as to its origin is required, we recommend additional functional testing of flow-mediated vasodilation and vascular distensibility coefficient in subjects with inexplicable arterial symptoms in absence of evident anatomical malformations, endofibrosis, or other intraluminal pathologies.

References

[1] F. G. R. Fowkes, E. Housley, E. H. H. Cawood, C. C. A. Macintyre, C. V. Ruckley, and R. J. Prescott, "Edinburgh artery study: prevalence of asymptomatic and symptomatic peripheral arterial disease in the general population," *International Journal of Epidemiology*, vol. 20, no. 2, pp. 384–392, 1991.

[2] G. Peach, G. Schep, R. Palfreeman, J. D. Beard, M. M. Thompson, and R. J. Hinchliffe, "Endofibrosis and kinking of the iliac arteries in athletes: a systematic review," *European Journal of Vascular and Endovascular Surgery*, vol. 43, no. 2, pp. 208–217, 2012.

[3] V. Aboyans, M. H. Criqui, P. Abraham et al., "Measurement and interpretation of the ankle-brachial index: a scientific statement from the American Heart Association," *Circulation*, vol. 126, no. 24, pp. 2890–2909, 2012.

[4] O. M. Pedersen, A. Aslaksen, and H. Vik-Mo, "Ultrasound measurement of the luminal diameter of the abdominal aorta and iliac arteries in patients without vascular disease," *Journal of Vascular Surgery*, vol. 17, no. 3, pp. 596–601, 1993.

[5] S. Shionoya, "Noninvasive diagnostic techniques in vascular disease," *International Angiology*, vol. 6, no. 3, pp. 213–221, 1987.

[6] L. Engelen, I. Ferreira, C. D. Stehouwer, P. Boutouyrie, and S. Laurent, "Reference intervals for common carotid intima-medi thickness measured with echotracking: relation with risk factors," *European Heart Journal*, vol. 34, no. 30, pp. 2368–2380, 2013.

[7] F. Londono, J. Bossuyt, L. Engelen et al., "A Simple calculator for the assessment of measurements of carotid-femoral pulse wave velocity and local arterial stiffness relative to the reference values database," *Journal of Hypertension*, vol. 33, supplement 1, no. 2, pp. e60–e, 2015.

[8] L. Engelen, J. Bossuyt, I. Ferreira et al., "Reference values for local arterial stiffness. Part a: carotid artery," *Journal of Hypertension*, vol. 33, no. 10, pp. 1981–1996, 2015.

[9] A. C. C. M. Van Mil, A. Greyling, P. L. Zock et al., "Impact of volunteer-related and methodology-related factors on the reproducibility of brachial artery flow-mediated vasodilation: analysis of 672 individual repeated measurements," *Journal of Hypertension*, vol. 34, no. 9, pp. 1738–1745, 2016.

[10] S. Holewijn, M. Den Heijer, D. W. Swinkels, A. F. H. Stalenhoef, and J. De Graaf, "Brachial artery diameter is related to cardiovascular risk factors and intima-media thickness," *European Journal of Clinical Investigation*, vol. 39, no. 7, pp. 554–560, 2009.

[11] E. H. B. M. Gronenschild, D. M. J. Muris, M. T. Schram, Ü. Karaca, C. D. A. Stehouwer, and A. J. H. M. Houben, "Semi-automatic assessment of skin capillary density: proof of principle and validation," *Microvascular Research*, vol. 90, pp. 192–198, 2013.

[12] R. J. Hinchliffe, F. D'Abate, P. Abraham, Y. Alimi, J. Beard, M. Bender et al., "Diagnosis and management of iliac artery endofibrosis: results of a delphi consensus study," *European Journal of Vascular and Endovascular Surgery*, vol. 52, no. 1, pp. 90–98, 2016.

[13] S. Shalhub, R. E. Zierler, W. Smith, K. Olmsted, and A. W. Clowes, "Vasospasm as a cause for claudication in athletes with external iliac artery endofibrosis," *Journal of Vascular Surgery*, vol. 58, no. 1, pp. 105–111, 2013.

[14] R. Joannides, W. E. Haefeli, L. Linder et al., "Nitric oxide is responsible for flow-dependent dilatation of human peripheral conduit arteries in vivo," *Circulation*, vol. 91, no. 5, pp. 1314–1319, 1995.

Permissions

All chapters in this book were first published in CRVM, by Hindawi Publishing Corporation; hereby published with permission under the Creative Commons Attribution License or equivalent. Every chapter published in this book has been scrutinized by our experts. Their significance has been extensively debated. The topics covered herein carry significant findings which will fuel the growth of the discipline. They may even be implemented as practical applications or may be referred to as a beginning point for another development.

The contributors of this book come from diverse backgrounds, making this book a truly international effort. This book will bring forth new frontiers with its revolutionizing research information and detailed analysis of the nascent developments around the world.

We would like to thank all the contributing authors for lending their expertise to make the book truly unique. They have played a crucial role in the development of this book. Without their invaluable contributions this book wouldn't have been possible. They have made vital efforts to compile up to date information on the varied aspects of this subject to make this book a valuable addition to the collection of many professionals and students.

This book was conceptualized with the vision of imparting up-to-date information and advanced data in this field. To ensure the same, a matchless editorial board was set up. Every individual on the board went through rigorous rounds of assessment to prove their worth. After which they invested a large part of their time researching and compiling the most relevant data for our readers.

The editorial board has been involved in producing this book since its inception. They have spent rigorous hours researching and exploring the diverse topics which have resulted in the successful publishing of this book. They have passed on their knowledge of decades through this book. To expedite this challenging task, the publisher supported the team at every step. A small team of assistant editors was also appointed to further simplify the editing procedure and attain best results for the readers.

Apart from the editorial board, the designing team has also invested a significant amount of their time in understanding the subject and creating the most relevant covers. They scrutinized every image to scout for the most suitable representation of the subject and create an appropriate cover for the book.

The publishing team has been an ardent support to the editorial, designing and production team. Their endless efforts to recruit the best for this project, has resulted in the accomplishment of this book. They are a veteran in the field of academics and their pool of knowledge is as vast as their experience in printing. Their expertise and guidance has proved useful at every step. Their uncompromising quality standards have made this book an exceptional effort. Their encouragement from time to time has been an inspiration for everyone.

The publisher and the editorial board hope that this book will prove to be a valuable piece of knowledge for researchers, students, practitioners and scholars across the globe.

List of Contributors

Marco Franchin, Matteo Tozzi and Gabriele Piffaretti
Vascular Surgery, Department of Surgery and Morphological Sciences, Circolo University Hospital, University of Insubria School of Medicine, Via Guicciardini 9, 21100 Varese, Italy

Federico Fontana and Filippo Piacentino
Interventional Radiology, Department of Surgery and Morphological Sciences, Circolo University Hospital, University of Insubria School of Medicine, Via Guicciardini 9, 21100 Varese, Italy

Kohei Hamamoto, Emiko Chiba, Tomohisa Okochi, Katsuhiko Matsuura and Osamu Tanaka
Department of Radiology, Saitama Medical Center, Jichi Medical University, 1-847 Amanuma-cho, Omiya-ku, Saitama 330-8503, Japan

Mitsunori Nakano
Department of Cardiovascular Surgery, Saitama Medical Center, Jichi Medical University, 1-847 Amanuma-cho, Omiya-ku, Saitama 330-8503, Japan

Kiyoka Omoto
Department of Laboratory Medicine, Diagnostic Ultrasound Division, Saitama Medical Center, Jichi Medical University, 1-847 Amanuma-cho, Omiya-ku, Saitama 330-8503, Japan

Masahiko Tsubuku
Department of Radiology, Maruyama Memorial General Hospital, 2-10-5 Hon-cho, Iwatsuki-ku, Saitama 339-8521, Japan

Sudheer Ambekar, Donald Smith and Hugo Cuellar
Department of Neurosurgery, Louisiana State University Health Sciences Center, 1501 Kings Highway, Shreveport, LA 71103, USA

Mayur Sharma
Center of Neuromodulation, Wexner Medical Center, The Ohio State University, Columbus, OH 43210, USA

Kimihiro Igari, Toshifumi Kudo, Takahiro Toyofuku and Yoshinori Inoue
Division of Vascular and Endovascular Surgery, Department of Surgery, Tokyo Medical and Dental University, 1-5-45 Yushima, Bunkyo-ku, Tokyo 113-8519, Japan

Vishal Dahya and Prasad Chalasani
Florida State University College of Medicine, 1115 West Call Street, Tallahassee, FL 32306-4300, USA

Nathan S. Anderson, Alexies Ramirez, Ahmad Slim and Jamil Malik
Cardiology Service, Brooke Army Medical Center, 3551 Roger Brooke Drive, San Antonio, TX 78234-6200, USA

J. Porter, Q. Al-Jarrah and S. Richardson
Department of Vascular Surgery, University Hospital of South, Manchester, Southmoor Road, Manchester M23 9LT, UK

Adam T. Marler, Jamil A. Malik and Ahmad M. Slim
Cardiology Service, San Antonio Military Medical Center, Fort Sam Houston, TX 78234, USA

John A. Stathopoulos
Columbia University, 30-10 38th Street, 2nd Floor, Astoria, NY 11103, USA

Klaus Hertting and Werner Raut
Department of Cardiology and Angiology, Krankenhaus Buchholz, 21244 Buchholz in der Nordheide, Germany

Salim Abunnaja, Marshall Clyde, Andrea Cuviello, Robert A. Brenes and Giuseppe Tripodi
The Stanley J. Dudrick Department of Surgery, Saint Mary's Hospital, 56 Franklin Street, Waterbury, CT 06706, USA

Francesca Fratesi, Ashok Handa, Raman Uberoi and Ediri Sideso
Department of Vascular Surgery, Oxford University Hospitals NHS Trust, Oxford OX3 9DU, UK

Luciano A. Sposato and Patricia M. Riccio
Vascular Research Institute, INECOFoundation, Pacheco deMelo 1860, Ciudad de BuenosAires (C1126AAB), BuenosAires, Argentina

Valeria Salutto, Diego E. Beratti and Claudio Mazia
Department of Neurology, Alfredo Lanari Institute of Medical Investigations, University of Buenos Aires, Buenos Aires, Argentina

PaulaMonti
Department of Medicine, Alfredo Lanari Institute of Medical Investigations, University of Buenos Aires, Ciudad de Buenos Aires, Argentina

Rainer Knur
Department of Cardiology and Angiology, Allgemeines Krankenhaus Viersen, Hoserkirchweg 63, 47147 Viersen, Germany

Handy Eone Daniel, Minka Ngom Esthelle, Bombah Freddy and Ngo Nonga Bernadette
Department of Surgery, Faculty of Medicine and Biomedical Sciences, University of Yaoundè I, Yaoundè, Cameroon

Ankouane Firmin
Department of Medicine, Faculty of Medicine and Biomedical Sciences, University of Yaoundè I, Yaoundè, Cameroon

Pondy O. Angele
Department of Pediatrics, Faculty of Medicine and Biomedical Sciences, University of Yaoundè I, Yaoundè, Cameroon

Christos Tourmousoglou, Efstratios Koletsis, Nikolaos Charoulis, Christos Prokakis, Panagiotis Alexopoulos, Emmanoil Margaritis and Dimitrios Dougenis
Cardiothoracic Department, University Hospital of Patra, 26504 Rio, Patra, Greece

Christina Kalogeropoulou
Department of Radiology, University Hospital of Patra, 26504 Rio, Patra, Greece

Fortune O. Alabi, Francis G. Christian, Fred Umeh and Maximo Lama
Department of Critical Care Medicine, Florida Hospital Celebration Health, Celebration, FL 34747, USA

Manuel Hernandez
Department of Radiology, Florida Hospital Orlando, Orlando, FL 32803, USA

Stephanie Thomas
Department of Microbiology, University Hospital of South Manchester, Wythenshawe Hospital, Southmoor Road, Manchester M23 9LT, UK

Jonathan Ghosh, Johnathan Porter and Adele Cockcroft
Department of Vascular Surgery, University Hospital of South Manchester, Wythenshawe Hospital, Southmoor Road, Manchester M23 9LT, UK

Riina Rautemaa-Richardson
Department of Microbiology, University Hospital of South Manchester, Wythenshawe Hospital, Southmoor Road, Manchester M23 9LT, UK
The University of Manchester, Manchester Academic Health Science Centre, Institute of Inflammation and Repair, Oxford Road, Manchester M13 9PT, UK

Chris Klonaris, Emmanouil Psathas, Athanasios Katsargyris, Stella Lioudaki and Theodore Karatzas
Second Department of Propaedeutic Surgery, University of Athens Medical School, "Laikon" Hospital, 17 Ag. Thoma Street, 11527 Athens, Greece

Achilleas Chatziioannou
Department of Radiology, University of Athens Medical School, "Areteion" University Hospital, 76 Vassilissis Sofias Str., 11528 Athens, Greece

Ahsan Syed Khalid
Saba University School of Medicine, Devens, MA 01434, USA

Omar M. Ghanem and Seyed Mojtaba Gashti
Medstar Union Memorial Hospital, Baltimore, MD 21218, USA

Alexander Hess, Britta Vogel, Benedikt Kohler, Oliver J. Müller, Hugo A. Katus and Grigorios Korosoglou
Department of Cardiology, Angiology and Pneumology, University of Heidelberg, Im Neuenheimer Feld 410, 69120 Heidelberg, Germany

Jan Hrubý, Robert Novotný, Miroslav Špalek, Petr Mitáš, Jaroslav Hlubocký, David Janák and Jaroslav Lindner
2nd Department of Cardiovascular Surgery, General Teaching Hospital, Prague and 1st Faculty of Medicine, Charles University, U Nnemocnice 2, 128 08 Prague 2, Czech Republic

Ctibor Povýšil
Department of Pathology, General Teaching Hospital, Prague and 1st Faculty of Medicine, Charles University, U Nemocnice 2, Prague 2, Czech Republic

Maher Kurdi
Pathology Department, Faculty of Medicine, King Abdulaziz University, Jeddah 21589, Saudi Arabia

Saleh Baeesa
Division of Neurological Surgery, Faculty of Medicine, King Abdulaziz University, Jeddah 21589, Saudi Arabia

Mohammed Bin-Mahfoodh
Neurosciences Department, King Faisal Specialist Hospital and Research Center, Jeddah 21499, Saudi Arabia

Khalil Kurdi
Radiology Department, King Faisal Specialist Hospital and Research Center, Jeddah 21499, Saudi Arabia

Keagan Werner-Gibbings and Steven Dubenec
Department of Vascular Surgery, Royal Prince Alfred Hospital, Sydney, NSW2006, Australia

Georgios Karaolanis, Viktoria Varvara Palla and Konstantinos Filis
1st Department of Surgery, Vascular Surgery Unit, Laikon General Hospital, Medical School of Athens, Athens, Greece

George Galyfos and Evridiki Karanikola
Division of Vascular Surgery, 1st Department of Propaedeutic Surgery, University of Athens Medical School, Hippokration General Hospital, Athens, Greece

Raad A. Haddad, Mazin Saadaldin, Binay Kumar and Ghassan Bachuwa
Department of Internal Medicine, Michigan State University, Hurley Medical Center, 1 Hurley Plaza, Flint, MI 48503, USA

Michele Arcopinto, Teresa Russo, Antonio Ruvolo, Antonio Cittadini, Luigi Saccà and Raffaele Napoli
Department of Translational Medical Sciences, School of Medicine, Federico II University, 5 Via Sergio Pansini, 80131 Napoli, Italy

Shamir O. Cawich, EmilMohammed, Marlon Mencia and Vijay Naraynsingh
Department of Clinical Surgical Sciences, University of theWest Indies, St. Augustine Campus, St. Augustine, Trinidad and Tobago

Arda Özyüksel
Medipol Üniversitesi Kalp ve Damar Cerrahisi Bölümü, TEM Otoyolu Göztepe Çıkışı, No. 1, Bağcılar, 34214 İstanbul, Turkey

RJza DoLan
Department of Cardiovascular Surgery, Hacettepe University, Ankara, Turkey

Sarah Kate Ryan
University of Queensland School of Medicine, Herston Road, Herston, Brisbane, QLD 4006, Australia

Maximilian Stephens and Roger Livsey
University of Queensland School of Medicine, Herston Road, Herston, Brisbane, QLD 4006, Australia
Department of Medical Imaging, Mater Misericordiae Hospital, Raymond Terrace, South Brisbane, QLD 4101, Australia

Yohei Kawatani, Yujiro Hayashi, Yujiro Ito, Hirotsugu Kurobe, Yoshitsugu Nakamura, Yuji Suda and Takaki Hori
Department of Cardiovascular Surgery, Chiba-Nishi General Hospital, 107-1 Kanegasaku, Matsudo-Shi, Chiba-ken 2702251, Japan

Mehmet Tasar, Nur Dikmen Yaman, Cahit Saricaoglu, Zeynep Eyileten, Bulent Kaya and Adnan Uysalel
Department of Cardiovascular Surgery, Heart Center, Ankara University School of Medicine, Dikimevi, 06340 Ankara, Turkey

Federico Bucci
Vascular Surgery Department, Sud Gironde Community Hospital, rue Langevin, 33210 Langon, France

Adriano Redler and Leslie Fiengo
General and Vascular Surgery Department, "Umberto I" University Hospital, Viale del Policlinico, 00186 Rome, Italy

Kimihiro Igari, Toshifumi Kudo, Takahiro Toyofuku and Yoshinori Inoue
Division of Vascular and Endovascular Surgery, Department of Surgery, Tokyo Medical and Dental University, 1-5-45 Yushima, Bunkyo-ku, Tokyo 113-8519, Japan

Takehisa Iwai
Tsukuba Vascular Center and Buerger Disease Research Institute, 980-1 Tatsuzawa, Moriya, Ibaraki 302-0118, Japan

Sherif Ali Eltawansy, Mana Rao and Sidney Ceniza
Department of Internal Medicine, Monmouth Medical Center, Long Branch, NJ 07740, USA

David Sharon
Department of Internal Medicine, Monmouth Medical Center, Long Branch, NJ 07740, USA
Department of Oncological Medicine, Monmouth Medical Center, Long Branch, NJ 07740, USA

E. Trautt, S. Thomas, J. Ghosh, P. Newton and A. Cockcroft
University Hospital of South Manchester, Manchester, UK

Tiwari Ashutosh, Kumar Nilesh, Varshney Ankur Nandan, Behera Dibyaranjan, Anand Arvind, Anand Ravi and N. K. Singh
Department of General Medicine, Institute of Medical Sciences, Banaras Hindu University, Uttar Pradesh, Varanasi 221005, India

Maheedhar Gedela
Department of Internal Medicine, University of South Dakota Sanford School of Medicine, Sioux Falls, SD, USA

Shenjing Li, Tomasz Stys and Adam Stys
Sanford Cardiovascular Institute, University of South Dakota Sanford School of Medicine, Sioux Falls, SD, USA

Naveen Swami
Department of Cardiothoracic Surgery, Heart Care Centre, Al Ahli Hospital, 2nd Floor, Bin Omran, P.O. Box 6401, Doha, Qatar

Georgey Koshy
Department of Cardiology, Heart Care Centre, Al Ahli Hospital, Doha, Qatar

Maan Jamal
Department of Radiology, Al Ahli Hospital, Doha, Qatar

Thair S. Abdulla
Department of Pulmonary Medicine and Intensive Care Unit, Al Ahli Hospital, Doha, Qatar

Abdulaziz Alkhulaifi
Department of Cardiothoracic Surgery, Heart Hospital, Hamad Medical Corporation, Doha, Qatar

Ata Firoozi, Jamal Moosavi, Omid Shafe and Parham Sadeghipour
Rajaie Cardiovascular Medical and Research Center, Iran University of Medical Sciences, Tehran, Iran Cardiovascular Intervention Research Center, Rajaie Cardiovascular Medical and Research Center, Iran University of Medical Sciences, Tehran, Iran

Stylianos Koutsias, Georgios Antoniou, Christos Karathanos, Vassileios Saleptsis and Athanasios D. Giannoukas
Department of Vascular Surgery, University Hospital of Larissa, University of Thessaly Medical School, 41000 Larissa, Greece

Konstantinos Stamoulis
Department of Anaesthesiology, University Hospital of Larissa, University of Thessaly Medical School, 41000 Larissa, Greece

Hiroshi Osawa, Daisuke Shinohara and Kouan Orii
Division of Cardiovascular Surgery, Shimada General Hospital, Higashi-cho 5-3, Choshi, Chiba 288-0053, Japan

Shigeru Hosaka and Shoji Fukuda
Department of Cardiovascular Surgery, National Center of Global Health and Medicine, Shinjuku, Tokyo 162-8655, Japan

Okihiko Akashi
Division of Cardiovascular Surgery, Ikegami General Hospital, Ota, Tokyo 146-8531, Japan

Hiroshi Furukawa
Department of Cardiovascular Surgery, Kawasaki Medical University, Kurashiki, Okayama 701-0192, Japan

Supatcha Prasertcharoensuk, Narongchai Wongkonkitsin, Parichat Tunmit and Su-a-pa Theeragul
Department of Surgery, Khon Kaen University, Khon Kaen, Thailand

Anucha Ahooja
Department of Radiology, Khon Kaen University, Khon Kaen, Thailand

Bedrettin Yildizeli
Department of Thoracic Surgery, Marmara University School of Medicine, Istanbul, Turkey
Mehmed Yanartaş
Department of Cardiovascular Surgery, Kartal Koşuyolu Training and Research Hospital, Istanbul, Turkey

Sibel Keskin
Department of Chest Diseases, Muğla Sıtkı Koçman University, Muğla, Turkey

Işik Atagündüz
Department of Hematology, Marmara University School of Medicine, Istanbul, Turkey

Ece Altinay
Department of Anaesthesia, Kartal Koşuyolu Training and Research Hospital, Istanbul, Turkey

Mona Laible, Werner Hacke, Peter Arthur Ringleb and Timolaos Rizos
Department of Neurology, University Hospital Heidelberg, 69120 Heidelberg, Germany

Martin Bendszus and Markus Möhlenbruch
Department of Neuroradiology, University Hospital Heidelberg, 69120 Heidelberg, Germany

Einar Dregelid
Department of Vascular Surgery, Haukeland University Hospital, Jonas Lies Vei 65, 5021 Bergen, Norway

Alireza Daryapeyma
Department of Vascular Surgery, Karolinska University Hospital, 171 76 Stockholm, Sweden

Özge AltJntaG, Azize Esra Gürsoy, Gözde Baran and Talip Asil
Department of Neurology, Medical Faculty, Bezmi Alem Vakıf University, Adnan Menderes Boulevard, Fatih, 34093 Istanbul, Turkey

ElnurMehdi
Department of Radiology, Medical Faculty, Bezmi Alem Vakıf University, Adnan Menderes Boulevard, Fatih, 34093 Istanbul, Turkey

Koki Takizawa and Hiroshi Osawa
Division of Cardiovascular Surgery, Shimada General Hospital, Choshi, Japan

Atsuo Kojima
Department of Vascular Surgery, Tomei Atsugi Hospital, Atsugi, Japan

Samuel J. K. Abraham
The Mary-Yoshio Translational Hexagon (MYTH), Nichi-In Center for Regenerative Medicine (NCRM), Chennai, India

Shigeru Hosaka
Department of Cardiovascular Surgery, National Center of Global Health and Medicine, Shinjuku, Japan

Kimihiro Igari, Toshifumi Kudo, Takahiro Toyofuku and Yoshinori Inoue
Division of Vascular and Endovascular Surgery, Department of Surgery, Tokyo Medical and Dental University, Tokyo, Japan

Tom Eisele, Benedikt M. Muenz and Grigorios Korosoglou
Department of Cardiology and Vascular Medicine, GRN Hospital Weinheim, 69469 Weinheim, Germany

Syed M. Asim Hussain and Thomas Joseph
North Cumbria University Hospitals NHS Trust, Cumberland Infirmary, Newtown Road, Carlisle, UK

Uygar Teomete
University of Miami Miller School of Medicine, Department of Radiology, Miami, FL 33136, USA

Rubee Anne Gugol and Ming-Lon Young
University of Miami Miller School of Medicine, Department of Pediatrics, Miami, FL 33136, USA

Holly Neville
Division of Pediatric Surgery, DeWitt Daughtry Family Department of Surgery, University of Miami Miller School of Medicine, Miami, FL 33136, USA

Ozgur Dandin
University of Miami Miller School of Medicine, Department of Surgery, Ryder Trauma Center, Miami, FL 33136, USA

Onur Saydam, Deniz Ferefli and Cengiz Sert
Tepecik Training and Research Hospital, Department of Cardiovascular Surgery, 35170 Izmir, Turkey

Mehmet Atay
Bakirkoy Dr. Sadi Konuk Training and Research Hospital, Department of Cardiovascular Surgery, 34147 Istanbul, Turkey

Nicole Ilonzo, Selena Goss, Chun Yang and Michael Dudkiewicz
Mount Sinai St. Luke's-West, New York, NY, USA

Owen S. Glotzer, Kathryn Bowser, F. Todd Harad and Sandra Weiss
The Heart and Vascular Center, Christiana Care, Newark, DE 19713, USA

Ciel Harris, Joseph Geffen, Keyrillos Rizg, Stuart Shah, Aaron Richardson and Cherisse Baldeo
Internal Medicine, University of Florida College of Medicine-Jacksonville, Jacksonville, FL, USA

Avinash Ramdass
Pulmonary, Sleep and Critical Care Medicine, University of Florida College of Medicine-Jacksonville, Jacksonville, FL, USA

Courtney Brooke Shires
Department of Otolaryngology, Head and Neck Surgery, University of Tennessee Health Science Center, 910 Madison Ave., Suite 430, Memphis, TN 38163, USA

Michael J. Rohrer
Department of Surgery, Division of Vascular and Endovascular Surgery, University of Tennessee Health Science Center, 910 Madison Ave., Second Floor, Memphis, TN 38163, USA

Himani Sharma and Abhinav Tiwari
Department of Internal Medicine, University of Toledo Medical Center, Toledo, OH, USA

Eleni I. Skandalou and Ilias D. Minasidis
Renal Unit "Therapeutiki", Thessaloniki, Greece

Fani D. Apostolidou-Kiouti and Ioannis K. Skandalos
Surgical Department, General Hospital "Agios Pavlos", Thessaloniki, Greece

NataliaMazuruc and Olga Belic
Department of Human Anatomy, State University of Medicine and Pharmacy "Nicolae Testemitanu", Chisinau, Moldova

Serghei Covantev
Laboratory of Allergology and Clinical Immunology, State University of Medicine and Pharmacy "Nicolae Testemitanu", Chisinau, Moldova

Xiaoye Li and Ying Xue
Department of Pharmacy, Zhongshan Hospital, Fudan University, Shanghai, China

Hongyi Wu
Department of Cardiology, Zhongshan Hospital, Fudan University, Shanghai, China

James O'Brien, Francesca Muscara, Aser Farghal and Irshad Shaikh
Department of General Surgery, Norfolk and Norwich University Hospital, Colney Lane, Norwich, Norfolk NR4 7UY, UK

Seth Stake
Sidney Kimmel Medical College, Thomas Jefferson University, Philadelphia, PA 19107, USA

Anne L. du Breuil and Jeremy Close
Department of Family and Community Medicine, Sidney Kimmel Medical College, Thomas Jefferson University, 833 East Chestnut Street, Suite 301, Philadelphia, PA 19107, USA

J. J. Posthuma and H. ten Cate
Laboratory for Clinical Thrombosis and Haemostasis, Department of Internal Medicine

Cardiovascular Research Institute Maastricht, Maastricht University Medical Centre, Maastricht, Netherlands

K. D. Reesink
Department of Biomedical Engineering, Maastricht University Medical Centre, Maastricht, Netherlands

M. Schütten
Department of Internal Medicine, Cardiovascular Research Institute Maastricht, Maastricht University Medical Centre, Maastricht, Netherlands

C. Ghossein and M. E. Spaanderman
Department of Obstetrics and Gynecology, Maastricht University Medical Centre, Maastricht, Netherlands

G. Schep
Department of Sports Medicine, M´axima Medical Centre, Veldhoven, Netherlands

Index

A

Abdominal Aortic Aneurysm, 1, 4, 15-16, 43, 46, 139, 141-142, 146, 149-150, 164-165

Adenocarcinoma, 59

Angulated Neck, 139-141

Arteriovenous Fistula, 5, 8-9, 55, 57, 97-98, 170, 173, 178-180, 209

Atherosclerosis, 23, 35, 41, 71, 80, 119, 169, 214-215, 218

Atrial Fibrillation, 2, 16, 47-50, 88, 166, 169, 206

B

Bacterial Endocarditis, 91, 93

Bd, 81, 83-84, 86, 108-110

Brachial Artery, 6, 35-38, 56-58, 95-97, 104, 171, 176, 183, 185-186, 217-219

Brachiocephalic Vein Stenosis, 194, 196

Buerger Disease, 110, 118-120

C

Cardiac Rehabilitation, 23

Catastrophic, 65, 67, 125-126, 209, 213

Cerebral Hyperperfusion Syndrome, 51-52, 54

Chimney-graft, 43-44, 46

Coil Embolization, 5-9, 22, 68-69, 75, 86-87, 106, 148, 162-164, 210

Computed Tomography, 1, 6, 16-18, 20-21, 27-31, 52, 54, 59-61, 71, 73, 81, 99, 112-115, 118-119, 122, 155, 158-159, 162-163, 174, 190, 201-202, 207-208

Congenital Heart Defects, 103

Cor Triatriatum Sinistrum, 62, 64

Coronary Artery, 26-31, 33, 111, 122, 129, 152-153, 203-205

Coronary Stent Graft, 77, 80

Critical Limb Ischemia, 35, 37, 108-110, 112

Cystic Adventitial Disease, 112, 116-117, 158-159, 161

D

Deep Vein Thrombosis, 41, 90, 122, 138, 152, 160, 193, 211, 214

E

Endovascular Repair, 1, 4-5, 19, 22, 43, 46, 73, 75-76, 104, 107, 139, 141-142, 146, 149-150, 157, 164, 166, 178

Evar, 1, 3-4, 43-46, 66, 139-142, 146, 148-149, 162, 164-165

F

Femoral Artery, 5, 10, 12, 15-16, 18-19, 21, 35-36, 38-40, 57, 73, 77-78, 82, 104, 158, 166-169, 173-174, 177-180, 217

Fibromuscular Dysplasia, 116, 118-119, 121

H

Hemodialysis, 1, 5-6, 94-98, 171, 173, 194-196

Hypertension, 1, 9, 16, 18, 24, 28, 30, 32-33, 39, 41, 43, 48, 51-52, 54, 60, 62, 64, 88, 110, 113, 118, 129, 140, 151, 153-154, 166, 170-173, 179, 181-185, 203, 207, 209, 219

I

Iatrogenic Femoral Arteriovenous Fistula, 173

Immune Thrombocytopenic Purpura, 151-152

In-stent Restenosis, 129, 131, 177

Inferior Pancreaticoduodenal Artery, 68, 71

Internal Jugular Vein, 5-9, 95, 122-125

Intracranial Aneurysms, 14, 81, 83-84, 86

Ischemic Stroke, 47-50

K

Kommerell's Diverticulum, 132, 134, 143-145, 187

M

Multiple Aneurysms, 68, 71, 81, 84, 161

Mynxgrip Closure Device, 35-36

N

No-touch Technique, 32, 34

Nutcracker Phenomenon, 99-102

O

Onyx Embolization, 11, 81, 83-84, 86

P

Paget-schroetter Syndrome, 88-90, 190, 193, 213-214

Papvc, 59-61

Papvr, 59-60

Periodontal Disease, 65-67

Peripheral Artery Disease, 77, 80, 166, 177, 216

Pipeline Embolization Device, 11, 13-14, 84

Popliteal Artery, 38, 78-79, 112-121, 158-161, 168-169, 178-179, 215

Posterior Tibial Artery, 118-119

Profunda Femoris Artery Aneurysms, 15-16, 19, 73, 75-76

Pruitt-inahara Shunt, 20

Pseudoaneurysm, 5, 8-14, 20-22, 55-57, 72-75, 84, 91-92, 150, 173-176, 206-210

Pulmonary Embolism, 39, 41-42, 124-125, 135, 161, 212-213

Pulmonary Endarterectomy, 151-153

R

Renal Artery Stenting, 32, 34, 131

Right Aortic Arch, 134, 143-145

Right Lower Bilobectomy, 59

S

Stent Graft, 19-22, 71, 76-77, 79-80, 103-104, 106, 140-141, 148, 165-166, 174-177, 187, 209

Subclavian Artery, 6-7, 9, 88, 103-107, 133-134, 143-145, 155-156, 174-177, 185-189, 213

Superficial Femoral Artery, 15, 18, 57, 78, 166, 168-169, 177-180

Superior Mesenteric Artery, 43, 69, 99-100, 142, 146, 148-149

Systemic Thrombolysis, 47-49, 214

T

Takayasu's Arteritis, 181, 183

Thromboangiitis Obliterans, 108, 110-111, 120-121

Traumatic Pseudoaneurysms, 11, 13

Type B Aortic Dissection, 103, 106, 157

U

Ultrasonography, 6, 8, 16, 68, 71, 80, 112-113, 161, 164, 172, 174, 193, 216-217

Upper Limb Ischemic Gangrene, 94

V

Variceal Bleeding, 62

Vascular Graft Infection, 65, 67, 126, 128

Vascular Ring, 132-134

Vascular Surgery, 1, 4, 19-20, 22, 37, 43, 46, 65, 67, 71-72, 76, 80, 88, 90, 97-98, 107-108, 110-111, 116-117, 139, 142, 150, 154, 161, 169, 181, 189, 196, 201, 214, 218-219

Venous Stasis Ulceration, 178-179

Venous Thrombosis, 37, 39, 41-42, 83, 88-89, 122, 124, 135, 138, 152, 190, 192-193, 211-212, 214

Visceral-anastomosis-first Approach, 154, 156

www.ingramcontent.com/pod-product-compliance
Lightning Source LLC
Chambersburg PA
CBHW080525200326
41458CB00012B/4331